Small Animal
Anesthesia Techniques

Small Animal Anesthesia Techniques

Amanda M. Shelby

Carolyn M. McKune

WILEY Blackwell

This edition first published 2014 © 2014 by John Wiley & Sons, Inc.

Editorial offices: 1606 Golden Aspen Drive, Suites 103 and 104, Ames, Iowa 50010, USA
The Atrium, Southern Gate, Chichester, West Sussex, PO19 8SQ, UK
9600 Garsington Road, Oxford, OX4 2DQ, UK

For details of our global editorial offices, for customer services and for information about how to apply for permission to reuse the copyright material in this book please see our website at www.wiley.com/wiley-blackwell.

Authorization to photocopy items for internal or personal use, or the internal or personal use of specific clients, is granted by Blackwell Publishing, provided that the base fee is paid directly to the Copyright Clearance Center, 222 Rosewood Drive, Danvers, MA 01923. For those organizations that have been granted a photocopy license by CCC, a separate system of payments has been arranged. The fee codes for users of the Transactional Reporting Service are ISBN-13: 978-1-1184-2804-7/2014.

Library of Congress Cataloging-in-Publication Data

Shelby, Amanda, author.
  Small animal anesthesia techniques / Amanda M. Shelby, Carolyn M. McKune.
     p. ; cm.
  Includes bibliographical references and index.
  ISBN 978-1-118-42804-7 (pbk.)
  I. McKune, Carolyn, author. II. Title.
  [DNLM: 1. Anesthesia–methods–Handbooks. 2. Anesthesia–veterinary–Handbooks. 3. Cats–Handbooks.
4. Dogs–Handbooks. 5. Pets–Handbooks. SF 914]
  SF914
  636.089'796–dc23
                                  2013045086

A catalogue record for this book is available from the British Library.

Wiley also publishes its books in a variety of electronic formats. Some content that appears in print may not be available in electronic books.

Cover images: ekg © Shevchuk Boris; cat © elenaleonova; dog sitting © druvo; dog laying down © aspenrock
Cover design by Matt Kuhns

Set in 10/12.5 pt TimesLTStd by Toppan Best-set Premedia Limited
Printed and bound in Singapore by Markono Print Media Pte Ltd

1 2014

Contents

Contributors

Nicole Fitzgerald, RVT, VTS-Anesthesia
Anesthesia Supervisor
Louisiana State University
Veterinary Teaching Hospital and Clinics

Carolyn M. McKune, **DVM DACVAA**
Mythos Veterinary LLC
Gainesville, Florida

Amanda M. Shelby, CVT, **VTS-Anesthesia**
Associate Clinical Specialist 3 (Anesthesia)
School of Veterinary Medicine
Louisiana State University
Baton Rouge, Louisiana

Preface

The purpose of this book is to provide an easily accessible guide to the veterinary professional, for development of a balanced anesthesia protocol with appropriate analgesia. The authors assume the reader is familiar with concepts of veterinary medicine; this book outlines the anesthetic process, gives example protocols for specific patients, and helps to anticipate anesthetic complications. The information, while supported by research where appropriate, is also reflective of the authors' personal preferences and experiences. It is recommended the anesthetist become familiar with healthy patients for routine procedures before attempting anesthesia in the critical patient.

Amanda M. Shelby
Carolyn M. McKune

Acknowledgments

While many veterinary professionals have and continue to be influential, I would like to give special acknowledgment to the following individuals who helped inspire my interests in anesthesia and the development of this work: L. Pablo, for your patience and guidance; J. Bailey, for encouraging improvement; A. Shih, for inspiring awe and speediness; S. Robertson, for your humility and compassion; T. Torres, for believing in me before anyone else; M. Fitzgerald, for your contributions, writing, and patience; C. McKune, for encouragement, reassurance, and professional guidance; A. daCunha and P. Queiroz-Williams, for capturing the great shots; and Thumbwars, for bathing the kids. Thank you.

A.S.

The efforts of many people resulted in the creation of this book, starting with the influence of Dr. Mike Mison, who reintroduced me to an academic setting where I would eventually go on to meet Ms. Amanda Shelby, veterinary technician extraordinaire, who would involve me in this project. However, a few folks along the way deserve a special acknowledgment: all of the anesthesia technicians and anesthesiologists at UC Davis College of Veterinary Medicine (particularly Dr. L. Barter, Dr. R. Brosnan, and Dr. P. Wong), who directly shaped the anesthesiologist I am today; Ms. Amanda Shelby, a brilliant mind with a hardworking mother's ethics; and Dr. Sheilah Robertson, a selfless mentor who is truly beyond her time. In addition, all of the students I have had the pleasure of working with since 2003 have taught me more about what it means to be a compassionate veterinarian than all of the formal instruction I've ever had.

However, no professional endeavor will succeed without a strong personal foundation. My rock in that respect is my wonderful husband, Dr. Michael J. Dark, without whom this would not have been possible. If I have to dedicate this book to someone, it is to the joys of my life: my children, Michael D. Dark and Elspeth L. Dark. You are the future and this book is for you.

C.M.

About the companion website

This book is accompanied by a companion website:

www.wiley.com/go/shelbyanesthesia

The website includes:

- Videos
- Images
- Worksheets for calculations

Chapter 1

Anesthetic process

Step 1: Preanesthetic assessment

The patient's primary veterinarian performs a complete physical examination (PE) and history, which is made available to the anesthetist. The anesthetist then reviews the patient's history, performs his or her own preanesthetic PE, and reviews or requests additional diagnostic information (such as blood work [BW] or radiographs). The preceding information is obtained and reviewed within 24 hours of anesthesia, to ensure the most recent and therefore most pertinent assessment of the patient. When all the necessary information is collected, the anesthetist assigns the anesthesia candidate an American Society of Anesthesiologists' (ASA) score.

A. History

Important components of patient history include identification of the chief complaint(s), supporting diagnostic information, time of last meal, previous anesthetic complications, known allergies, vaccination records, and current medications. Each of these components plays a vital role in the anesthetist's ability to advocate for the patient. For example, identifying the chief complaint of the patient will ensure the appropriate analgesia is selected, correct area is prepared for surgery, appropriate fluids are chosen, necessary supportive measures (such as inotropes) are prepared in advance, and so on. The time of the last meal is a key determinant if fasting duration is appropriate (although this is not always possible in the emergent situation), to reduce the incidence of regurgitation and possible esophageal stricture. Previous anesthesia concerns and known allergies allow the anesthetist to appropriately tailor drugs to avoid combinations that would result in serious consequences (such as a patient that has allergies to eggs receiving propofol, which contains an egg lecithin). Vaccination records are important to control contagious disease and to protect from zoonotic diseases (such as rabies). Current medications also influence the anesthetic protocol; a good rule of thumb is to ask a client what passes through the pet's mouth other than food or water. Often, clients forget herbs or vitamins that are considered medications.

Small Animal Anesthesia Techniques, First Edition. Amanda M. Shelby and Carolyn M. McKune.
© 2014 John Wiley & Sons, Inc. Published 2014 by John Wiley & Sons, Inc.
Companion website: www.wiley.com/go/shelbyanesthesia

B. PE guidelines

The primary veterinarian performs a complete PE prior to electing anesthesia for a patient. However, the anesthetist systematically performs his or her own PE on every patient in his or her care. Developing a consistent approach to the PE increases the likelihood of recognizing abnormal findings. If possible, this exam is performed prior to any administration of drugs. A quiet, stress-limited environment for patient evaluation is ideal. The following is a rough guide for the anesthetic PE:

1. Overall observation

(a) Disposition: Is the patient nervous, calm, anxious, or aggressive?

(b) Gait: Is the patient lame or neurologic? Does the patient have a head tilt?

(c) Level of consciousness: Is the patient bright or quiet? Is it alert and responsive or depressed and obtunded?

(d) Pain assessment: Does the patient display any outward signs of discomfort or pain? A preemptive pain evaluation will assist in postoperative pain assessment and includes assessment of the patient's demeanor, attention and response to palpation of areas considered painful, desire or reluctance to move, and posture (1).

(e) Observation of respiratory effort and abdomen: Does the abdomen look distended? Is there an abdominal component to the patient's breathing?

2. Head to tail evaluation

(a) Head: Starting at the head, look at the overall symmetry of the eyes, nose, lips, mandible, and maxilla. Is discharge from the eyes or nose present? Are the eyes "sunken in"? Determine capillary refill time (CRT) by lifting the patient's lip and pressing on a section of pink gingiva. Take note of the mucous membrane color (MMC) and moistness. If possible, open and examine the mouth. Does anything prohibit straightforward intubation?

(b) Neck: Palpate the size of the trachea to assist with endotracheal (ET) tube selection.

(c) Body: Auscultate the thorax. Listen for lung and heart sounds. Determine the heart rate (HR) and rhythm. Palpate the abdomen for fluid, enlarged organs, or masses that might make ventilation under anesthesia challenging. Palpate femoral pulses while ausculting heart sounds to feel for pulse variations. Perform skin tenting to establish hydration status. Obtain body temperature (Table 1.1).

C. Blood work guidelines

BW is important in helping the anesthetist determine the patient's hydration status as well as roughly predicting drug metabolism and elimination. Minimum BW for young, healthy patients undergoing routine/elective procedures includes packed cell volume (PCV), total solids (TS), and an Azo-Stick to assess renal function within 24 hours of anesthesia. A complete blood count (CBC) and chemistry (CHEM) within 2 weeks of

Table 1.1   Physical examination: normal findings for the canine and feline.

Species	Heart rate (beats/min)	Respiratory rate (breath/min)	Temperature (F)	CRT (s)	Mucous membrane color
Canine	80–160	16–24	99.5–102.0	<2	Pink or pigmented
Feline	160–240	40–60	99.5–102.5	<2	Pink

Table 1.2   Normal blood work for canine and feline patients.

CBC	Canine	Feline
PCV (%)	37–55	25–45
TP (g/dL)	6–7.5	6–7.5
Hb (g/dL)	13.3–20.5	10.6–15.6
PLTS ($\times 10^{-3}$/mL)	177–398	175–500
WBC ($\times 10^{-3}$/mL)	5.3–19.8	4.04–18.70
RBC ($\times 10^{-6}$/mL)	5.83–8.87	6.56–11.20
CHEM[a]		
ALT (U/L)	16–91	33–152
ALP (U/L)	20–155	22–87
AST (U/L)	23–65	1–37
BUN	9–30	10–25
Creatinine (mg/dL)	0.7–1.8	1.0–2.0
TP (g/dL)	5.4–7.1	6.0–8.6
Total bilirubin (mg/dL)	0.3–0.9	0.1–0.8
Albumin (g/dL)	2.5–3.7	2.4–3.8
Ionized calcium (mmol/L)	1.25–1.5	1.1–1.4
Total calcium (mg/dL)	9.8–11.7	9.1–11.2
Sodium (mEq/L)	140–150	146–157
Potassium (mEq/L)	3.9–4.9	3.5–4.8
Chloride (mEq/L)	109–120	116–126
Lactate (mmol/L)	0.5–2.0	0.5–2.0
Glucose (mg/dL)	65–112	67–168
Azo-Stick	5–15	5–15
Urine-specific gravity (SG)	1.018–1.050	1.018–1.050
Coagulation test parameters		
PT (s)	6.8–10.2	9.6–13.2
PTT (s)	10.7–16.4	12.6–15.7
ACT (s)	60–125	60–125
BMBT (min)	2–3	2–3

Source: Reference 2.
[a]Reference ranges are specific to the analyzer and laboratory being used.

the anesthetic assessment are recommended for nonelective procedures, geriatric patients, and patients with any abnormal findings on PE. If the patient has any indication of changes in PE or abnormalities on previous BW, the CBC and CHEM are repeated prior to anesthesia. Additional BW such as clotting profiles, blood typing, cross matching, and blood gas and electrolyte analysis are indicated based on the procedure or disease process (Table 1.2 and Table 1.3).

Table 1.3 Normal blood gas values for canine and feline patients.[a]

pH	7.35–7.45
$PaCO_2$ (mmHg)	35–45
PaO_2[b] (mmHg)	80–100
HCO_3 (mEq/L)	17–26
BE (mEq/L)	(–4) to 0, 0–4

Source: Reference 2.
Note: Reference values will vary slightly with the analyzer and laboratory being used.
[a]Felines are more acidic when compared with canines, with slightly lower pH normal ranges and lower HCO_3.
[b]Normal range for PaO_2 is dependent on inspired oxygen content (FiO_2). This table lists the value of PaO_2 for a patient breathing room air, with a FiO_2 of 21%. Under anesthesia, FiO_2 increases to 100%, bringing up PaO_2 to 400–500 mmHg.

Table 1.4 Physical status classification system (3).

ASA Physical Status 1	A normal healthy patient
ASA Physical Status 2	A patient with mild systemic disease
ASA Physical Status 3	A patient with moderate systemic disease
ASA Physical Status 4	A patient with severe systemic disease
ASA Physical Status 5	A moribund patient that is not expected to survive without the operation or intervention
ASA Emergency	Accompanies the assigned ASA status to denote urgency

D. Physical status

Assignment of physical status is based on the patient's overall signalment, PE, diagnostics, and anesthetic urgency. The ASA's assignment of physical status is used to classify patients based on the preanesthetic assessment of intraoperative and postoperative risks (Table 1.4).

Step 2: Premedication

Premedication is performed with the goals of providing sedation to facilitate restraint and intravenous (IV) catheterization, providing preemptive analgesia, and reducing dosage requirements of induction and maintenance drugs. Depending on the drug(s) selected, premedication is typically given intramuscularly (IM) (see Figure 1.1), but may be administered subcutaneously, orally/buccally, or IV. Additionally during this phase of the anesthetic process, the patient is catheterized (see Table 1.6), preoxygenated for at least 3–5 minutes with 100% oxygen up to the point of induction and intubation, and pre-instrumented if deemed necessary. See Table 1.5.

Step 3: Induction

Induction is the process of initiating anesthesia to facilitate intubation. Typically, this involves giving an induction drug intravenously either as a bolus or "to effect." See Table 1.7 for a list of commonly used drugs.

Table 1.5 Premedication drugs.

Drug	Dose (mg/kg)	Route	Sedation	Analgesia	Benefits	Disadvantages
Acepromazine	0.01–0.05	IV, IM, SQ	Moderate	None	Antiarrhythmic, antiemetic, antihistamine	Vasodilation, reduction in cardiac output
Buprenorphine	0.01–0.03	IV, IM, SQ	Minimal	Partial mu agonist	Minimal cardiovascular side effects, analgesia, euphoria in cats, reversible	No reduction in inhalant requirement
Butorphanol	0.1–0.4	IV, IM, SQ	Moderate	Kappa agonist, Mu antagonist	Minimal cardiovascular effects, reversible	Antagonizes effects of mu opioids; minimally effective for severe pain
Dexmedetomidine	0.001–0.015	IV, IM, SQ	Profound	Moderate analgesic	Reversible	Cardiovascular effects (initial vasoconstriction, bradycardia, reduced cardiac output)
Diazepam	0.1–0.5	IV, IM	Moderate sedation for neonate, geriatric, and debilitated patients	None	Reversible, minimal cardiovascular effects	IM absorption inconsistent; may cause excitement in healthy patients
Hydromorphone	0.05–0.2	IV, IM	Moderate	Full mu agonist	Reversible, minimal cardiovascular effects	May cause vomiting
Ketamine	2–20	IM, IV, PO	Immobilization	Somatic analgesic	Useful as part of an injectable technique	Muscle rigidity, pain on injection
Meperidine	5	IM only	Moderate	Full mu agonist	Mild anticholinergic action, reversible	Histamine release, short acting
Methadone	0.1–0.5	IM, IV	Minimal	Full mu agonist, NMDA antagonist	Reversible, no vomiting	Minimal sedation
Midazolam	0.1–0.5	IM, IV	Moderate for neonate, geriatric, and debilitated patients	None	Reversible, minimal cardiovascular side effects, water soluble	Unpredictable in healthy patients
Morphine	0.1–0.5	IM	Moderate	Full mu agonist	Reversible, minimal cardiovascular effects	Histamine release, vomiting
Oxymporphone	0.05–0.1	IM, IV	Moderate	Full mu agonist	Reversible, minimal cardiovascular effects	Expensive

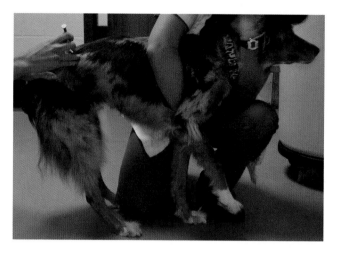

Figure 1.1 IM premedication in the epaxial muscles of a dog. Palpate dorsal spinal processes of lumbar spine; epaxial muscles lie laterally on either side. Insert needle and aspirate to ensure placement in muscle. Inject. Courtesy of Patricia Queiroz-Williams.

Table 1.6 IV catheter placement.

> **Materials:** Clippers with 40 blade, scrub, gauze, tape, over-the-needle catheter, T-port or injection cap, heparinized saline (flush)
>
> **Techniques:**
> 1. Select IV site to catheterize. Typical sites include cephalic, lateral saphenous (canine), or medial saphenous (feline) veins. Based on observation and palpation of the vessel, select the largest size catheter that will fit.
> 2. Clip and aseptically prepare area over vessel.
> 3. Assistant is responsible for restraining patient, especially the head, and holding off the vessel of choice (see Figure 1.2). If the catheter is placed in the right cephalic vein, the assistant restrains the patient's head from the patient's left side with his or her left arm and holds off the vessel with the right.
> 4. The anesthetist's nondominant hand holds the distal aspect of the limb intended for catheterization. The dominant hand places the catheter.
> 5. Insert the over-the-needle catheter through the skin over the vessel. Keep the catheter parallel to the vessel.
> 6. Look for a flash of blood in the stylet's chamber; once flash occurs, insert the entire catheter slightly further into the vessel to ensure the end of the catheter is well seated. Blood should continue to flow if the catheter has remained in the vessel.
> 7. Advance catheter off the stylet. If in the vessel, there is minimal resistance to advancing of the catheter.
> 8. Once the catheter is in place, and the injection cap or T-port is placed, flush with heparinized saline. Proper placement in the vessel is confirmed by aspiration of blood or palpating the pulsing of flush in the vessel.
> 9. Tape catheter in place. Use a narrow piece of tape, sticky side up under the catheter. Fold the tape sticky side to sticky side with the hub of the catheter between (see Figure 1.3). Wrap the remainder of the tape around the limb, securing the catheter to the patient. Additional pieces of tape are placed around the catheter to keep hair away from the injection port and to provide additional support and security.

Chapter 1

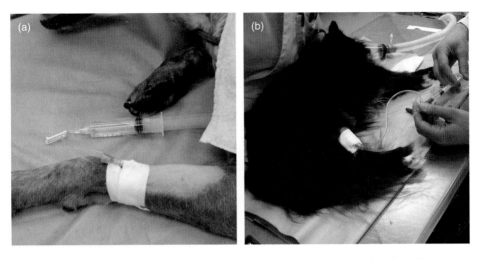

Figure 1.2 (a) Cephalic IV catheter. (b) Saphenous IV catheter in a canine patient.

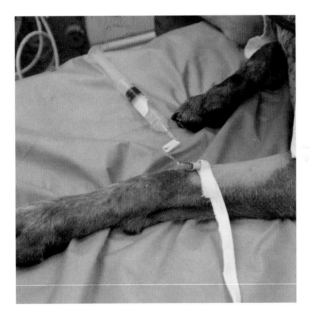

Figure 1.3 Taping a cephalic catheter in place. With tape sticky side up placed under the catheter hub, fold tape over the catheter hub, allowing the tape to adhere sticky side to sticky side. Wrap the remaining length of tape securely around patient's limb. Courtesy of Anderson da Cuhna.

A. Selecting an ET tube

There are several ways to select an appropriately sized ET tube. One can palpate the trachea, using the thumb and index finger to feel the lateral edges to gauge width. Another method is to assess the diameter of the space between the nares and to select an ET tube of that width. This method may over- or underestimate ET tube size depending on species and breed variation. One may also use previous experience to choose an appropriate size of ET tube. Whatever method is chosen, prior to inducing the patient, have three ET tubes available (the size believed to fit, a size smaller, and a size larger). Brachycephalic breeds (i.e., pugs or bulldogs) often use smaller ET tubes than expected. Sight hounds and dachshunds typically use larger ET tubes than expected. Cats will typically use 3.5- to 5-mm internal diameter (ID) ET tubes. Determining the length of ET tube is also important prior to inducing the patient. Hold the ET tube next to the patient, with the tip at the thoracic inlet (see Figure 1.4). This measurement helps to avoid endobronchial intubation. ET tubes are commonly reused in the veterinary setting. The ET tube is cut to a suitable length; excessively long ET tubes increase resistance and dead space. ET tubes come with two different types of cuff systems: high-pressure/low-volume cuffs or low-pressure/high-volume cuffs. The high-pressure/low-volume cuff adheres well to the ET tube, resulting in little additional diameter to the tube. However, it requires a high intracuff pressure to achieve a seal; in addition, this high pressure occurs with relatively little volume delivered into the pilot balloon, which is deceiving for the anesthetist, who may administer more volume to "fill" the pilot balloon, resulting in tracheal damage. This seal is in contact with only a small portion of the tracheal wall, forming a tight, high-pressure seal only at a pinpoint location. These cuffs are associated with adverse events such as tracheal rupture and tears in cats (4). The authors discourage their use. Low-pressure/high-volume cuffs add some bulk to the ET tube, making them potentially more difficult to place. However, they exert a much lower pressure while still achieving

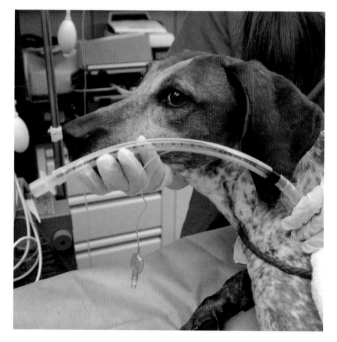

Figure 1.4   Sizing the length of ET tube on a patient prior to inducing. Courtesy of Anderson da Cuhna.

Table 1.7 Induction drugs.

Drug	Dose (mg/kg)	Route	Advantages	Disadvantages
Etomidate	1–2	IV	Minimal cardiovascular effects, short acting Given to "effect"	If patient is not sufficiently premedicated, it may vomit at induction (5); laryngeal tone is not reduced (lidocaine may facilitate intubation). Adrenocortical suppression occurs, which is detrimental in septic and Addisonian patients.
Isoflurane	3–5% in 100% oxygen	Mask or chamber	Given to "effect" No venous access necessary. Anesthetist is not in direct contact with fractious patients when using a chamber.	Dose-dependent vasodilation, cardiac and respiratory depression, environment, and personnel exposure.
Ketamine	5–7	IM, IV	Fast onset, short acting, increases HR and BP, provides analgesia	Muscle rigidity (use with benzodiazepine). Avoid in patients with seizures.
Neuroleptic induction (opioid and benzodiazepine)	a. Opioid options: Fentanyl 0.005–0.01 or Hydromorphone 0.1 b. Benzodiazepine options: Midazolam or Diazepam 0.2–0.3	IV	Minimal cardiovascular effects	May cause dysphoria in healthy patients.
Propofol	2–6	IV	Given to "effect" Fast onset, short acting Recovery is smooth. No venous access necessary. Anesthetist is not in direct contact with fractious patients.	Apnea, vasodilation (preoxygenation is advised).
Sevoflurane	5–8% in 100% oxygen	Mask or chamber	Given to "effect" Quicker and less odiferous than isoflurane (typically better tolerated)	Dose-dependent vasodilation, cardiac and respiratory depression, environment and personnel exposure. Expensive.

HR, heart rate; BP, blood pressure.

9

Table 1.8 Intubation of canine or feline patient.

Materials: Laryngoscope, variety of ET tubes, lubricant, stylets, tie to secure tube, 4 × 4 gauze square to hold the tongue.

Techniques:

1. Induction agent is appropriately administered until jaw is lax and lateral palpebral reflex is absent.
2. The patient is placed in sternal recumbency, if possible. The assistant opens the mouth of the patient by placing one hand over the snout, holding behind the maxillary canine teeth and using the other hand to withdraw the tongue between the mandibular canine teeth. Slight hyperextension of the head and neck helps the anesthetist visualize the larynx (see Figure 1.5).
3. The anesthetist places the laryngoscope blade on the base of the tongue under the epiglottis. It is important to place the tip of the blade under the epiglottis on the base of the tongue to avoid damaging this sensitive tissue, which could contribute to airway obstruction at extubation. Applying pressure on the base of the tongue will help displace the epiglottis and allow visualization of the larynx. A brief examination of the larynx is performed every time a patient is induced.
4. Once the anesthetist visualizes the larynx, the ET tube is advanced between the arytenoids. In dogs, when resistance is encountered, a slight twist of the ET tube helps facilitate advancement. In brachycephalic patients, an elongated soft palate often obstructs visualization of the arytenoids. The tip of the ET tube is used to displace the soft palate. In cats, laryngeal spasms and rigid arytenoids make intubation more difficult. For cats, a drop of lidocaine on each arytenoid is helpful to minimize laryngeal spasms (see Figure 1.6). Position the end of the ET tube over the arytenoids, be patient, and wait for the patient to take a breath. If the patient is not taking decent breaths, the assistant may try pinching a toe to stimulate a deep breath. At inspiration, the arytenoids will open slightly. With a gentle, determined motion, insert the ET tube between the arytenoids. Slight rotation may help facilitate intubation if resistance is encountered. However, feline laryngeal tissue is easily damaged, and therefore, applying any force during intubation is highly discouraged.
5. Once intubated, the patient is immediately attached to the breathing circuit with an appropriate flow rate of 100% oxygen. The anesthetist visually confirms proper intubation. The ET tube cuff is inflated, while the anesthetist attempts to "hold" a 20–25 cmH$_2$O breath. The ET tube cuff is inflated only if a leak is present! Once the cuff is sealed, the inhalant anesthetics are initiated.

Note: Although typically the preferred position for intubation is sternal, patients are also intubated in lateral or dorsal recumbency. For patients in lateral recumbency, the head is hyperextended until it forms a straight line with the spine. Dorsal recumbency is a difficult position for intubation and is performed only if necessary (e.g., a patient is accidentally extubated during a surgical procedure).

an adequate seal. In addition, the seal is formed along the entire length of the cuff, rather than at one specific point. In all, this type of cuff, while more cumbersome, provides the safest seal. See Table 1.8 for information on intubating a patient.

Step 4: Maintenance phase

This phase typically involves gas inhalants or total intravenous anesthesia (TIVA). Close, continual patient monitoring is key. See Table 1.9 for agents routinely used to maintain anesthesia.

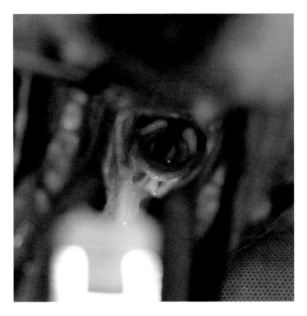

Figure 1.5 Canine larynx. Courtesy of Anderson da Cuhna.

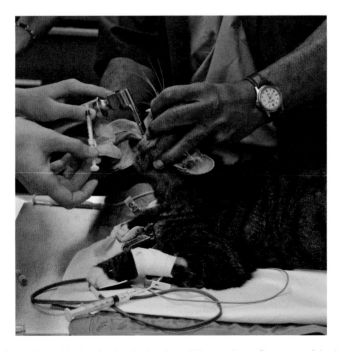

Figure 1.6 Sternal positioning for intubation in a feline patient. Courtesy of Anderson da Cuhna.

11

Table 1.9   Routine maintenance anesthetics.

Agent	Dose/MAC	Advantages	Disadvantages
Isoflurane	Dog: 1.3% Cat: 1.6%	Quickly titratable, no venous access is required; however, it is recommended.	Dose-dependent cardiovascular and respiratory depression
Sevoflurane	Dog: 2.3% Cat: 2.6%	Quickly titratable, less soluble than isoflurane, no venous access is required; however, it is recommended.	Dose-dependent cardiovascular and respiratory depression, expense
Propofol constant rate infusion (CRI)	0.2–0.4 mg/kg/min	Smooth recovery, no ET tube is required although it is recommended when possible, airway is available to clinician for procedures.	Apnea, vasodilation

MAC, minimum alveolar concentration.

Step 5: Recovery/postoperative phase

The recovery phase begins with the discontinuation of the maintenance anesthetic agent and includes extubation and at least the first 3 hours postextubation. The postoperative phase includes any period during which the patient requires continual management and observation. A patient is extubated only when it can maintain its own airway. Typically, this occurs when the patient swallows and lifts its head. The ET tube cuff is deflated only after the patient can swallow (unless otherwise indicated). Most anesthetic mortalities that occur in the recovery phase will happen in the first 3 hours (6). Continuous observation is recommended during this phase, and it is important to provide adequate analgesia and pain assessment. Pain scoring techniques are helpful in assessing the patient (see Appendix A).

References

1. Morton C, Reid J, Scott E, Holton L, Nolan A. Application of a scaling model to establish and validate an interval-level pain scale for assessment of acute pain in dogs. Am J Vet Res. 2005;66(12):2154–66.
2. Silverstein D, Hopper K. Small Animal Critical Care Medicine. St. Louis, MO: Saunders Elsevier; 2008.
3. ASA Physical Status Classification System (April 9, 2013). Available at: http://www.asahq.org/Home/For-Members/Clinical-Information/ASA-Physical-Status-Classification-System.
4. Mitchell SL, McCarthy R, Rudloff E, Pernell RT. Tracheal rupture associated with intubation in cats: 20 cases (1996–1998). J Am Vet Med Assoc. 2000;216(10):1592–5.
5. Muir WW, Mason DE. Side effects of etomidate in dogs. J Am Vet Med Assoc. 1989;194(10):1430–4.
6. Brodbelt D. Perioperative mortality in small animal anaesthesia. Vet J. 2009;182(2):152–61.

Chapter 2

Anesthesia equipment and monitoring

This chapter details proper anesthesia equipment and how to safely set up an anesthetic machine (1). In addition, it outlines tools to assist the anesthetist in monitoring patient vital signs and anesthetic depth. Descriptions of monitoring equipment, equipment uses, advantage and disadvantages of the devices, and how to properly place equipment on the patient are provided. Normal wave forms and vital parameters are depicted.

I. Anesthesia machine

This critical piece of equipment functions to produce a gas mixture with variable composition of precisely selected gases (2). The machine has three systems:

A. High pressure system

1. Receives gases at cylinder pressure and then serves to decrease that pressure and make it constant.
2. Yoke or yoke block connects the machine to the compressed gas source (pipeline or cylinder).
3. Cylinder pressure gauge uses a bourdon tube to indicate how much pressure the remaining compressed gas in the tank exerts, as an indicator of how much supply is available (see Equation 2.1).

$$\text{psi} \times 0.3 = \text{L} \qquad (2.1a)$$

$$\text{psi} \times 1.7 = \text{L} \qquad (2.1b)$$

Equation 2.1 is used to determine the volume of oxygen remaining in the cylinder from pounds per square inch of pressure. Equation 2.1a is for "E" cylinder, and Equation 2.1b is for "H" cylinder.

4. Pressure regulator reduces pressure (which fluctuates with temperature and content) to 50 psi and maintains constant flow of compressed gas to the anesthetic system.

Small Animal Anesthesia Techniques, First Edition. Amanda M. Shelby and Carolyn M. McKune.
© 2014 John Wiley & Sons, Inc. Published 2014 by John Wiley & Sons, Inc.
Companion website: www.wiley.com/go/shelbyanesthesia

B. Intermediate pressure system

1. Receives gases from the regulator or pipeline, which are made constant. From there gases pass to the flowmeter and oxygen flush valve.
2. Pipeline inlet allows access to a hospital pipeline system if present.
3. Oxygen pressure failure device attempts to protect the patient in case of delivery of a hypoxic gas mixture, and will either alarm or cut off non-oxygen gases should supply of oxygen pressure drop considerably.
4. Flowmeter assembly controls and measures the amount of gas flow in liters per minute (L/min). Gas flow is measured at the largest point on the indicator (e.g., if a ball is used, it is measured at the center of the ball). Each flowmeter will depict where an indicator is read on the flowmeter.

C. Low pressure system

1. Gases at this point move from the flowmeter to the machine outlet (where breathing circuits are connected).
2. A vaporizer, a device uniquely customized for each anesthetic agent, converts an agent from liquid to vapor form.
3. The common gas outlet is where all gases from the machine arrive at. Depending on the machine, a separate common gas outlet for a rebreathing (RB) system and non-rebreathing (NRB) system may be present.

D. Other critical components of the anesthesia machine

1. Adjustable pressure limiting (APL) valve (or "pop-off" valve) limits or allows gas to remain or exit the breathing circuit, depending on its degree of closure.
2. An oxygen flush valve rapidly delivers oxygen into the circuit (bypassing the vaporizer) (see Figure 2.1).

II. Setting up the anesthesia machine

A. Selecting a breathing system

1. NRB systems (see Figure 2.2) are typically reserved for patients less than 7 kg. Required oxygen flow rates are 200–300 mL/kg/min with a minimum acceptable flow of 0.5 L/min.
2. RB systems (see Figure 2.3) are typically selected for patients more than 7 kg. Recommended oxygen flow rates are 10–30 mL/kg/min (see Table 2.1).

B. Reservoir bag

1. Reservoir bag allows manually assisted ventilation by the anesthetist. To deliver a breath, close the APL, compress reservoir bag to desired size breath by watching the manometer (less than 20 cmH₂O in dogs and cats), and do not forget to open the APL valve.

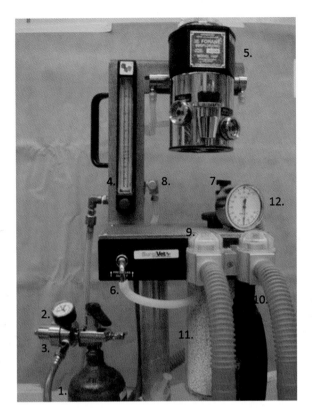

Figure 2.1 Anesthesia machine with circle system labeled: 1. oxygen "E" cylinder; 2. cylinder pressure gauge; 3. pressure regulator; 4. oxygen flowmeter; 5. vaporizer; 6. common gas outlet; 7. APL or "pop-off" valve; 8. oxygen flush valve; 9. unidirectional valves; 10. reservoir bag connection; 11. CO_2-absorbent canister; 12. pressure manometer.

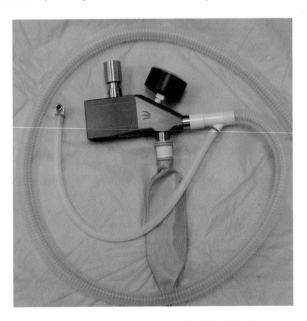

Figure 2.2 Non-rebreathing system (modified Bain circuit) with adaptor.

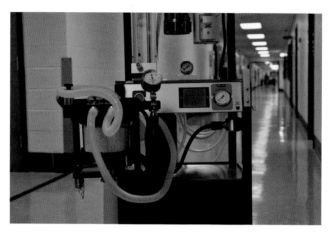

Figure 2.3 Rebreathing system connected to anesthesia machine. Courtesy of Anderson da Cuhna.

Table 2.1 Comparison of breathing systems.

Non-rebreathing system		Rebreathing system	
Advantages	*Disadvantages*	*Advantages*	*Disadvantages*
Minimal resistance	High oxygen flows,	Low oxygen flow	Increased resistance in
Less dead space	heat loss, water	rates, less	circuit (unidirectional
Light weight	loss, more	expensive	valves and carbon
High oxygen flow	expensive	Less body heat	dioxide absorber)
rates allow rapid	If oxygen flow is	loss	More components of
change in inspired	too low, patient	Closed circuit is	anesthetic machine
anesthetic	will rebreathe	performed if	can lead to risk of
concentration	expired gases.	desired	malfunction
		Rebreathing of	"Y" piece adds dead
		expired carbon	space
		dioxide difficult if	Large volume of
		all components	breathing circuit
		are operational	requiring longer time
			between changes in
			inspired anesthetic
			concentration
			More maintenance
			(changing CO_2
			absorbent)
			Bulkier system

2. The reservoir bag is equal to or larger than the calculated size:

$$\text{Weight (kg)} \times \text{minute volume} \times V_T = \text{bag size} \qquad (2.2)$$
$$\text{Example: } 20\,\text{kg} \times 6 \times 10 = 1200\,\text{mL. (Use a 2-L bag.)}$$

Typical ranges for minute volume and tidal volume are 3–6 L/min and 10–20 mL/kg, respectively. The example shows that a 20-kg patient would require a 2-L reservoir bag.

Table 2.2   Pressure checking the anesthesia machine.

Technique:
1. Turn on oxygen tank or connect to oxygen source. 2. Connect the breathing circuit appropriate for the patient. Ensure the fresh gas outlet is connected. 3. Connect the reservoir bag. 4. Close the pop-off valve or APL valve. 5. Occlude the patient end of the breathing circuit. 6. Turn on the oxygen flowmeter and fill the breathing circuit with oxygen until the manometer reaches 30 cmH$_2$O. Turn off the flowmeter. 7. Hold this pressure for 20–30 seconds.[a] 8. Open the pop-off valve to relieve pressure from the circuit.

[a]If the pressure doesn't hold, leaks are present. See "Troubleshooting Leaks."

C. Pressure checking the anesthesia machine

Table 2.2 details a common method for pressure checking both the RB and NRB systems. However, this method of pressure checking the breathing system does not check the integrity of the inspiratory tube of a modified Bain system.

D. Troubleshooting leaks

1. Ensure pop-off valve is closed completely.
2. Replace the breathing circuit and/or reservoir bag.
3. If using an RB system, check the soda sorb canister and unidirectional valves for proper placement or cracks.
4. Ensure fresh gas outlet is connected to the circuit in use.

III. Monitoring patient depth

The most accurate determinant of anesthetic depth is the patient itself. Heart rate (HR), respiratory rate (RR), and blood pressure (BP) will change with anesthetic depth but are also influenced by other factors. Table 2.3 lists clinical signs of anesthetic depth.

Table 2.3   Monitoring anesthetic depth.

	Too light	**Surgical plane**	**Too deep**
Palpebral reflex	Present	Absent	Absent
Jaw tone	Tight	Loose	Absent
Pupil position	Central	Ventral medial	Central
Corneal reflex	Present	Present	Absent
Anal tone	Tight, blinking[a]	Absent, lax	Absent

[a]Blinking implies when stimulated with a thermometer or a pinch, the patient responds with closing the anal sphincter.

Chapter 2

IV. Mechanical ventilation (MV) or intermittent positive pressure ventilation (IPPV)

A. Mechanical ventilation

MV is useful in cases where the patient is not ventilating adequately due to respiratory depression, disease, or paralysis (e.g., use of neuromuscular blockers). MV exerts positive pressure, and, while useful, it is important to recognize that IPPV has negative effects on cardiac output (CO) by decreasing venous return to the heart, decreasing CO_2, and increasing delivery of inhalant anesthetic. Only experienced personnel should operate a mechanical ventilator; caution is exercised in patients with hypovolemia and cardiopulmonary disease. Basic concepts of commercial ventilators are similar in function; however, the terminology or labeling may vary. It is important to understand how adjustments to the ventilator settings will affect ventilation before using it on a patient. Thorough review of the manufacturer's operation manual prior to using a ventilator is advised to ensure proper and safe use.

B. Classification of ventilators

There are three basic characteristics of ventilators: the mechanism by which they are controlled, the mechanism by which they are cycled from inspiration to expiration, and the mechanism that triggers the ventilator to begin a breath. Ventilators are classified as volume- or pressure-controlled; this refers to how the ventilator delivers its flow. In the case of volume-controlled ventilation, flow is administered to a certain volume, regardless of the amount of pressure delivered. In the case of pressure-controlled ventilation, flow is administered to a certain pressure, regardless of how much volume is administered. As the reader can deduce, pressure-controlled ventilation is likely to result in less barotrauma. Ventilators are cycled by time, volume, or flow. This is the mechanism by which the ventilator moves from inspiration to expiration. In a time-cycled ventilator, inspiration occurs for a set period of time (e.g., 1.5 seconds are spent in inspiration before the ventilator moves to expiration). Time-cycled ventilation is how the vast majority of veterinary anesthesia ventilators function. In a volume-cycled ventilator, achieving a target volume moves the ventilator from inspiration to expiration. In a pressure-cycled ventilator, achieving a target pressure moves the ventilator from inspiration to expiration. These latter two cycling mechanisms are common applications of ventilators intended for use in the critically ill patient (i.e., long-term ventilation). Finally, the ventilator trigger is what tells the ventilator to begin inspiration: time or pressure. A time-triggered ventilator uses the time to initiate a cycle based on the RR the anesthetist has selected; this is the way most veterinary anesthesia mechanical ventilators function. A pressure-triggered ventilator waits for feedback from the patient (usually in the form of an attempted breath) to trigger the beginning of a cycle, a feature important in critically ill patients a clinician is trying to wean from the ventilator but often impractical in anesthetized animals.

Ventilators are further classified as having ascending or descending bellows. Ascending bellows, which are most commonly used, compress down during inspiration and ascend during expiration. Leaks are easily detected in these ventilators because the bellows fall when a leak is present (a distinct advantage). Descending bellows compress upward during inspiration and descend during expiration.

C. Terminology and adjustable parameters

1. Inspiratory time to expiratory time (I:E) ratio is the relationship between time of inspiration and expiration. Normal I:E ratios are 1:2–1:3.5. Increasing the I:E ratio (i.e., 1:5) decreases inspiratory time, whereas decreasing I:E ratio (i.e., 1:1) gives the patient longer inspiratory times.
2. Peak inspiratory pressure (PIP) is the maximum pressure during the inspiratory phase or breath. In healthy small animal patients, PIP of 10–20 cmH$_2$O is enough to provide a "normal" breath for adequate ventilation. Rarely is a PIP greater than 20 cmH$_2$O needed or recommended for the small animal patient.
3. Tidal volume (V$_T$) is the volume of breath the patient receives. Normal V$_T$ is between 10 and 20 mL/kg. Graduations typically located on the bellow casing allow the anesthetist to estimate V$_T$; however, these graduations may be inaccurate. A spirometer is an accurate reflection of tidal volume, if available.
4. RR is the number of breaths per minute the patient receives. Normal RR for anesthetized canine patients is between 6 and 12; for feline patients, between 8 and 16.
5. Inspiratory flow is the speed of the flow of air during the inspiratory phase or breath. It is expressed in milliliters per second. Adjustments in inspiratory flow on many ventilators will linearly influence the V$_T$ and PIP.
6. Inspiratory time is the length of time a breath is given during the inspiratory phase. Increasing inspiratory time may increase the V$_T$ and PIP.
7. Expiratory time is the time allowed between inspirations. Some ventilators use expiratory time as a means to set the RR. Expiratory time is inversely related to the RR, meaning an increase in expiratory time decreases RR.
8. A pressure relief valve is not present on all ventilators as an adjustable feature; however, this allows the release of excessive pressure or sets off an alarm to notify the anesthetist that the maximum PIP has been exceeded. It is recommended that this valve is set to 5 cmH$_2$O over the maximum PIP.
9. Peak end-expiratory pressure (PEEP) valve is not present on all ventilators but allows the anesthetist to hold positive pressure at the end of the expiratory phase. This technique is used for specific situations where the patient may experience severe atelectasis. PEEP over 10 cmH$_2$O is typically not recommended. PEEP valves of fixed pressures are available for application to an anesthetic machine or ventilator. They are attached to the pop-off valve of the anesthetic machine or the exhaust valve of a ventilator. The anesthetist observes the manometer to ensure the PEEP valve is functional.
10. Inspiratory hold (breath hold) is not present on all ventilators; however, this button allows the anesthetist to hold a breath with the lungs inflated at a desired PIP (see Table 2.4).

Table 2.4   General setup of a mechanical ventilator.

Technique:
1. Connect ventilator's driving gas to source. While any pressurized gas will drive the ventilator, typically the driving gas is oxygen.
2. If the ventilator requires electrical power, plug in to outlet.
3. Ensure ventilator settings are set appropriately or turned to the lowest delivery pressure to avoid barotrauma when turned on. Depending on the make and model of the ventilator (see Figure 2.4), this involves reducing the inspiratory time, inspiratory flow, or volume controls.
4. Evacuate the reservoir bag on the anesthetic machine to avoid personnel exposure to waste anesthetics.
5. Replace the reservoir bag with the breathing line from the ventilator.
6. Close the pop-off (APL) valve on the anesthetic machine.
7. Connect the ventilator's scavenging hose to a scavenging system.
8. To inflate the bellows, increase the oxygen flow on the anesthetic machine. Reduce flow to appropriate rate for patient and breathing circuit when bellows are full.
9. Turn on ventilator; watch the patient's V_T, PIP, and $EtCO_2$. Adjust to ensure adequate ventilation.

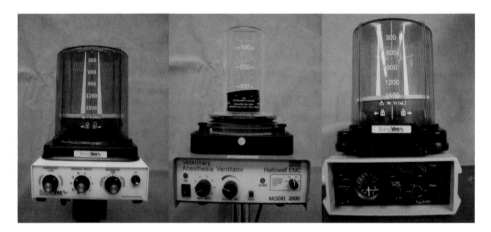

Figure 2.4   Selection of ventilators.

D. Troubleshooting common problems of a mechanical ventilator

1. Leaks

An ascending bellow that will not fill or gradually loses volume indicates the presence of a leak.

(a) Check to ensure that the drive gas source is connected.
(b) Ensure breathing circuit did not become disconnected from patient and connection of ventilator is secure.
(c) Ensure bellow casing is secured and no tears are present in the bellow.

(**d**) Ensure adequate oxygen flow from the anesthetic machine.
(**e**) Make sure pop-off (APL) valve is closed.

2. Hypoventilation

Adjustment of these following parameters may address hypoventilation (decrease $EtCO_2$). Additionally, several of these maneuvers increase oxygenation:

(**a**) Increasing inspiratory time (affects V_T)
(**b**) Increasing PIP (affects V_T)
(**c**) Increasing inspiratory flow (affects V_T)
(**d**) Increasing RR (or decrease expiratory time).

3. EtCO₂ increase

Manipulation of the following parameters will allow an increase in $EtCO_2$:

(**a**) Decreasing RR (increase expiratory time)
(**b**) Decreasing inspiratory time (affects V_T; see above description)
(**c**) Decreasing inspiratory flow (affects V_T)
(**d**) Decreasing PIP (affects V_T)
(**e**) V_T can be decreased but is not decreased below 10 mL/kg.

4. Sudden change in PIP or V_T

(**a**) Changes in lung compliancy or elasticity and resistance may be the result of possible anesthetic complications such as a spontaneous pneumothorax (see Chapter 6, "Pneumothorax") or anaphylactic reaction (see Chapter 6, "Anaphylaxis/Anaphylactoid Reaction" section).
(**b**) An airway or ET tube obstruction will cause an increase in PIP and decrease in V_T.

V. Monitoring equipment

Table 2.5 shows the vital parameters to be monitored under anesthesia.

A. Blood pressure monitoring

1. Direct or invasive blood pressure (IBP) monitoring

IBP monitoring via arterial line is useful in debilitated or critically ill patients (ASA III–V) because of its accuracy. Common arteries for catheterization include the dorsal pedal, auricular, deep lingual, metacarpal, and coccygeal. A variety of equipment is used to measure arterial pressure (Figure 2.5 and Figure 2.6). A simple aneroid manometer is used to measure mean arterial pressure (MAP) directly, or a transducer can give direct

Table 2.5 Normal vital parameters under anesthesia.

	Canine	Feline
HR (bpm)	60–160	100–250
RR (breaths/min)	6–12	8–16
SAP (mmHg)	90–180	90–180
DAP (mmHg)	45–55	45–55
MAP (mmHg)	60–80	60–80
Temperature (F)	96–98	96–98
$EtCO_2$ (mmHg)	35–45	35–45
SpO_2 (%)	97–100	97–100

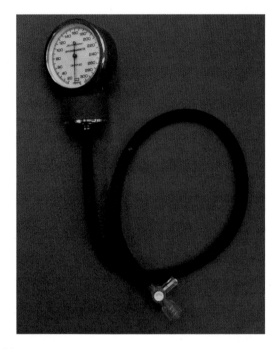

Figure 2.5 Aneroid manometer.

systolic, diastolic, and mean pressures. Regardless of the equipment used to measure direct arterial pressure, the arterial catheter is flushed periodically to avoid clotting and maintain patency. Placement of the aneroid manometer or pressure transducer should be leveled with the apex of the heart to ensure accurate values. See Table 2.6 for directions on setup of IBP monitoring. If the aneroid manometer or pressure transducer is below the apex of the heart, values are falsely high. Conversely, if the transducer is above the heart, values are falsely low. An example of a classical arterial tracing is depicted in Figure 2.7.

(a) Advantages: IBP monitoring is the most accurate and provides continuous monitoring of arterial BP. Arterial pressure is truly measured (as opposed to calculated) and therefore

Table 2.6 Placement of arterial catheter and setup of methods to measure IBP.

Materials: Over-the-needle catheter, aseptic prep, noncompliant pressure tubing, transducer or aneroid manometer, tape, clippers, syringe of heparinized saline; optional: T-port[a] or injection cap, pressure bag with heparinized saline (1–2 units/mL) when using a continuous flush transducer

Technique:

1. Palpate the artery. An artery that is not palpable is almost impossible to catheterize.
2. Clip and aseptically prepare site for catheterization.
3. Select size of catheter (often based on the size of the patient); for example, a large dog may take a 20-g catheter and cat may take a 22-g catheter. In general, the arterial catheter in the dorsal pedal artery is typically one size smaller than the cephalic venous catheter. Catheters larger than 20 g (even for an animal as large as a horse!) are unnecessary.
4. The skin is either left intact or nicked at the chosen site of entrance (operator preference).
5. Insert the catheter at a 45-degree angle to the skin to begin; the catheter is inserted distal to where the pulse is palpated. It is helpful to continue to palpate the pulse as a guide while placing the catheter. Arteries spasm, clot quickly, and have thick vascular walls, which make them more difficult than veins to catheterize. Often, the anesthetist must be mildly aggressive to achieve success (this is a skill that takes several attempts to develop proficiency).
6. Once blood is present in the stylet, advance the over-the-needle catheter slightly farther into the artery and slide the catheter off the stylet. It is important to use the stylet as a guide, leaving it in place until the catheter is completely fed into the artery.
7. Remove the stylet. Arterial blood is bright red and should be pulsing. Place the T-port, injection cap, or pressure tubing on the catheter and secure with tape similar to techniques used for IV catheters (see Table 1.6).
8. Once the catheter is correctly placed, connect the transducer to the arterial catheter using noncompliant pressure tubing (tubing that has limited elasticity) filled with heparinized saline. If an injection cap is used on the arterial catheter, a needle of the same size is used to connect pressure tubing. Alternatively, a three-way stopcock can be added to serve as a port for sampling.
9. The next step depends on whether an aneroid manometer or an automated system is used to determine IBP:

Automated System	*Aneroid Manometer*
The appropriate transducer (check manufacturer's specifications) is connected to the transducer cable. The catheter is zeroed to atmospheric pressure at the automated monitoring system. This is accomplished by turning the three-way stopcock off to the patient and open to room air. Once a baseline zero has registered, turn the stopcock off to the atmosphere, and an arterial BP appears along with a distinct waveform (see Figure 2.6). For an accurate pressure, the transducer is level with the apex of the heart.	With the stopcock off to the patient, disposable tubing (often an extension set) is connected to the aneroid manometer to prevent contamination of the manometer. This tubing is then connected to the stopcock and is filled approximately halfway with heparinized saline. The meniscus of the waterline is placed at heart level and taped in place on a fixed object (e.g., an IV pole). The stopcock is then turned off to the atmosphere, and the waterline will reset itself in accordance with the animal's pressure. The gauge of manometer will register the MAP and moves with each heartbeat (i.e., the anesthetist can obtain HR as well from this device).

Note: Placing arterial lines is an advanced skill that requires practice.
[a]Luer lock T-ports, injection caps or pressure tubing should be used when attached to the arterial catheter to ensure that accidental loss of blood from the catheter does not occur. The use of T-ports, injection caps, or needles to connect the pressure tubing will cause dampening of the pressure waveform; however, they allow sampling access.

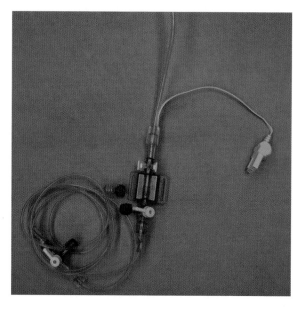

Figure 2.6 Arterial blood pressure continuous flush transducer for use with an automated system.

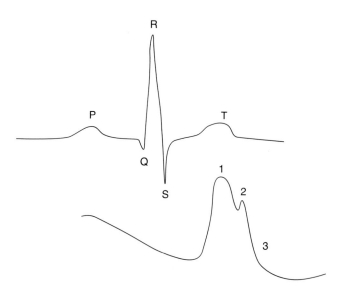

Figure 2.7 ECG with correlating arterial wave form. ECG waves are labeled P, Q, R, S, and T. 1. Systolic blood pressure. 2. Dicrotic notch. 3. Runoff during diastole.

can serve as a reliable tool on which to base intraoperative management decisions. In patients anticipated to require a fair amount of intraoperative adjustments (ASA III–V patients), having a direct arterial line provides a sound basis for alternations to the anesthetic plan. Additionally, a direct arterial line is useful for sampling: the arterial line is used to collect samples for blood gas assessment, electrolytes, packed cell volume/total solids (PCV/TS), blood glucose, and so on, which will also help with modifications of the intraoperative plan. The arterial waveform helps with assessment of volume status. Systolic arterial pressure (SAP) variations (changes in the arterial wave form secondary to IPPV) are correlated to states of hypovolemia (3). In cases of a cardiac arrest, observing pulse pressure waves tells the anesthetist the effectiveness of chest compressions as well as when it is necessary to rotate personnel performing compressions.

(b) Disadvantages: IBP monitoring requires advanced skills. Because the arterial line is often out of sight of the anesthetist, dislodgement results in a significant amount of hemorrhage before it is noticed. Direct pressure applied for no less than 5 minutes is necessary once the arterial line is removed to prevent hematoma formation at the site of catheterization. Arterial lines, especially in the feline, are not intended for long-term use, as the semi-occlusion of an artery by a catheter may result in poor limb perfusion. Although arterial lines do not require a tremendous amount of additional equipment, there is an initial investment of noncompliant tubing and a BP measurement device.

2. Indirect or noninvasive blood pressure (NIBP) monitoring

(a) Doppler, cuff, and sphygmomanometer: Using a Doppler, cuff, and sphygmomanometer allows continuous audible HR assessment, and obtains indirect SAP. The Doppler in tandem provides additional assurance that BP obtained with an oscillometric monitor is accurate (see Table 2.7, Figure 2.8, and Figure 2.9).

(b) Oscillometric BP monitoring: There are many oscillometric units available, but most operate under the same principles. A distensible cuff is inflated and obstructs blood flow through the artery. As the cuff deflates, the oscillations are detected and reported as systolic, diastolic, and mean BP (Figure 2.10). The methods with which these three pressures are derived vary from manufacturer to manufacturer, but it is safe to say that not every value is actually measured—some are calculated, increasing the room for error and inaccuracy. In general, MAP is usually measured and systolic/diastolic pressures are calculated with a proprietary algorithm.

B. Capnograph and agent analysis

The capnograph allows evaluation of ventilation and circulation by a display of $EtCO_2$ and assists with error identification, such as obstructions of the airway, leakage of the endotracheal (ET) tube cuff, and RB of CO_2 secondary to equipment malfunctions (see Figure 2.11). When $EtCO_2$ is compared with arterial CO_2 ($PaCO_2$/$PEtCO_2$ gradient), the anesthetist has information regarding alveolar perfusion, ventilation to perfusion (V/Q) mismatching, and venous admixture. Monitoring $EtCO_2$ is also useful in evaluating cardiopulmonary resuscitation (CPR) efforts. Often, one has the option to purchase an agent analyzer that commonly functions as a capnograph. The agent analyzer gives the anesthetist inspired and expired inhalant and oxygen concentrations (Table 2.8). This assists in the fine-tuning of changes in the anesthetic plane based on expired inhalant

Table 2.7 Obtaining an NIBP.

Materials: Clippers, Doppler, BP cuff, ultrasound gel, tape, sphygmomanometer or oscillometric unit

Technique:
1. Clip area over artery (common areas include metacarpal, the dorsal pedal, or coccygeal artery).
2. Fill the crystal (concave side of the Doppler probe) with ultrasound gel; at this point, it is useful to test the Doppler on the anesthetist to ensure it is properly functioning prior to placing the Doppler on patient.
3. Place the crystal over artery and secure in place with tape. Turn on Doppler to hear audible heartbeat. If audible heartbeat is not heard, feel for a pulse to confirm patient has heartbeat, and then slight manipulation of the probe under the tape may facilitate an audible sound.
4. Select a BP cuff with a width that is 30–40% of the circumference of the patient's limb and place on the limb proximal to the Doppler (see Figure 2.9).
5. For obtaining a BP using a sphygmomanometer, connect the sphygmomanometer to the BP cuff and inflate cuff until the arterial flow is obstructed (heart sounds are no longer audible on Doppler). Ideally, the inflation pressure is no less than 20–30 mmHg higher than anticipated BP. While watching the gauge, slowly release the sphygmomanometer's pressure until audible heart sounds (arterial flow) are heard. This value is the SAP.
6. For obtaining a BP using an oscillometric unit, following placement of the cuff on the patient's limb proximal to the Doppler (see Figure 2.10), connect the oscillometric unit to the cuff. In some cases, only the cuff supplied by the manufacturer is compatible for use with the oscillometric device. Activate the oscillometric unit by pressing start or inflate. When the BP cuff is inflated, the Doppler noise should disappear, reappearing as pressure is released from the cuff. The complete occlusion of the artery, resulting in cessation of the Doppler heart sounds, is essential for accuracy in oscillometric units. Typically, the anesthetist has the option of selecting an interval (stat, every minute, every three minutes, etc.). An oscillometric unit reports systolic, diastolic, and mean arterial pressures.

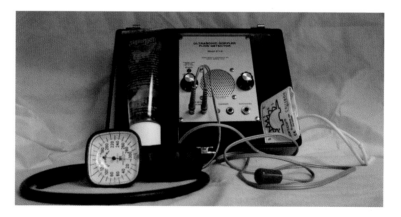

Figure 2.8 Doppler, sphygmomanometer, and blood pressure cuff for obtaining NIBP.

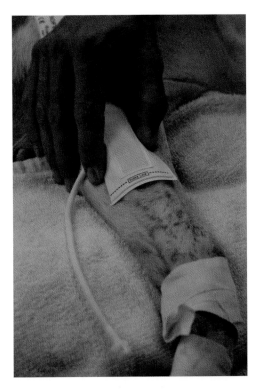

Figure 2.9   Patient with Doppler placed on front limb. The anesthetist is demonstrating how to properly size a BP cuff for the front limb of a canine patient.

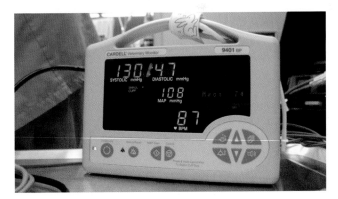

Figure 2.10   Cardell oscillometric BP monitor.

concentrations that most closely correspond to alveolar concentrations. This also assesses the accuracy of the vaporizer.

C. Electrocardiography (ECG)

ECG allows evaluation of the heart's electrical activity and arrhythmia detection but does not assess structural function of the heart (see Table 2.9). Additionally, the ECG allows

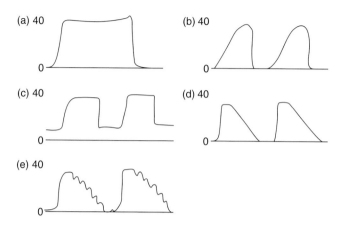

Figure 2.11 Normal (a) capnograph waveform and common abnormal capnograph waveforms, (b) obstructive waveform, (c) rebreathing CO_2, (d) leaks within the breathing circuit or ET tube, (e) cardiac oscillations.

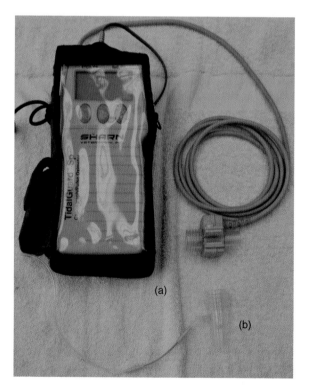

Figure 2.12 (a) Mainstream and (b) sidestream CO_2 analyzers.

Table 2.8 Comparison of mainstream and sidestream capnograph units.

Mainstream		Sidestream	
Advantages	*Disadvantages*	*Advantages*	*Disadvantages*
"Real" time	Bulky unit placed	Minimal bulk to	Delay in display
Does not produce	on the end of	the end of	secondary to sampling
waste gas, does not	the ET tube	the ET tube	Increased possibility of
require scavenging	Adaptor is	Adaptor is	sample contamination
Easy to calibrate	expensive to	inexpensive	Requires scavenging of
Respiratory secretions	replace	Submersible for	waste gas
are not an issue	Difficult to clean	easy cleaning	Difficult to calibrate
due to the use of			in-house
infrared technology			Requires respiratory
measuring CO_2			secretions to be
levels			trapped in Nafion
			tubing or a water trap
			to avoid inaccuracies
			or failure of the system

Chapter 2

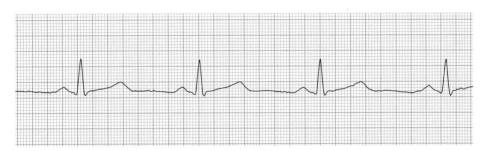

Figure 2.13 Normal ECG lead 2 at 25 mm/s.

the anesthetist to determine the patient's HR (Figure 2.13 and Figure 2.14). First, the anesthetist must know the paper speed at which the ECG was run. At a 50-mm/s speed, 10 "big" boxes equal 1 second. At a 25 mm/s speed, five "big" boxes equal 1 second. The simple way to estimate HR is to take a standard pen and lay it across the ECG. At a 50-mm/s speed, one pen equals approximately 3 seconds; count the number of complexes that run the length of the pen and multiple by 20 to get the beats per minute. At a 25-mm/s speed, one pen equals 6 seconds. Count the number of complexes that run the length of the pen and multiple by 10 to calculate the number of beats per minute.

D. Esophageal stethoscope

An esophageal stethoscope is used to audibly quantitate the heartbeat and assess cardiac rhythm (Table 2.10 and Figure 2.15).

E. Pulse oximetry

Pulse oximetry is commonly referred to as SpO_2. The pulse oximeter uses red and infrared light to measure oxygen saturation of hemoglobin (Hb). Pulse oximeters are available

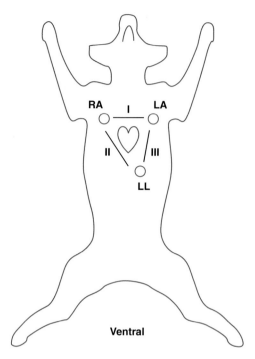

Figure 2.14   Diagram of patient showing electrode placement of a traditional ECG leads I, II, III.

Table 2.9   Placement of three-lead ECG.

Materials: ECG pads or leads with alligator clips, monitoring unit, conduction gel (ultrasound) or alcohol
Technique:
1. (See Figure 2.14) White lead = right arm (RA) Black lead = left arm (LA) Red lead = left leg (LL)
2. RA and LA leads are placed at their respective locations on the leg or axial region of the front limb, and the LL is placed caudal to the apex of the heart or on the left hind limb.
3. Leads need adequate contact with the skin. If electrode pads are used, they may be placed on the carpal pad of the paws; otherwise, a section of hair is shaved and lead is applied. Alligator clips are used, but attention should be paid to placement to avoid traumatic damage to the patient's skin. A conductive gel or alcohol is used with alligator clips.
4. Lead II is the routinely evaluated lead (see Figure 2.13).

as convenient portable patient side monitors or as part of a multiparameter monitoring system. Normal values are above 92%. Low readings indicate improper probe placement, hypoxemia, vasoconstriction, methemoglobinemia, or extreme hypotension. It is also possible for the pulse oximeter to read within a normal range in a patient experiencing carbon monoxide poisoning, although the oxygen saturation is actually low. Readings

Table 2.10 Esophageal stethoscope placement.

Technique:
1. Insert esophageal stethoscope into the mouth of the anesthetized intubated patient. The stethoscope will pass into the esophagus smoothly if the tongue is pulled forward.
2. Use earpieces to auscult for a heartbeat as the anesthetist continues to insert the esophageal probe. Continue to advance the probe until the strongest heart sounds are heard.
3. Secure the esophageal probe to the ET tube to avoid dislodgement. The HR and rhythm can be continuously monitored by wearing the ear piece or attaching it to an audio box (see Figure 2.15).

Table 2.11 Placement of the pulse oximeter.

Technique:
1. Ensure the probe is operational by looking for the red light on the probe.
2. Place probe over nonpigmented skin. Typical areas used are the tongue, webbing between toes, lip, ear, vulva, or prepuce.
3. Pulse oximeters with a plethysmographic display of the pulse amplitude allow the user to visualize the presence of a pulse, ensuring the oximeter is reading accurately.

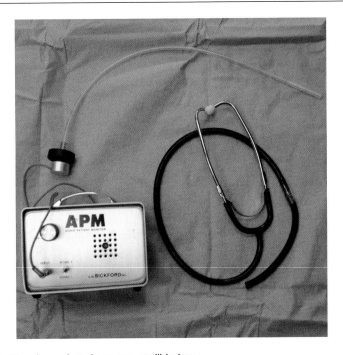

Figure 2.15 Esophageal stethoscope, audible box.

are also affected by patient motion, external light sources, and prolonged placement of probe in one location (Table 2.11 and Figure 2.16).

F. Temperature probe

Esophageal temperature probes work nicely to give continuous, accurate monitoring of core body temperature. Rectal temperature probes work well; however, continuous

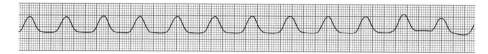

Figure 2.16   Pleth waveform from an automated monitoring system.

Table 2.12   Esophageal temperature probe placement.

Technique:
1. Once the ET tube is securely in place, the tongue of the patient is drawn rostral.
2. The temperature probe is guided into the esophagus. There should be little to no resistance until the gastroesophageal sphincter is encountered; the anesthetist need not advance the probe beyond the distal third of the esophagus. Further advancement may increase the potential for regurgitation.

monitoring is not as easily accomplished due to fecal accumulation and difficult access during a surgical procedure (Table 2.12).

G. Central venous pressure (CVP)

Measurement of CVP allows assessment of venous return (preload) and cardiac function (especially in the face of right-sided heart failure), as well as a point of care for hydration assessment (Table 2.13, Figure 2.17, and Figure 2.18).

H. Blood gas analysis

Blood gas (or acid–base) analysis allows the anesthetist to evaluate the pH of the patient and partial pressure of important respiratory gases (oxygen and carbon dioxide). Blood gas analysis allows identification of V/Q mismatch or shunting (see Chapter 6, "Hypoxemia/Inappropriate P:F Ratio" section). Depending on the machine used to perform this analysis, additional information such as electrolytes, glucose, hematocrit, and lactate is also obtained (see Table 1.2, Table 1.3, and Figure 2.19).

1. Collecting a blood sample

To obtain a blood sample for evaluation of oxygenation, arterial sampling is necessary. For most other parameters, a venous sample is adequate. If an arterial sample is not obtained to assess oxygenation, use a blood sample from the lingual vasculature; arterial and venous anastomosis is present. This is not entirely representative but gives more useful information than a venous sample in regard to oxygenation. The syringe is heparinized to avoid clot formation, which damages the analyzer and gives inaccurate results. Make sure air bubbles are removed from the sample, and it is capped to avoid exposure to air. Run the sample according to analyzer's manufacturer directions. If electrolytes are analyzed, use a lithium heparin syringe.

Table 2.13 Placement and setup of a central line catheter to measure CVP.

Materials: Central venous catheter kit (MILA®, Mila International, Erlanger KY; Arrow®, Arrow International, Inc., Cleveland, OH), aseptic prep, clippers, tailors measuring tape, sterile drape, sterile gloves, suture material
Optional materials: towel or fluid bag under the shoulders, ECG, #11 scalpel blade, sterile gauze

Technique:
1. The patient is placed in lateral recumbency. Placing a rolled up towel or fluid bag under the cranial edge of the shoulder and mild extension of the neck may help visualize the jugular vein.
2. Measure from the proposed point of catheter insertion in the jugular vein to just prior to the level of the heart with a measuring tape. The location of the heart is often approximated by pulling the elbow of the patient dorsally and parallel with the costochondral junction of the ribs.
3. Clip and aseptically prepare an area over the jugular vein. The field is sterilely draped if the jugular catheter is intended to remain in place after anesthesia, and the anesthetist should wear sterile gloves.
4. An assistant will hold off both jugular vessels, below the drape.
5. The skin is sufficiently nicked at the proposed site of entry.
6. An introducer over-the-needle catheter, to allow guide wire placement, is first placed in the vessel. Make sure this catheter fits the guide wire! For example, there is no use placing a 24-g over-the- needle catheter when the anesthetist must place a 20-g guide wire through this catheter.
7. Once the introducer catheter is placed, remove the stylet and insert the guide wire through the catheter into the jugular.
8. Withdraw the catheter over the guide wire (leaving the guide wire in place). Always keep a hand on the guide wire!
9. Place the dilator over guide wire to the level of the skin. Grip both the dilator and guide wire firmly. Steadily and aggressively push through the skin to dilate the vessel. This is difficult! Twisting the dilator during pushing may assist advancement.
10. Remove the dilator. The vessel may bleed; place sterile gauze 4 × 4 over this area as the dilator is removed (leaving the guide wire in place). Gentle pressure may help avoid excessive bleeding or hematoma formation.
11. Place the indwelling jugular catheter over the guide wire. It is important when advancing the catheter into the vessel that the anesthetist holds the guide wire so it is *never* lost. The anesthetist will slowly back out the guide wire while inserting the catheter. Insert the catheter to the premeasured length and withdraw guide wire. If a significant amount of the catheter remains outside the patient, a small jacket for securing the catheter is available in most jugular catheter kits.
12. Secure the catheter in place by suturing to patient. Additionally, a wrap is placed loosely around the neck to protect the catheter.
13. When measuring CVP, connect the pressure tubing, three-way stopcock, and transducer to catheter if using an automated system. A water column is also used to measure CVP. With an automated system, zero the transducer by turning the three-way stopcock off to the patient and open to atmospheric pressure. Zero to atmospheric pressure. Once zeroed, turn the stopcock off to the atmosphere. Normal CVP in the conscious patient is usually less than 10–14 cmH$_2$0; however, in the anesthetized patient, CVP can vary significantly, depending on things such as volume status, cardiac output, and the use of mechanical ventilation.

Note: An ECG is often monitored in conjunction with the placement of a jugular catheter. The presence of abnormal rhythms or heartbeats indicates the jugular catheter is contacting the myocardium.

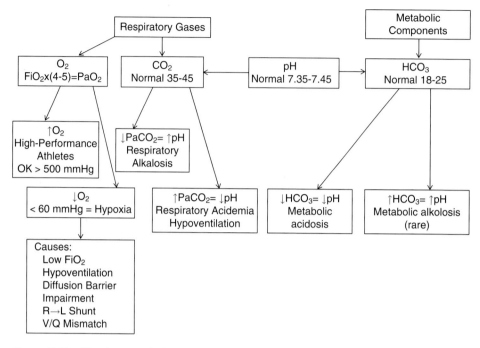

Figure 2.20 Blood gas analysis and oxygenation.

Table 2.14 Blood gas compensation rules for dog.

Primary (simple) problem	Expected compensatory response
Acute respiratory acidosis	$HCO_3 \uparrow$ 1.5 mEq/L for every 10 mmHg $\uparrow$ in pCO_2
Chronic respiratory acidosis	$HCO_3 \uparrow$ 3.5 mEq/L for every 10 mmHg $\uparrow$ in pCO_2
Acute respiratory alkalosis	$HCO_3 \downarrow$ 2.5 mEq/L for each 10 mmHg $\downarrow$ in pCO_2
Chronic respiratory alkalosis	$HCO_3 \downarrow$ 5.5 mEq/L for each 10 mmHg $\downarrow$ in pCO_2
Metabolic acidosis	$pCO_2 \downarrow$ 0.7 mmHg for every 1 mEq/L $\downarrow$ in HCO_3
Metabolic alkalosis	$pCO_2 \uparrow$ 0.7 mmHg for every 1 mEq/L $\uparrow$ in HCO_3

Source: de Morais H, DiBartola S. Ventilatory and metabolic compensation in dogs with acid–base disturbances. J Vet Emerg Crit Care. 1991;1:39–49.

(III) HIGH pH: The patient is alkalotic. Look for low PCO_2: respiratory alkalosis (see Chapter 6). If the HCO_3 is high: metabolic alkalosis (see Chapter 6).

(c) Step 3: Determine if there is adequate compensation (see Table 2.14). The patient should have adequate compensation when a primary problem exists. In a mixed problem, compensation will be inadequate.

References

1. Dorsch J, Dorsch S. Understanding Anesthesia Equipment. Second ed. Baltimore, MD: Williams & Wilkins; 1975.
2. Eger E, Epstein R. Hazards of anesthetic equipment. Anesthesiology. 1964;25(4):490–504.
3. Eichhorn V, Trepte C, Richter HP, Kubitz JC, Goepfert MS, Goetz AE, et al. Respiratory systolic variation test in acutely impaired cardiac function for predicting volume responsiveness in pigs. Br J Anaesth. 2011;106(5):659–64.

Chapter 2

Anesthetic drugs and fluids

Introduction

The drugs covered in this chapter are commonly used in anesthetic protocols during the anesthetic process. Many drugs are grouped and listed in tables with relevant information the anesthetist should know before their administration. Otherwise, drugs are listed in alphabetical order in the remaining pages of this chapter.

I. Acepromazine (see Table 3.11)

II. Albuterol: Intermediate-acting beta$_2$-adrenergic agonist

A. Indication

Bronchodilator, helpful in reducing V/Q mismatch.

B. Dosage

Two puffs of 90 mcg/puff by metered dose inhaler (inhalation), separated by 1–5 minutes.

C. Duration

Four hours.

D. Characteristics

1. Possible increase in heart rate (HR)
2. Decrease in potassium (K$^+$)
3. Causes hyperglycemia
4. Tremors may result from beta-receptor stimulation in the muscles
5. Protection from light.

40

Table 3.1 Anticholinergics.

Drug	Dose	Duration	Characteristics	Contraindications
Atropine	0.02–0.05 mg/kg IM, IV, SQ	Varies among species Rapid onset, short duration	1. Competitively binds muscarinic cholinergic receptors in place of acetylcholine. 2. Antagonizes parasympathetic nervous system effects (prevents bradycardia, decreases GI motility, decrease salivation, causes mydriasis). 3. Promotes bronchodilation. 4. May increase the incidence of arrhythmias, tachycardia, increased myocardial workload, and oxygen consumption. 5. Can result in some sedation, as it crosses the blood–brain barrier. 6. Low doses may cause an idiosyncratic second degree AV block. Repeat dose.	Patients with 1. HCM, tachycardia because of increase in myocardial workload and oxygen consumption 2. Glaucoma 3. Ileus is a concern
Glycopyrrolate	0.01 mg/kg IV, IM, SQ	30–45 min duration. Effects are similar to atropine but longer lasting with slower onset (may take up to 5–10 min.)	1. Blocks acetylcholine at the muscarinic receptors. 2. Promotes bronchodilation and smooth muscle relaxation. 3. Decreases vagal tone/response. 4. Does not cross the placental or blood–brain barrier; therefore, no sedation is expected. 5. Decreases salivation and GI motility. 6. Low doses may cause an idiosyncratic second degree AV block. Repeat dose.	Same as atropine

HCM, hypertrophic cardiomyopathy.

Table 3.2 Blood pressure support.

Drug name	Classification	Dosage	Duration	Characteristics	Contraindications	Additional notes
Dobutamine	Positive inotrope	0.12–1.2 mg/kg/h IV as CRI	Short acting	1. Beta$_1$ stimulation increases myocardial contractility to improve SV and CO. 2. High doses may cause hypertension, tachycardia, and arrhythmias. 3. Minimal B$_2$ agonist stimulation results in some smooth muscle relaxation (this may cause decrease in BP although CO is likely increasing).	Patients with 1. HCM 2. Ventricular hypertrophy 3. Ventricular arrhythmias 4. Endogenous catecholamine overproduction	1. Common dilution for administration is 1 mg/mL. 2. Refrigeration recommended after opening; dilutions should be used within 24 h.
Dopamine	Positive inotrope	0.12–1.2 mg/kg/h IV as a CRI	Short acting	1. Action at beta$_1$, alpha, and dopaminergic receptors. 2. Action at various receptors depends on dose (although exact doses are controversial). Low doses (<0.18 mg/kg/h) may increase renal profusion in dogs at dopaminergic receptors. At mid-range doses (0.18–0.6 mg/kg/hr), beta$_1$ receptor stimulation increases myocardial contractility. At higher doses, alpha receptor is stimulated, increases SVR by vasoconstriction.	Patients with 1. Endogenous catecholamine overproduction (e.g., pheochromocytomas), ventricular tachyarrhythmias 2. HCM 3. Ventricular hypertrophy	1. Common dilution = 1 mg/mL. 2. Dilutions are used within 24 h and discarded if solution changes color. 3. Refrigerate bottle after opening. 4. Protect bottle and dilutions from light. 5. High doses or administration of undiluted product can cause arrhythmias, hypertension, and tachycardia.

(Continued)

Table 3.2 (Continued)

Drug name	Classification	Dosage	Duration	Characteristics	Contraindications	Additional notes
Phenylephrine	Vasopressor	0.01–0.05 mg/kg IV, CRI 0.03–0.06 mg/kg/h	A single bolus may last up to 20 min.	1. Potent alpha₁ agonist with no beta activity. 2. Results in smooth muscle contraction causing vasoconstriction. 3. Constriction of veins is greater than that of arteries. 4. May result in hypertension with a reflex bradycardia.	Patients with 1. Hypertension 2. Valvular cardiovascular disease (e.g., MR)	1. Useful to manage hypotension in patients where increasing HR or workload is undesirable (i.e., patients with HCM or valvular stenosis). 2. Because profound vasoconstriction results in decreased perfusion, it is prudent to monitor lactate levels. Increasing lactate levels may indicate that this drug is worsening perfusion in spite of improved BP. 3. Extravasation may result in sloughing or necrosis of surrounding skin. 4. Used intranasally (1% nasal solution is available) to reduce bleeding after a rhinoscopy 5. Protect from light.

| Vasopressin | Vasopressor | 0.4–0.8 units/kg IV; CRI 0.02–0.04 units/kg/h | 10–20 min | 1. Synthetic antidiuretic hormone which increases renal permeability to water and helps maintain plasma osmolarity.
2. Acts at vasopressin receptors to cause vasoconstriction.
3. Recommended in refractory or asystolic cardiac arrest as a one-time dose instead of epinephrine (see Appendix C, "CPR"). | Patients with
1. Hypertension
2. Pregnancy due to uterine smooth muscle contraction | 1. Doses of vasopressin used to manage hypotension are considered supraphysiologic; this results in profound vasoconstriction of blood vessels in splanchnic circulation and ultimately sloughing of the GI mucosa. The authors like to use lowest effective dose starting at 0.04 units/kg.
2. Safest when used only in cases refractory to traditional BP management.
3. Administer only once during CPCR due to the drug's prolonged half-life.
4. Reflex bradycardia occurs secondary to increased vascular tone.
5. Protect from light. |

SV, stroke volume; CO, cardiac output; BP,blood pressure; HR, heart rate; CNS, central nervous system; CRI, constant rate infusion; HCM, hypertrophic cardiomyopathy; AHA, American Heart Association; CPCR, cardiopulmonary cerebral resuscitation; SVR, systemic vascular resistance; MR, mitral regurgitation.

Table 3.3 Common crystalloid fluids for anesthetic management.

Crystalloid	Buffer	pH	Osmolarity (mOsmol/L)	Electrolytes (mEq/L)	Contraindications	Practical notes
Lactated Ringer's solution (LRS)	Lactate	6.5	273	Calcium: 2.7 Chloride: 109 Lactate: 28 Potassium: 4 Sodium: 130	Do not deliver in the same catheter with blood products (contains Ca++ which will chelate with the anticoagulant in blood products).	Lactate buffer is broken down by the liver to bicarbonate, resulting in an alkalinizing effect.
Normosol	Acetate	6.6	294	Acetate: 27 Chloride: 98 Gluconate: 23 Magnesium: 3 Potassium: 5 Sodium: 140		1. There is a report of a single dog becoming hypotensive secondary to bolus of Normosol-R. 2. Safe to administer with blood products.
Plasma-lyte 148	Acetate	5.5	294	Acetate: 27 Chloride: 98 Gluconate: 23 Magnesium: 3 Potassium: 5 Sodium: 140		Because this product contains magnesium instead of calcium, it is safe to administer with blood products.

	pH	Osmolarity	Electrolytes (mEq/L)	Contraindications	Comments
Sodium chloride 0.9%	5.5	308	Chloride: 154 Sodium: 154	Patients with severe acidosis.	1. This product is safe to administer with blood products. 2. Slightly acidifying solution is useful in patients with alkalosis.
Sodium chloride 7.5% (hypertonic saline)		2464	Chloride: 1232 Sodium: 1232	1. Patients' with uncontrolled hemorrhage, dehydration, preexisting electrolyte imbalances such as hyponatremia or hypernatremia. 2. May cause pulmonary edema if patient has preexisting heart disease.	1. Administration of this solution is not intended as an end unto itself, but rather to provide the clinician time to institute other maneuvers to restore volume. 2. Rapidly expands intravascular volume for a short duration and transiently decreases afterload. 3. Follow with administration of isotonic crystalloid solutions.

Note: Dogma surrounding conventional anesthesia fluid rates has recently been challenged (4). Current recommendations for fluid rates in anesthetized animals are less than 10 mL/kg/h, in order to avoid hypervolemia. Davis and colleagues recommend beginning anesthesia fluids at 5 mL/kg/h in the canine and 3 mL/kg/h in the feline. Routine maintenance for the un-anesthetized patient is 2–3 mL/kg/h. Shock doses are between 50 and 60 (feline) and 90 (canine) mL/kg bolus. Isotonic crystalloids will rapidly redistribute outside the vascular space within 15 min of administration. Hypertonic fluids are typically reserved for treatment of shock (hypovolemic/hemorrhagic) and are used concurrently with isotonic crystalloids. Dosage for hypertonic saline 7.5% in the canine patients is 4–8 mL/kg IV and feline patients 1–4 mL/kg IV over 5 min. To reduce intracranial pressure, hypertonic saline can be given at 4 mL/kg over 5 min; 7.5% hypertonic saline has a duration of 30–60 min.

Table 3.4 Common colloid fluids for anesthetic management.

Colloid (common products available)	Dosage	Duration	Characteristics	Contraindication	Practical notes
Dextran (70)	Canine 20–40 mL/kg/day	24 h or longer	1. High molecular weight option is Dextran 70 (most commonly available preparation). 2. Increases colloidal oncotic pressure. 3. May result in coagulopathies.	Patients with 1. Prolonged clotting profiles or clotting disorders (e.g., von Willebrand's disease). 2. Oliguric/anuric, normo or hypervolemic and CHF.	
Hydroxyethyl starch (6% hetastarch in 0.9% NaCl, 6% hetastarch in balanced electrolyte solution, and 10% pentastarch in 0.9% saline)	1. Canine IV bolus 2–5 mL/kg, volume support not to exceed 10–20 mL/kg/day 2. Feline bolus 2–3 mL/kg, volume support not to exceed 5–10 mL/kg/day	12–24 h	1. Retained in vasculature longer than crystalloids due to larger molecular size, which maintains intravascular volume and prevents tissue edema. 2. May dilute clotting factors and perpetuate bleeding.	1. Patients with clotting/bleeding disorders or active hemorrhage. 2. Patients with pulmonary edema or congestive heart failure. 3. Oliguric or anuric renal failure patients. 4. Normo or hypervolemic patients.	1. This fluid is not a substitute for maintenance fluids. 2. The patient's Total protein (TP) value may decrease, but hetastarch helps maintain oncotic pressure; monitoring with colloid oncotic pressure (COP) monitoring is advised.

Note: Colloids are used for volume expansion, in the treatment of hypotension, or to help maintain oncotic pressure in the hypoproteinemic patient. CHF, congrestive heart failure.

Table 3.5 Common inhalants.

Inhalant	MAC in dog and cat	Duration	Blood/gas partition coefficient	Oil/gas partition coefficient	Vapor pressure (mmHg)	Characteristics
Desflurane	Ranging from 7.2% (canine) to 9.8% (feline)	Short acting (shorter than isoflurane and sevoflurance)	0.42	18.70	700	1. CNS depressant; prevention of movement is likely mediated at the level of the spinal cord. 2. Dose-dependent cardiovascular and respiratory depression. 3. Decreased SVR. 4. Requires a precision vaporizer with an external heat source (requires electricity to function).
Isoflurane	Well conversed between species at 1.2 (canine) and 1.4% (feline)	Based on exposure (longer acting than sevoflurane or desflurane)	1.4	91	240	1. CNS depressant; prevention of movement is likely mediated at the level of the spinal cord. 2. Dose-dependent cardiovascular and respiratory depression. 3. Decreased SVR thus causing hypotension. 4. Requires a precision vaporizer.
Sevoflurane	Well conversed between species at 2.3 (canine) and 2.6% (feline)	Based on exposure (shorter acting than isoflurance).	0.68	47	160	1. CNS depressant; prevention of movement is likely mediated at the level of the spinal cord. 2. Dose-dependent cardiovascular and respiratory depression. 3. Decreased SVR. 4. Requires a precision vaporizer. 5. Less soluble than isoflurane, although clinically this difference is insignificant. 6. Results in by-products when used with soda-lime, including fluoride ions that may be toxic to the kidney. 7. Odor of sevoflurane is not pungent; it works well to mask or box down patients.

SVR, systemic vascular resistance; CNS, central nervous system.

Table 3.6 Common induction agents.

Induction agent	Classification	Dosage	Duration	Characteristics	Contraindications	Practical notes
Alfaxalone	Synthetic neuroactive steroid	1–4 mg/kg IV to effect (over 60 s) as a single bolus Constant rate infusions of 4.2–6 mg/kg/h are reported (5, 6).	Single bolus duration is dependent on dose; 5–30 min is reported (7).	1. The current formulation does not have the Cremophor emulsifier, which was responsible for anaphylactoid reactions resulting in market withdrawal. 2. Current formulation has a HPCD base that is not associated with reactions. 3. Acts via GABA receptors. 4. Smooth induction. 5. Standard induction doses do not appear to elicit hypotension (8) when given slowly to effect. 6. Respiratory depression is a common side effect, especially if alfaxalone is administered quickly (9). 7. While recovery is typically smooth, there are incidences of agitation and noise sensitivity (10). 8. Acceptable induction for young animals (under 12 weeks of age)(11). 9. No pain on injection noted (12). 10. Rapid plasma clearance with little accumulation after repeated administration (7, 8).	Respiratory depression may worsen outcome in patients with neurologic disease.	1. When ultra-short recovery is the target goal, propofol is possibly superior (10). 2. When used as the sole anesthetic, MV is often required (6).

| Etomidate | Imidazole derivative | 0.5–2.0 mg/kg IV to effect | Promptly redistributed away from the brain, although metabolism may take between 2 and 5 h. | 1. Minimal cardiovascular and respiratory depression.
2. No histamine release.
3. Decreases $CMRO_2$ consumption.
4. Inhibits adrenal steroidogenesis and stress response to surgery at 1/100th of the dose required to induce anesthesia.
5. Contains propylene glycol.
6. Causes hemolysis.
7. No analgesia. | 1. Critically ill patients suspected of adrenal exhaustion.
2. Long-term infusions.
3. Patients with Addison's disease.
4. Patients (especially cats) with renal failure, due to propylene glycol and resultant hemolysis. | 1. Ideal for cardiovascularly compromised patients.
2. Ideal for neurological or neurosurgical patients.
3. When given without sedation or in a healthy patient, etomidate can cause myoclonus and vomiting at induction and requires high doses.
4. Best when given in sedated patients or with a dose of midazolam 0.2 mg/kg IV. |
| Ketamine | NMDA antagonist and dissociative anesthetic | 1. Induction dosage in sedated patient: 3–5 mg/kg IV
2. IM induction dosage of 5–10 mg/kg
3. Buccal dose 5–20 mg/kg for sedation/ immobilization | Duration is dependent on route of administration, but single IV boluses are expected to last less than 5 min with a rapid onset between 60 and 90 s. | 1. Causes indirect stimulation of cardiovascular system through catecholamine reuptake inhibition (increases BP and HR and thus CO, increases myocardial O_2 requirements).
2. Canines completely metabolize ketamine; however, the feline metabolizes ketamine to norketamine, an active metabolite which may contribute to altered feline recovery.
3. May result in apneustic breathing pattern.
4. Patients induced with ketamine exhibit a catatonic state (mydriasis, nystagmus, swallowing, and muscle movement/rigidity). | 1. Patients with seizures or neurologic problems, especially if there is suspicion of increased in ICP.
2. Ocular injuries and glaucoma.
3. HCM.
4. Cats with significant renal insufficiency. | 1. Administer with a muscle relaxant such as benzodiazepine or alpha$_2$ agonist.
2. Induction dose acts as the loading dose if a CRI is immediately started.
3. Used at 1 mg/kg to reduce propofol induction dose.
4. Lubricate eyes, although animal may still blink.
5. Cats may exhibit emergence delirium.
6. Controlled, Schedule III. |

(Continued)

Table 3.6 (*Continued*)

Induction agent	Classification	Dosage	Duration	Characteristics	Contraindications	Practical notes
				5. In privileged sites such as the central nervous system (secondary to the protection of the blood–brain barrier), vasodilation and thus an increase in ICP occur. 6. Increased extraocular muscle tone results in an increase in IOP. 7. May result in hyperthermia due to increased muscle tone. 8. Decreases MAC of gas inhalants up to 40%. 9. Painful on IM injection due to low pH.		
Pentobarbital	Barbiturate	1. Anesthetic dose: 20–30 mg/kg IV 2. To control seizures 5–15 mg/kg IV	Effect terminates rapidly, but may take up to 8 h to clear from the body.	1. Highly protein bound. 2. Redistributes quickly (effect terminates shortly after administration), but hepatic metabolism and renal clearance are necessary for elimination. 3. As with most induction agents, will cross the placental barrier. 4. Cardiovascular and respiratory depression are common. 5. If used as an anesthetic, excitement may occur during recovery. 6. The very alkalotic pH of pentobarbital will cause sloughing if extravasation of the drug occurs.	1. Patients with hypoalbuminemia or liver insufficiencies will have profound and prolong effect. 2. Not recommended for C-sections with viable fetuses. 3. Use with caution in patients with renal insufficiencies.	1. Do not use to treat seizures secondary to lidocaine toxicity. 2. Sometimes used to control seizures following myelograms. 3. Manufactured at 390 mg/mL as euthanasia agent; dose is 120 mg/kg IV. 4. Controlled substance.

| Propofol | Injectable sedative-hypnotic anesthetic | 1. 2.0–6.0 mg/kg IV; 2–4 mg/kg IV to effect in patients with appropriate premedication
2. TIVA: 6–24 mg/kg/h IV | 10–20 min as a single bolus; prolonged exposure to propofol (e.g., as a CRI) can result in prolonged duration of sedation in the feline. | 1. Acts via $GABA_A$ receptors.
2. Smooth inductions and recoveries.
3. Noncumulative.
4. Rapidly redistributes; metabolized both hepatically and extrahepatically (e.g., in the muscle, lung, and kidney).
5. Decreases ICP, $CMRO_2$, and CBF. There is no change in cerebral autoregulation.
6. Anticonvulsant.
7. May suppress the sympathetic nervous system to a greater extent than the parasympathetic nervous system. Asystole may result if given rapidly to patients with high vagal tone.
8. Systemic vasodilation after administration may result, although HR is often unchanged.
9. Apnea occurs when administered rapidly.
10. Muscle twitching and paddling (myoclonus) have been observed.
11. May result in Heinz body formation and toxic changes in RBCs in cats with repeated administration.
12. No analgesia. | 1. Patients with allergies to eggs.
2. Patients with increased triglycerides or cholesterol.
3. Because propofol can result in hypoventilation, ventilation status must be carefully maintained in patients with neurologic disease.
4. CRI infusions in cats may result in prolonged recoveries; use only standard formulation of propofol for cat CRIs. | 1. Ideal for patients with liver insufficiencies.
2. Best administration technique is slowly to effect.
3. Preoxygenation may reduce the effects of apnea at induction (12).
4. In healthy patients, preinduction bolus of isotonic fluids (5 mL/kg) helps reduce the effects of vasodilation.
5. Ideal alternative to inhalant anesthetic for neurological patients as TIVA. It is imperative to maintain an airway and administer oxygen.
6. Two formulations are currently available:
  (a) Propofol which comes as a single dose vial.
  (b) Propofol 28 which has a shelf life of 28 days. Contains benzyl alcohol which is not recommended for use as a CRI in cats.
7. Pain on injection occurs in humans when using small vessels or catheters that have been left in place for greater than 24 h. This may occur in animals.
8. Extravascular administration is not associated with adverse events.
9. Can be used to control seizures but anesthetist should be ready to intubate if respiratory depression occurs.
(Continued) |

Table 3.6 (Continued)

Induction agent	Classification	Dosage	Duration	Characteristics	Contraindications	Practical notes
Tiletamine and Zolazepam (Telazol)	Injectable anesthetic combination of dissociative agent and benzodiazepine	2–4 mg/kg IV, 6–10 mg/kg IM	Varies by dose, route, and species. Surgical anesthesia lasts less than 30 min, but it may take up to 4 h before drug effect subsides completely.	1. Combination of a dissociative agent (tiletamine) and a benzodiazepine (zolazepam) as a 1:1 ratio. 2. Cats have prolonged recoveries due to the slower metabolism of zolazepam. In short procedures, dogs may have rough recoveries because of metabolism of zolazepam before tiletamine. 3. Patients appear in a catatonic state including central, fixed, and dilated pupils. 4. Similar effects as ketamine.	Patients with 1. Seizures or increased in ICP. 2. Ocular injuries and glaucoma. 3. HCM. 4. Cats with significant renal insufficiency.	1. Typical reconstitution is 100 mg/mL. 2. Useful in aggressive animals IM as chemical restraint and induction. 3. Controlled substance, Schedule III. 4. Works well in exotic patients as a means of induction or chemical restraint. 5. Lube the eyes as minimal blinking may occur.

$CMRO_2$, cerebral metabolism rate of oxygen; BP, blood pressure; HR, heart rate; CO, cardiac output; CBF, cerebral blood flow; ICP, intracranial pressure; TIVA, total intravenous anesthesia; IOP, intraocular pressure; NMDA, N-methyl-D-aspartate.

Table 3.7 Common Local Anesthetics.

Local anesthetic	Dosage	Toxic dose	Duration	Characteristics	Contraindications	Practical notes
Bupivacaine	1. Regional: 1–1.5 mg/kg in dogs, 1 mg/kg in cats 2. Epidural dosage: 0.5–1.0 mg/kg	1. Dogs: 3 mg/kg 2. Cats: 2 mg/kg	3–5 h, slow onset (may take up to an hour epidurally, regionally 10 min)	1. Inhibits conduction of noxious stimulus by blocking sodium channels; at least three nodes of Ranvier must be inhibited to provide effect. 2. Loss of motor function when used in epidural or brachial plexus block. 3. Highly protein bound (caution with dosage in hypoalbuminemic animals).	IV administration	1. If multiple blocks are used, ensure total dosage for patient does not exceed the toxic dose. 2. In an epidural, use preservative-free formulations. 3. Do not dilute concentration to less than 2.5 mg/mL or block may not be effective.

(Continued)

Table 3.7 (*Continued*)

Local anesthetic	Dosage	Toxic dose	Duration	Characteristics	Contraindications	Practical notes
Lidocaine	1. Dogs: 0.5–2 mg/kg IV or as regional/infiltrative block. 2. Cats: Regional/infiltrative block 0.5–1.5 mg/kg.	1. Dogs: 6 mg/kg 2. Cats: 3 mg/kg	60–90 min, quick onset (2–5 min regionally)	1. Na⁺ channel blocker. 2. Inhibits conduction of noxious stimulus by blocking sodium channels if at least three nodes of Ranvier are inhibited. 3. Loss of motor function when used in epidural or brachial plexus block. 4. Highly protein bound.	1. Cats have increased sensitivity to local anesthetics. 2. Avoid IV use in patients with AV block, sick sinus syndrome, or escape rhythms. 3. Patients with liver dysfunction or hypoproteinemia may have prolonged effect when given IV.	1. Used for regional and epidural (use preservative free) anesthesia. 2. Commonly combined with longer lasting local anesthetics for regional blockade. 3. Often preparations for regional blocks contain epinephrine; use with caution in peripheral limbs. 4. Used IV as a CRI to control ventricular arrhythmias and as a visceral analgesic in dogs.
Mepivacaine	1. Dogs: do not exceed 3 mg/kg. 2. Cats: do not exceed 1.5 mg/kg.	1. Dogs: 6 mg/kg 2. Cats: 3 mg/kg	1.5–3 h with quick onset (2–5 min regionally).	1. Na⁺ channel blocker. 2. Slightly longer lasting than lidocaine, shorter duration than bupivacaine.	1. Avoid IV use.	1. Useful for dental blocks due to quick onset and length of duration.
Proparacaine 0.5%	Two drops administered one minute apart	Unknown	Dogs: Up to 55 min Cats: Up to 30 min	1. Na⁺ channel blocker for ophthalmic use.	None	1. Keep refrigerated. 2. Protect from light.

Note: Toxic sign for local anesthetics are as follows: first signs of toxicity are usually GI in nature (nausea, vomiting). As the toxicity worsens, neurologic signs evolve (tremors, twitches, and seizures). As toxicity progresses, cardiovascular depression and arrest will follow. Doses noted as "toxic" in this chart suggest the dose at which GI signs may begin to manifest.

Table 3.8 Neuromuscular blocking (NMB) agents.

NMB	Dosage	Duration	Characteristics	Contraindications
Atracurium	0.1–0.2 mg/kg slow IV	Onset occurs within 3–5 min and effect lasts 20–30 min	1. Competes to bind the cholinergic receptor at the neuromuscular junction which prevents muscle contractions of skeletal muscle (paralysis). 2. Few cardiovascular side effects. 3. Results in histamine release when given rapidly in high doses (resulting in hypotension and tachycardia). 4. Metabolized by Hofman elimination in plasma (metabolism is dependent upon patient's pH and body temperature). 5. Protect from light and refrigerate drug.	1. Patients with a history of adverse reactions (histamine release).
Cisatracurium	0.1 mg/kg IV bolus, CRI 0.03–0.24 mg/kg/h IV	20–35 min	1. Cleared primarily by Hofmann elimination (metabolism is dependent upon patient's pH and body temperature). 2. Minimal cardiovascular side effects (cisatracurium does not induce histamine release). 3. Protect from light and refrigerate drug.	
Pancuronium	0.05–0.1 mg/kg IV	40–60 min	1. Competes with acetylcholine at the neuromuscular junction which prevents muscle contractions of skeletal muscle (paralysis). 2. Longer duration of action than atracurium. 3. Does not result in histamine release. 4. Inhibition of cardiac muscarinic receptors (especially those of the sinoatrial node) may result in an increase in HR, BP, and CO. 5. Dependent on renal excretion, as most is eliminated unchanged in the urine (>80%). 6. Must be refrigerated.	1. Patients with renal insufficiency or failure. 2. Patients with CHF or HCM.

Note: NMB are indicated where muscle paralysis is required. They are most commonly used for ophthalmology procedures when the eyes must remain central. Reversals for NMBs are edrophonium or neostigmine (see Table 3.13). Before administration of NMB, a peripheral nerve stimulator (PNS) and ventilator should be placed on the patient. A train of four (TOF) twitches are monitored to evaluate the effect of the NMB. At least two twitches must be present prior to administration of reversal agent. Diligent monitoring of the patient to ensure adequate ventilation prior to extuabtion is also required. Monitoring with a capnograph and pulse oximeter is beneficial during recovery. Patients may relapse or have residual paralytic effects and are continuously monitored until completely recovered. See Chapter 4, "Ocular Surgeries" section, for more extensive discussion on NMB. CHF, congestive heart failure; HCM, hypertrophic cardiomyopathy; HR, heart rate; BP, blood pressure; CO, cardiac output.

Chapter 3

Table 3.9 Non-opioid analgesia.

Analgesic	Classification	Indication	Dosage	Duration	Characteristics	Contraindications	Practical notes
Amantadine	NMDA antagonist	Adjunctive analgesic for osteoarthritis in the canine.	3–5 mg/kg PO	24 h	1. Oral NMDA antagonist. 2. Originally developed and still used as an antiviral drug. 3. Due to amantadine's effects on release and reuptake of dopamine, caution is warranted for use in patients receiving other drugs that may alter neurotransmitter release (e.g., tramadol). 4. May cause dysphoria or confusion in older patients.	Patients on tramadol.	Sole usage of the drug is unlikely to provide substantial analgesia, but the drug may be useful to enhance the benefits of NSAIDs for dogs with chronic pain.

| Dexmedetomidine | Alpha₂ agonist | Analgesia, sedation, common premedication. | 1. Premedication: 0.0005–0.003 mg/kg IV, 0.003–0.015 mg/kg IM
2. CRI 0.0005–0.003 mg/kg/h IV for sedation and analgesia in recovery or supplemental intraoperative analgesia. | Relatively short onset when given IM (10–20 min), Duration of up to 2–3 h | 1. Profound sedation and (especially if combined with an opioid).
2. Moderate analgesia (potentially synergistic action when used with opioids).
3. Initial hypertension with a reflex bradycardia, secondary hypotension due to a reduction in CO and centrally mediated bradycardia.
4. Arrhythmias including second-degree AV block and ventricular premature beats are common.
5. Patients often develop a transient hyperglycemia.
6. Diuresis is common.
7. Reversible with atipamezole (see Table 3.13). | 1. Patients with cardiovascular disease including valvular regurgitation or arrhythmias.
2. Renal insufficiencies, anuria, or a blocked urinary system.
3. Liver disease. | 1. Most effective when administered to a patient that is allowed 5–10 min in a quiet, darkened room.
2. Sedation is enhanced when combined with an opioid.
3. Continuously monitor patient after premedication. Ensure reversal dose is calculated and is available if needed.
4. Reversal is only to be given IM (see Table 3.13).
5. Vasoconstriction may cause pale or blue MMC, and the pulse oximeter may have difficulty obtaining a measurement.
6. Low doses (0.001–0.003 mg/kg) work nicely as premedication in cats with HCM.
(Continued) |

Table 3.9 (Continued)

Analgesic	Classification	Indication	Dosage	Duration	Characteristics	Contraindications	Practical notes
Gabapentin	Analgesic	Neuropathic pain	5–10 mg/kg q 8–10 h PO	While often dosed every 12–24 h, pharmacokinetic studies in the canine suggest that the dosage frequency may more suitably be every 4–6 h (13).	1. Exact mechanism of analgesia is unknown, but an increase in GABA synthesis is suspected. 2. Anticonvulsant. 3. Eliminated by the kidney largely unchanged with minimal hepatic metabolism. 4. Seizures may result with abrupt discontinuation; taper dose when withdrawing. 5. Profound sedation may occur when beginning this therapy. 6. Protect from light.	Sudden withdrawal of drug. Patients must be tapered off.	

| Ketamine | NMDA antagonist and dissociative anesthetic | Somatic Pain | 1. CRI for intraoperative analgesia 0.6–1.8 mg/kg/h
2. Postoperative CRI 0.18–0.3 mg/kg/h IV
3. Loading dose for CRI 0.5 mg/kg IV | Onset of action is between 60 and 90 s. Short duration, single bolus less than 30 min. | (see Table 3.6)
1. While the canine will completely metabolize ketamine, the feline only metabolizes ketamine to norketamine, an active metabolite which may contribute to altered recovery.
2. Decreases central sensitization and prevents "wind-up" pain through its effects on the dorsal horn of the spinal cord; this drug may also reduce opioid tolerance.
3. Decreases MAC of gas inhalants up to 40%.
4. Dosage of ketamine necessary for analgesia is approximately one-tenth the dose necessary for induction of anesthesia (e.g., subanesthetic). | 1. Patients with seizures or neurologic problems, especially if there is an increase in ICP.
2. Ocular injuries and glaucoma.
3. HCM.
4. Cats with significant renal insufficiency. | 1. In place of a loading dose, the patient is induced with ketamine immediately followed by a CRI.
2. Controlled drug, Schedule III. |

(Continued)

Table 3.9 (Continued)

Analgesic	Classification	Indication	Dosage	Duration	Characteristics	Contraindications	Practical notes
Lidocaine	Local anesthetic, Na$^+$ channel blocker	Possible anti-inflammatory, visceral analgesic.	1. Dogs 0.5–2 mg/kg IV or as regional/infiltrative block. 2. Cats 0.5–1.5 mg/kg as regional/infiltrative block. 3. In dogs: CRI 1.5–3 mg/kg/h IV. Intraoperative CRI rates usually range from 2–3 mg/kg/h IV, whereas postoperative CRI rates are usually 1.5 mg/kg/h IV. 4. Antiarrhythmic dosages are 3.0–4.5 mg/kg/h following a loading dosage of 2 mg/kg; use caution with dosages >6 mg/kg as toxicity results.	As a regional block, 60–90 min.	1. Anti-inflammatory. 2. Class 1B anti-arrhythmic for ventricular dysrhythmias such as VPC and ventricular tachycardia. 3. Ideal analgesia for neurological cases (e.g., dogs with disk disease) due to Na$^+$ channel blockade reducing neuron firing. 4. Useful analgesic for GI surgeries were endotoxemia is suspected (inhibits endotoxin release) or when promoting GI motility is important. 5. Free radical scavenger. 6. MAC sparing (18%) when given as CRI. 7. Highly protein bound.	1. In the feline, administration as a CRI decreases CO (14) and is discouraged. 2. Methemoglobinemia, while rare, can result from the administration of lidocaine. 3. *Do not* administer to patients with third-degree AV block, sick sinus syndrome, or patients with escape beats. 4. Patients with extreme liver dysfunction will have prolonged effect of systemically administered lidocaine.	1. 0.1 mL dropped on larynx of cats reduces laryngeal spasms and assists with intubation. 2. Commonly combined with longer lasting local anesthetics like bupivacaine for regional blockade. 3. Often preparations for regional blocks contain epinephrine; use with caution in peripheral limbs.

8. Signs of toxicity are usually GI in nature (nausea, vomiting) initially. As the toxicity worsens, neurologic signs evolve (tremors, twitches, and seizures). Eventually, cardiovascular depression and arrest will follow. *If GI signs are present, discontinue any lidocaine administration immediately.*

| Maropitant | Neurokinin receptor antagonist | Antiemetic and adjunctive analgesia for visceral pain. | 1 mg/kg SC, 2 mg/kg PO | 24 h | 1. Novel work suggests there may be a role for NK-1 and associated substance P antagonism in visceral pain.
2. Protein bound; use with caution in animals receiving drugs that are also protein bound (e.g., NSAIDs). | Patients with possible gastrointestinal obstruction. | 1. While studies looking at this drug in the feline are available (15), this drug is currently only labeled for use in the dog.
2. Work suggesting this drug's use as an analgesic is preliminary. |

(Continued)

Table 3.9 (*Continued*)

Analgesic	Classification	Indication	Dosage	Duration	Characteristics	Contraindications	Practical notes
Xylazine	Alpha$_2$ agonist	Profound sedation, muscle relaxation, analgesia.	0.5–2 mg/kg IM, 0.2–1 mg/kg IV.	Onset of 10–15 min when given IM. Duration of 30–120 min depending on dose and route.	1. Mild to moderate albeit short-lived analgesia. 2. Initial hypertension with a reflex bradycardia, after which secondary hypotension due to a reduction in CO and centrally mediated bradycardia results. 3. Arrhythmias including second-degree AV block and ventricular escape beats. 4. Causes vomiting in 60% of dogs and 90% of cats. 5. Patients often develop a transient hyperglycemia due to insulin resistance. 6. Diuresis is common. 7. Vasoconstriction results in pale or blue MMC, the pulse oximeter may have difficulty obtaining a measurement. 8. Reversible with Yohimbine (see Table 3.13).	1. Patients that have cardiovascular disease including valvular insufficiency or arrhythmias. 2. Patients with renal insufficiencies, anuria, or a blocked urinary system. 3. Patients with liver disease, as this drug is highly dependent on hepatic metabolism. 4. Avoid in geriatric, diabetic, pregnant, pediatric, sick, or debilitated patients.	1. Effect of alpha$_2$ agonists is most notable when administered to a patient that is then allowed 5–10 min in a quiet, darkened room. 2. Effect of sedation is enhanced when combined with an opioid. 3. Continuously monitor patients after premedication. Ensure reversal dose has been calculated and is available. 4. Reversal should only be given IM. 5. Do not use if avoidable in blocked cats due to diuresis. 6. Not recommended when another drug is available.

Sources: References 14 and 15.

CO, cardiac output; HCM, hypertrophic cardiomyopathy; MCRO$_2$, myocardial requirement of oxygen; VPC, ventricular premature contraction; MMC, mucous membrane color.

Table 3.10 NSAIDs.

NSAID name	Dosage	Duration	Characteristics	Contraindications	Practical notes
Carprofen	1. Dog 2.2 BID or 4.4 mg/kg SID PO, SQ, IV. 2. The authors cannot recommend carprofen in cats due to its unpredictable metabolism in this species.	12–24 h (depending on dose used)	1. Preferentially inhibits COX-2. 2. Antipyretic and anti-inflammatory. 3. Highly protein bound. 4. May compromise renal blood flow. 5. Rare side effect of hepatic toxicity in dogs (16). 6. Reduces healing time of gastric ulcers, and can cause other gastrointestinal side effects such as vomiting, anorexia and diarrhea.	1. In patients known to have renal failure use at the lowest effective dose or avoid. 2. Preemptive evaluation of liver function and liver enzymes, as well as periodic rechecks of liver values, is warranted in any patient where long term use is indicated. 3. Patients that are predisposed to or experience intraoperative hypotension may have compromised renal blood flow. It is the authors' recommendation to avoid this drug for the first 24 h post anesthesia in these patients.	1. Although there are some benefits to administering carprofen prior to an inflammatory event, caution is advised using this drug preoperatively. 2. Injectable and oral formulation available. 3. Typically used postoperatively 2.2–4.4 mg/kg SQ.
Deracoxib	1. Postoperative pain in dogs 3–4 mg/kg. 2. Osteoarthritis pain in dogs 1–2 mg/kg.	24 h	1. Selective COX-2 inhibitor. 2. Highly protein bound. 3. May compromise renal blood flow. 4. Reduces healing time of gastric ulcers and can cause other gastrointestinal side effects such as vomiting, anorexia, and diarrhea.	1. In patients known to have renal failure, this is best used at lowest possible dose or avoided. 2. Patients that are predisposed or experience intraoperative hypotension may have compromised renal blood flow. It is the authors' recommendation to avoid this drug for the first 24 h post anesthesia in these patients.	

(Continued)

Table 3.10 (Continued)

NSAID name	Dosage	Duration	Characteristics	Contraindications	Practical notes
Ketoprofen	Cats and dogs initial dose 2 mg/kg followed by 1.0 mg/kg for up to 5 days	24 h	1. Nonselectively inhibits both COX-1 and COX-2. 2. Increases bleeding times. 3. Antipyretic and anti-inflammatory. 4. May result in gastric ulcers bleeding and vomiting. 5. Highly protein bound.	1. Use with caution in patients already receiving highly protein-bound drugs (e.g., warfarin, heparin) or patients that are hypoproteinemic. 2. Avoid in patients with ulcers. 3. If used in patients experiencing hypotension within the previous 24 h, it may compound renal damage. 4. Not recommended for long-term use due to gastric ulceration.	
Meloxicam	1. Dog: 0.2 mg/kg SC as the first dose, following doses 0.1 mg/kg PO. 2. Cats: 0.1 mg/kg SC or PO once. This dosage is recommended in compliance with the FDA's black box warning about repeated dosing of meloxicam in this species.	24 h	1. COX-2 preferential. 2. Metabolized by oxidation in the cats; this is the preferred route of metabolism for drugs used in this species, as cats do not glucuronidate effectively. 3. Renal failure has been documented in individual feline case studies, although it cannot be duplicated in large population studies. For this reason, meloxicam should not be disregarded as useful NSAID for the feline. 4. Synergistic effect when combined with an opioid for analgesia.	1. Patients with hepatic or renal insufficiencies. 2. Patients prone to GI ulcers. 3. Use caution in patients that are hypotensive during the anesthetic period.	1. If given prior to anesthesia (either with the premedication or orally in the morning), ensure the patient is normotensive throughout the anesthetic period. If one cannot be certain, *do not* administer meloxicam until the animal is stabilized in the postoperative period. 2. Common NSAID for small breed dogs and cats. 3. Injectable and oral formulations are available. 4. Common postoperative dose is 0.1 mg/kg SQ.

Note: NSIADs are used for decreasing inflammation and pain due to inflammatory mediators and osteoarthritis. It is important to allow 3-5 days "wash out" between NSAIDs or following administration of steroids.

Table 3.11 Non-opioid sedatives/premedications.

Drug Name	Classification	Dosage	Duration	Characteristics	Contraindications	Practical notes

Acepromazine	Phenothiazine tranquilizer	1. Healthy patients in combination with opioid: 0.03–0.05 mg/kg IM
		2. 0.01–0.03 mg/kg is routinely given IV pre- and postoperatively for sedation
			Slow onset (up to 30 min when given IM), duration of 2–3 h or longer, may last substantially longer in patients with hepatic dysfunction	1. Reduces MAC of inhalants.
				2. Because the drug is long lasting, postoperative recoveries are often smooth.
				3. Inhibition of dopaminergic receptors of the brain causes sedation.
				4. Metabolized by the liver and excreted by the kidneys.
				5. No reversal agent.
				6. Cardiovascular characteristics.
				  (a) Alpha₁ blockade results in peripheral vasodilation.
				  (b) Reduction in SV, CO, and afterload resulting in hypotension, which may result in a mild increase in HR.
				  (c) Antiarrhythmic properties.
				7. Hypothermia may result as a consequence of catecholamine depletion in the thermoregulatory center of the brain.
				8. Antiemetic.
				9. Decrease in PCV by up to one-third secondary to splenic engorgement.
				10. Decreased platelet aggregation although hemostasis is not altered.
					1. Hypovolemic or hypotensive patients.
					2. Patients with severe liver dysfunction.
					3. Splenectomy.
					4. Caution in patients with HCM, valvular stenosis or DCM.
						Commonly diluted to 1 mg/mL with 0.9% saline or sterile water.

(Continued)

Table 3.11 (Continued)

Drug Name	Classification	Dosage	Duration	Characteristics	Contraindications	Practical notes
Dexmedetomidine	Alpha₂ agonist	1. Premedication: 0.0005–0.003 mg/kg IV, 0.003–0.015 mg/kg IM. 2. CRI 0.0005–0.003 mg/kg/h IV for sedation and analgesia in recovery or supplemental intraoperative analgesia.	Relatively short on set when given IM (10–20 min). Duration of up to 2–3 h	1. Profound sedation (especially if combined with an opioid). 2. Moderate analgesia (potentially synergistic analgesia action when used with opioids). 3. Initial hypertension with a reflex bradycardia, after which secondary hypotension due to a reduction in CO and centrally mediated bradycardia. 5. Arrhythmias including second-degree AV block and ventricular escape beats are common. 6. Patients often develop a transient hyperglycemia due to insulin resistance. 7. Diuresis is common. 8. Reversible with atipamezole (see Table 3.13)	1. Patients with cardiovascular disease including valvular regurgitation or arrhythmias. 2. Renal insufficiencies, anuria, or a blocked urinary system. 3. Liver disease.	1. Most effective when administered to a patient that is allowed 5–10 min in a quiet, darkened room. 2. Should continuously monitor the patient after premedication. Ensure reversal dose has been calculated and is available if needed. 3. Reversal is given IM (see Table 3.13). 4. Vasoconstriction may cause pale or blue MMC, and the pulse oximeter may have difficulty obtaining a measurement. 5. Low doses work nicely as premedication in cats with HCM.

| Diazepam | Benzodiazepine | In dogs half-life is less than 1 h. In cats half-life can be up to 5 h. | Premedication: Dogs and Cats 0.1–0.4 mg/kg IV, IM 2. Seizures: 0.5–1 mg/kg IV, CRI 0.2–0.5 mg/kg/h | 1. Central acting CNS depressant via the $GABA_A$ receptor binding site. 2. When used alone as a premedication, the drug may cause minimal sedation, dysphoria, or enhanced sedation depending on the patient's temperament and health. 3. Relaxes skeletal muscle. 4. Minimal adverse cardiovascular and respiratory effects. 5. Propylene glycol-based and highly lipid soluble, making it incompatible with many drugs and painful on IM or SQ injection as well as inconsistently absorbed. 6. Protect from light. 7. Highly protein bound. 8. Metabolized by the liver. 9. Appetite stimulant. 10. Reversible with flumazenil (see Table 3.13). | 1. Patients with liver insufficiencies will have prolonged effect. 2. Avoid in patients with hepatic encephalopathy. 3. Crosses the placental barrier and may result in respiratory depression in neonates. | 1. Controlled drug, schedule IV. 2. Most predictable sedation in debilitated, geriatric or neonatal patients. 3. May enhance sedation of other premedication agents such as an opioid. 4. Commonly combined (equal volumes or at 0.2–0.3 mg/kg) with ketamine for induction. |
| Midazolam | Benzodiazepine | 30–45 min | 1. Premedication/sedation: 0.1–0.3 mg/kg IM, IV; 2. Seizures: 0.5–1 mg/kg IV | 1. Central-acting CNS depressant via the $GABA_A$ receptor binding site. 2. When used alone as a premedication, this drug may result in minimal sedation, dysphoria, or enhanced sedation depending on the patient's temperament and health. 3. Relaxes skeletal muscle. 4. Minimal adverse cardiovascular and respiratory effects. 5. Protect from light. 6. Highly protein bound. 7. Metabolized by the liver. 8. Reversal is flumazenil (see Table 3.13). 9. Water soluble and reliably absorbed when given IM. | 1. Patients with liver insufficiencies will have prolonged effect. 2. Avoid in patients with hepatic encephalopathy. 3. Crosses the placental barrier and may result in respiratory depression in neonates. | 1. Most predictable sedation in debilitated, geriatric, or neonatal patients. 2. May enhance sedation of other premedication agents such as opioids. 3. Used to reduce induction dose of propofol. 4. Effective sedation for most small mammals and avian species. 5. Works well intranasal in rabbits or pigs. 6. Controlled drug, Schedule IV. |

(Continued)

Table 3.11 (*Continued*)

Drug Name	Classification	Dosage	Duration	Characteristics	Contraindications	Practical notes
Xylazine	Alpha₂ agonist	0.5–2 mg/kg IM, 0.2–1 mg/kg IV	Quick on set when given IM (10–15 min) with duration of 30–120 min depending on dose and route	1. Mild to moderate, albeit short-lived, analgesia. 2. Initial hypertension with a reflex bradycardia, after which secondary hypotension is due to a reduction in cardiac output and centrally mediated bradycardia. 3. Vasoconstriction may cause blue or pale MMC, and the pulse oximeter may have difficulty obtaining a measurement. 4. Arrhythmias including second-degree AV block and ventricular escape beats are common. 5. Causes vomiting in 60% of dogs and 90% of cats. 6. Patients often develop a transient hyperglycemia due to insulin resistance. 7. Diuresis is common. 8. Metabolized by the liver. 9. Reversible with yohimbine (see Table 3.13)	1. Cardiovascular disease including valvular regurgitation or arrhythmias. 2. Patients with renal insufficiencies, anuria, or a blocked urinary system. 3. Liver disease. 4. Avoid in geriatric, diabetic, pregnant, pediatric, sick, or debilitated patients.	1. Reversal should only be given IM. 2. Not recommended for use when another drug is available.

SV, stroke volume; CO, cardiac output; AV, atrioventricular; HCM, hypertrophic cardiomyopathy; DCM, dilated cardiomyopathy; HR, heart rate; CNS, central nervous system.

Table 3.12 Opioids.

Opioid	Indication/uses	Dosage	Duration	Characteristics	Contraindications	Practical notes
Buprenorphine	Mild to moderate analgesia and sedation	1. 0.01–0.03 mg/kg IM, SQ, IV, or in cats, buccally. 2. Epidural 0.004 mg/kg preservative free formulation.	6–8 h	1. Partial mu agonist. 2. Difficult to reverse due to extremely high affinity for mu receptors. 3. Does not cause vomiting or histamine release. 4. Ceiling effect. 5. May cause euphoria in cats making them more cooperative. 6. Protect from light. 7. Reversible with naloxone (see Table 3.13) 8. Metabolized by the liver. 9. Causes miosis in the canine and mydriasis in the feline.		1. Ideal premedication in cats; however, has minimal sedation in dogs. 2. Controlled, Schedule III 3. Buccal is ideal for fractious cats especially when combined with ketamine. 4. In cats, buprenorphine has been shown to be as effective as morphine in treating moderate to severe pain (17).
Butorphanol	Mild visceral pain, sedation and antitussive	0.1–0.4 mg/kg IM, SQ, IV	60–180 min	1. Semisynthetic agonist/antagonist (kappa agonist via which mediates its analgesic actions and mild mu antagonist). 2. Minimal cardiovascular and respiratory side effects. 3. Antitussive and reduces bronchospasms. 4. Protect from light. 5. Metabolized by the liver.		1. Partial reversal for full agonists at 0.1 mg/kg IV. 2. Controlled, Schedule IV.

(Continued)

Table 3.12 (*Continued*)

Opioid	Indication/uses	Dosage	Duration	Characteristics	Contraindications	Practical notes
Fentanyl	Intraoperative management of noxious stimuli, postoperative analgesic, common component of a neuroleptic analgesic induction	1. IV: Bolus 0.002–0.010 mg/kg, CRI 0.012–0.04 mg/kg/h (18) 2. Postoperative CRI 0.002–0.005 mg/kg/h 3. Transdermal delivery: 25 mcg/h for patients under 10 kg, 50 mcg/h for patients 10–20 kg, 75 mcg/h for patients 20–30 kg, and 100 mcg/h for patients greater than 30 kg	Dependent on delivery method. IV bolus in dogs and cats 20–45 min. Transdermal onset 12 h.	1. Full mu agonist. 2. May cause bradycardia and hypoventilation at high doses. 3. Significantly reduces MAC when used as a CRI during anesthesia. 4. Reversible with naloxone (see Table 3.13). 5. May cause sedation. 6. May cause dysphoria when given IV to healthy, unsedated patients. 7. Metabolized by the liver. 8. Causes miosis in the canine and mydriasis in the feline.	1. Patients with head trauma or increased ICP if not supporting ventilation.	1. Ideal for older or cardiovascularly compromised animal to reduce MAC. 2. Controlled, Schedule II. 3. "Wooden chest" phenomena is described in human patients subsequent to the use of fentanyl and other opioids. This refers to muscle rigidity of the thorax and abdomen, preventing adequate ventilation. While not commonly seen in veterinary species, should this occur, reversal of the opioid, neuromuscular blockade, and mechanical ventilation may be necessary. 4. Heat can increase the rate of delivery and absorption of transdermal fentanyl patches. 5. Transdermal fentanyl patches may result in skin irritation. 6. Some formulations of transdermal fentanyl patches cannot be cut. If patch is dispensing more fentanyl than the patient requires, cover half the patch (allow half the patch to have contact with the skin). 7. Hair must be shaved over area the patch will be attached and skin clean.

Drug	Indication	Dose	Duration	Pharmacology/Effects	Contraindications
Hydromorphone	Sedation, premedication for painful procedures, intraoperative noxious stimuli management, postoperative analgesic	0.05–0.1 mg/kg IV, 0.1–0.2 mg/kg IM	4 h	1. Full mu agonist. 2. When given IM, will likely cause vomiting and panting. 3. High doses may cause bradycardia and slight respiratory depression. 4. May increase ICP secondary to hypoventilation. 5. Minimal cardiovascular side effects, although it may cause bradycardia at high doses. 6. Metabolized by the liver. 7. Reversible with naloxone (see Table 3.13). 8. Causes miosis in the canine and mydriasis in the feline. 9. Histamine release may occur but is unlikely.	1. Patients with head trauma or increased ICP if ventilation is not supported. 2. Avoid if possible in patients predisposed to histamine release (MCT, heart worm extractions). 3. Patients with severe liver dysfunction may have prolonged duration.	1. Up to 69% of cats may experience hyperthermia secondary to hydromorphone (21), especially if intraoperative hypothermia occurs (22).
Meperedine	Mild analgesia, sedation, useful as premedication specifically in young patients.	1. Canine: 5–10 mg/kg IM 2. Feline: 3–5 mg/kg IM	45 min	1. Full mu agonist. 2. Histamine release possible (especially when given IV), which may result in hypotension and facial edema. 3. Has anticholinergic effects (e.g., increase in HR). 4. Synergistic action with sedatives may cause profound sedation. 5. Vomiting may occur. 6. Excitement possible when used alone. 7. Metabolized by the liver. 8. Reversible with naloxone (see Table 3.13). 9. Causes miosis in the canine and mydriasis in the feline. 10. May block sodium channels, similar to local anesthetics. 11. May also possess alpha$_2$ agonist activity.	1. Patients prone to histamine release (MCT, heart worm extractions). 2. Patient receiving monoamine oxidase inhibitors (MAOI) (e.g., selegiline). 3. Patients with head trauma or increased ICP if ventilation is not supported.	1. Ideal for young patients with patent ductus arteriosus (PDA) or portosystemic shunt (PSS) as premedication. 2. This drug is extremely short acting and thus has limited usefulness in most veterinary practices. 3. In human patients, the combination of a meperidine and an MAOI has reportedly caused serotonin syndrome—a potentially fatal reaction. While this is not documented in veterinary medicine, the possibility exists. 4. Controlled drug, schedule II.

Chapter 3

(Continued)

Table 3.12 (Continued)

Opioid	Indication/uses	Dosage	Duration	Characteristics	Contraindications	Practical notes
Methadone	Premedication, minimal sedation, intraoperative management noxious stimuli reduction, and postoperative analgesia	0.1–0.5 mg/kg IV, IM, SQ	4 h	1. Full mu agonist opioid but also possesses NMDA antagonist properties. 2. Does not cause vomiting. 3. High doses may result in bradycardia and respiratory depression. 4. Metabolized by the liver. 5. Reversible by naloxone (see Table 3.13). 6. Causes miosis in the canine and mydriasis in the feline.		1. Ideal for painful patients where vomiting needs to be avoided (patients with increased ICP, IOP, GI foreign bodies etc.). 2. Ideal postoperative analgesic where nausea or sedation is undesirable. 3. May reduce central sensitization due its NMDA antagonist properties. 4. Controlled substance, Schedule II
Morphine	Premedication, sedation, intraoperative management, and postoperative analgesia	1. 0.1–1.0 mg/kg SC, IM; CRI 0.1–0.3 mg/kg/h IV 2. Epidural: 0.1 mg/kg preservative free formulation	Onset of action may take up to 30 min. Duration of IM systemic, single dose administration is 2–4 h; epidural duration is 12–24 h.	1. Prototype mu agonist opioid, to which all other opioids are compared. Morphine also works at delta and kappa receptors. 2. While morphine will not eliminate the feeling of pain, the tolerance to pain is significantly increased with this drug. 3. Poor lipid solubility results in prolonged duration of epidural analgesia. 4. Morphine is metabolized in the liver to several metabolites; the active metabolite (which results in analgesia) is morphine-6-glucuronide. 5. Decreased MAC up to 45% (19). 6. Vomiting and panting likely when given IM, as well as other signs of nausea (excessive salivation). 7. Vomiting will increase ICP and IOP.	1. Patients predisposed to histamine release (MCT, heart worm extraction). 2. Patients with head trauma, increased ICP, or IOP. 3. Patients with biliary disease. 4. Avoid in patients where vomiting is undesirable.	1. The highly overrated phenomena of excitement in cats have been reported. The study responsible for this rumor used doses of up to 20 mg/kg to cause dysphoria (23). Most cats actually experience euphoria secondary to morphine administration at clinical doses. 2. The authors advise gentle bladder expression or catheterization of any animal which receives morphine epidurally prior to recovery, as well as good nursing care documenting normal urination.

8. May result in histamine release, especially with high doses given rapidly IV.
9. Respiratory depression and bradycardia is possible at high doses.
10. Initially increases peristaltic motility followed by prolonged period of GI stasis, which may result in constipation.
11. Morphine, among other opioids, causes contracture of the Sphincter of Oddi (common biliary duct), increasing gall bladder pressure.
12. Causes miosis in the canine and mydriasis in the feline.
13. When given alone, possible dysphoria, excitement, and increase responsiveness to noise may result.
14. Works synergistically with sedatives.
15. Reversible with naloxone (see Table 3.13).
16. Consistent with the effects of most opioids, there is a decrease in tracheal sensitivity after the administration.
17. Systemic and epidural morphine results in a release of antidiuretic hormone.

3. Controlled substance, Schedule II.
4. Useful in an animal with prolonged intubation due to the reduction in tracheal stimulation.
5. Express bladder and monitor for bladder distention following the use of morphine.
6. Used by some veterinarians intra-articularly to target the peripheral mu opioid receptors.

(Continued)

Table 3.12 (*Continued*)

Opioid	Indication/uses	Dosage	Duration	Characteristics	Contraindications	Practical notes
Oxymorphone	Premedication, sedation, intraoperative, and postoperative analgesia	0.05–0.2 mg/kg IV, IM, SQ	2–4 h	1. Full mu agonist. 2. More lipid soluble than morphine, resulting in a faster onset of action. 3. Decreases MAC up to 40% (20). 4. Vomiting is less likely with this drug than morphine. 5. Does not result in histamine release. 6. May result in panting when given IM. 7. Respiratory depression and bradycardia is possible at high doses. 8. Causes miosis in the canine and mydriasis in the feline. 9. When given alone, possible dysphoria, excitement, and increased responsiveness to noise may result. 10. Works synergistically with sedatives. 11. Reversible with naloxone (see Table 3.13). 12. Metabolized by the liver.	Patients with head trauma or increased ICP if ventilation is not supported.	Controlled, Schedule II.

| Remifentanil | Intraoperative and postoperative analgesic | IV: Bolus 0.002–0.005 mg/kg, CRI 0.012–0.042 mg/kg/h. | Seconds regardless of duration of exposure | 1. Full mu agonist.
2. May cause bradycardia and hypoventilation at high doses.
3. Significantly reduces inhalant requirement when used as a CRI during anesthesia.
4. Highly lipid soluble.
5. Metabolized by plasma esterase. | Patients with head trauma or increased ICP if ventilation is not supported. | 1. Postoperatively, an alternative opioid is likely more suitable for analgesia due to remifentanil's short duration.
2. Commonly used for patients with liver failure, hepatic shunts, or extremely critical patients.
3. Often used in the older or cardiovascularly compromised animal to reduce MAC.
4. Formulation available must be reconstituted.
5. Controlled, Schedule II. |
| Tramadol | Oral analgesic | Canine 2.5–5 mg/kg PO, Feline 2 mg/kg PO | 4–12 h | 1. Central-acting analgesic with weak mu opioid receptor agonist.
2. Inhibits reuptake of norepinephrine and serotonin; may actually stimulate serotonin release.
3. May result in sedation.
4. Protect from light.
5. Works well for mild to moderate pain; the drug is only one-fifth to one-tenth as potent as morphine. The active metabolite, O-desmethyltramadol, is responsible for some of the analgesia. | 1. Avoid use in patients currently on monoamine oxidase inhibitors (e.g., selegiline).
2. Caution in patients with renal disease or seizures. | 1. Only available as an oral formulation in the United States.
2. Useful with NSAIDs to control postoperative pain.
3. Currently, Tramadol is not a controlled substance. |

Sources: References 21, 22, and 23.

Table 3.13 Reversal agents.

Reversal	Reversal for	Dosage	Duration	Characteristics	Contraindications	Practical notes
Atipamezole	Alpha$_2$ agonists (e.g., dexmedetomidine)	Dogs: equal volume as dexmedetomidine IM Cats: equal to 0.5 volume of dexmedetomidine IM	2–3 h	1. Antagonizes alpha$_2$ agonists by binding to the alpha$_2$ receptors. 2. May decrease BP. 3. May cause excitement. 4. May have gastrointestinal side effects, such as vomiting or diarrhea.	IV injection results in severe hypotension due to action at the peripheral alpha$_2$ receptors.	1. If alpha$_2$ agonists are the sole means of analgesia and pain is anticipated after recovery, consider administering other analgesics prior to reversal. 2. Signs of reversal occur in 5–10 min following IM injection.
Edrophonium	Nondepolarizing NMB reversal (atracurium, cisatracurium, and pancuronium)	0.25–0.5 mg/kg slow IV	Difficult to determine; generally less than 1 h.	1. Inhibits acetylcholinersterase to increased acetylcholine concentrations at the neuromuscular junction. 2. Give slowly to reduce impact of bradycardia, secondary to edrophonium's cholinergic effect. 3. Protect from light.		1. If a preexiting bradycardia is present, or if patient is predisposed to bradycardia, administering an anticholinergic (atropine or glycopyrrolate) prior to edrophonium is warranted. 2. Only administer edrophonium when at least two twitches are present on the PNS. Preferably, all four twitches are present in a TOF prior to reversal. 3. Before extubating patient, ensure patient is breathing adequately (capnography is a helpful tool in this regard). 4. Monitor patient after extubation for any relapse in neuromuscular paralysis.
Flumazenil	Reversal of benzodiazepine	0.02–0.1 mg/kg IV	30–60 min	1. Protect from light. 2. Administered IV.		To reverse benzodiazepines, calculate full dose of reversal and dilute 10-fold. Give slowly until desired reversal effect is achieved.

Drug	Indication	Dose	Duration	Effects	Contraindications	Notes
Naloxone	Used to reverse opioid full and partial agonists	0.01–0.04 mg/kg IV	60 min	1. Antagonizes both exogenous and endogenous opioids. 2. May result in hypertension and excitement. 3. Short duration may necessitate repeated dosing, depending on duration of the opioid reversed.		1. Reversal of opioid agonists may leave the patient painful! Always have alternative analgesia on board prior to beginning reversal. 2. Commonly used to reverse opioid affects when they contribute to a prolonged or dysphoric recovery. 3. Calculate dose and dilute 1:10 with saline; give in increments until desired reversal is achieved for nonemergent situations. 4. Emergency situation or anesthetic arrest: full dose of naloxone is given IV when an opioid was administered and repeated every hour for the duration of opioid agonist.
Neostigmine	Nondepolarizing NMB reversal (atracurium, cisatracurium, and pancuronium)	0.01–0.03 mg/kg IV given slowly over 20 min	4–6 h	1. Increases the amount of the neurotransmitter acetylcholine at the neuromuscular junction (favoring binding of acetylcholine). 2. Does not cross the blood–brain barrier or placenta. 3. May result in bradycardia. 4. Increases smooth muscle tone of the bladder. 5. Results in peristalsis (diarrhea) and increased secretions.	Patients with urinary or GI obstruction.	Give anticholinergic (atropine or glycopyrrolate) prior to giving neostigmine, to prevent the muscarinic effects which may otherwise result (e.g., bradycardia).
Yohimbine	Reversal of $alpha_2$ agonists, specific for xylazine	0.1 mg/kg IM, IV	2 h	1. Reversal will occur within a matter of moments. 2. May result in hypotension. 3. At high doses, may result in seizures.		Reversal of $alpha_2$ agonists' sedative and analgesic effects; prior to reversal, an alternative analgesic should be systemically administered to the animal.

BP, blood pressure; NMB, neuromuscular blocking; PNS, peripheral nerve stimulator; TOF, train of four.

E. Contraindications

1. Patients with cardiac disease (patients with preexisting tachyarrhythmia)
2. Caution in end-stage pregnancy, as beta stimulation can relax the uterine tissue.

F. Practical notes

1. Use a chamber that facilitates proper particle dispersion for full effect
2. When administering this drug to an intubated patient, a significant amount of the drug (50–70%) will reside within the endotracheal (ET) tube (1). Therefore, the doses delivered may be increased when administering albuterol to an intubated patient.

III. Alfaxalone (see Table 3.6)

IV. Amantadine (see Table 3.9)

V. Atenolol: Beta$_1$-adrendergic antagonist

A. Indication

Slows sinus rate and is antihypertensive.

B. Dosage

0.1–0.5 mg/kg IV slowly (over 5 minutes).

C. Duration

Twelve hours.

D. Characteristics

1. Negative inotrope and negative chronotrope
2. Little to no hepatic metabolism; clearance dependent on renal function, as it is eliminated by the kidneys
3. May cause bradycardia and bradyarrhythmias.

E. Contraindications

1. Uncontrolled heart failure patients
2. Patients with existing bradyarrhythmias
3. Use conservatively in patients with renal failure
4. Asthmatic patients.

F. Practical notes

1. Commonly used in patients with hypertrophic cardiomyopathy (HCM) or hyperthyroidism
2. This drug is not typically used under anesthesia to decrease the sinus HR.

VI. Atipamezole (see Table 3.13)

VII. Atracurium (see Table 3.8)

VIII. Atropine (see Table 3.1)

IX. Bupivacaine (see Table 3.7)

X. Buprenorphine (see Table 3.12)

XI. Butorphanol (see Table 3.12)

XII. Calcium gluconate: Calcium supplement

A. Indications

1. Treatment for hyperkalemia, hypocalcemia, and Ca^{2+} channel blocker toxicity
2. Positive inotrope
3. Administer after large amounts of blood products (e.g., if more than one unit of blood is administered).

B. Dosage

0.2–0.4 mg/kg IV over 30 minutes.

C. Characteristics

1. Positive inotrope action improves contractility of myocardium, which may improve CO and BP
2. Protect from light.

D. Contraindications

1. Cardiac arrhythmias, such as ventricular fibrillation
2. Hypercalcemia.

E. Practical notes

1. Always administer slowly
2. Ensure an ECG is placed on the patient and monitor HR
3. Administered separately from other drugs and blood products.

XIII. Carprofen (see Table 3.10)

XIV. Cisatracurium (see Table 3.8)

XV. Dantrolene: Muscle relaxant

A. Indications

Malignant hyperthermia (MH).

B. Dosage

1.0 mg/kg IV.

C. Duration

Eight hours.

D. Characteristics

1. No discernible effects on respiratory and cardiovascular systems
2. Results in muscle weakness
3. Protect from light.

E. Contraindications

1. Can cause drowsiness and dizziness
2. Hepatoxicity is possible; use with caution in patients with hepatic disease.

F. Practical notes

1. Drug is very expensive and frequency of MH is rare. If there is preemptive suspicion that a patient may have an MH episode, often this is obtained from a local human hospital prior to anesthesia.
2. Once reconstituted only stable for 6 hours.
3. Reconstitute per manufacturer instructions.

XVI. Deracoxib (see Table 3.10)

XVII. Desflurane (see Table 3.5)

XVIII. Desmopressin (DDAVP): Related to antidiuretic hormone (vasopressin)

A. Indications

Used in patients with von Willebrand's disease to increase the release of von Willebrand's factor (Factor VIII).

B. Dosage

1–4 mcg/kg SQ.

C. Duration

Two hours; however, additional dosage within 24 hours will not result in a greater effect (2).

D. Characteristics

1. Acts as an antidiuretic similar to antidiuretic hormone (ADH) causing reabsorption of water in the kidney
2. Results in less vasoconstriction than vasopressin
3. Results in a dose-dependent increase in von Willebrand's factor (Factor VIII).

E. Contraindications

Hypercoagulable patients.

F. Practical notes

Effects are short-lived, but drug is useful for administration prior to a surgical event in a patient with Von Willebrand's disease.

XIX. Dexamethasone SP (dexamethasone sodium phosphate): Glucocorticoid

A. Indication

Anti-inflammatory, immunosuppressive.

B. Dosage

0.1–2.0 mg/kg IV, IM or PO.

C. Duration

Twelve to twenty-four hours.

D. Characteristics

1. Suppresses inflammatory mediators
2. May reduce intracranial pressure (ICP) and edema
3. Protect from light.

E. Contraindications

1. Do not use in patients currently receiving nonsteroidal anti-inflammatory drugs (NSAIDs).
2. Caution in diabetics and patients with renal insufficiencies.
3. Do not use in patients with gastrointestinal ulcers (GI) ulcers or GI compromise.

F. Practical notes

1. Long-term use results in adrenocortical dependency; if a patient has received dexamethasone, especially at high doses, an Addisonian crisis may manifest under anesthesia (see Chapter 5). Patients tapered slowly off the drug are unlikely to have this effect.
2. An increase in urination and water consumption may result from a high dosage of this drug.
3. It may cause GI ulcers.
4. Immunosuppressive features may precipitate delayed wound healing and secondary infections.
5. Has no mineralocorticoid activity.
6. Commonly referred to as Dexmethasone SP 4 mg/mL.

XX. Dexmedetomidine (see Table 3.9 and Table 3.11)

XXI. Dextrans (see Table 3.4)

XXII. Dextrose: Fluid supplement

A. Indication

Hypoglycemic patients, diabetic ketoacidosis, neonates, adjunctive treatment for hyperkalemia.

B. Dosage

1. IV bolus for profound hypoglycemia 0.5 mg/kg (diluted 1:4 with isotonic fluids)
2. Fluid additives: Add appropriate amount to yield a 2.5–5% solution. See Appendix B, "Creating Dilutions and Reconstituting Solutions."

C. Duration

Often given as a component of a constant rate infusion (CRI) to prolong transient effect.

D. Characteristics

Extremely hypertonic requiring dilution prior to administration.

E. Contraindications

Hyperglycemic patients.

F. Practical notes

1. Common dilutions for anesthesia are 2.5–5% in crystalloid solutions.
2. Monitor blood glucose (BG) from an independent catheter.
3. High concentrations of dextrose cause tissue irritation (especially when given peri-vascular) due to its hypertonic nature.

XXIII. Diazepam (see Table 3.11)

XXIV. Diphenhydramine: Antihistamine

A. Indication

Patients with conditions that predispose the patient to histamine release: mast cell tumors (MCTs), anaphylaxis, and heart worm extractions.

B. Dosage

0.5–2.0 mg/kg IM, IV.

C. Duration

6–8 hours.

D. Characteristics

1. Blockade of histamine$_1$ (H$_1$) receptors
2. May result in sedation and prevent vomiting.

E. Practical notes

1. In patients with histamine release, there are decreased symptoms of reaction; however, this will not reverse a reaction.

2. Use as premedication in patients that are expected to have histamine release (heart worm extractions, MCT).

XXV. Dobutamine (see Table 3.2)

XXVI. Dopamine (see Table 3.2)

XXVII. Doxapram: Respiratory stimulant

A. Indication

Used to stimulate respiration typically in neonates.

B. Dosage

2–5 mg/kg IV or 1–2 drops under tongue of newborn.

C. Duration

Usually administered only once, as additional dosages may have a decrease in effectiveness.

D. Characteristics

1. Stimulates respiration by action on the carotid chemoreceptors, resulting in an increase in V_T rather than RR
2. May increase CO
3. Repeated dosages may result in undesirable CNS stimulation
4. Contains benzyl alcohol
5. Protect from light.

E. Contraindications

1. Use cautiously in neonates due to benzyl alcohol.
2. Do not use if patients are receiving any other CNS stimulants.

F. Practical notes

Used as respiratory stimulant most commonly in newborns; very rarely used in adult patients

XXVIII. Edrophonium (see Table 3.13)

XXIX. Ephedrine (see Table 3.2)

XXX. Epinephrine (see Table 3.2)

XXXI. Eutetic mixture of local anesthetic (EMLA) cream (AstraZeneca, London)

A. Indication

Topical anesthetic.

B. Dosage

Minimal amount to cover area of anticipated insult.

C. Duration

Dependent on contact time, but may exceed 2 hours (3).

D. Characteristics

1. Contains lidocaine 2.5% and prilocaine 2.5% (both local anesthetics), which penetrate the skin's full thickness
2. Onset of action depends on contact with skin
3. Heat may decrease onset time
4. Minimal to immeasurable systemic absorption.

E. Contraindications

None.

F. Practical notes

1. Recommendations for application include clipping hair and applying cream. Cover. Onset may take 45–60 minutes.
2. The authors find covering the area where cream is applied with plastic such as an examination glove to "trap" body heat may decrease onset up to a total time of 10–20 minutes.
3. This works well to assist in the placement of catheters in neonates or critical patients to avoid or minimize sedation.
4. This is used over areas of incision in place of a line block.

XXXII. Esmolol: Beta receptor antagonist

A. Indication

Prevention of tachycardia and hypertension.

B. Dosage

0.05–0.1 mg/kg IV, CRI 3–12 mg/kg/h.

C. Duration

10 minutes.

D. Characteristics

1. $Beta_1$ antagonist that results in decrease in HR; high doses result in myocardial depression, reduction in CO, and bradycardia
2. Metabolized by plasma esterases
3. Protect from light.

E. Contraindications

1. Bradyarrhythmias such as AV block, escape rhythm
2. Beta antagonists are not used if there is a suspected catecholamine-induced nidus for hypertension or tachycardia (e.g., pheochromocytoma), unless appropriate alpha blockade is already present; unopposed alpha stimulation may prove fatal for the patient.

XXXIII. Etomidate (see Table 3.6)

XXXIV. Famotidine: H_2 receptor antagonist

A. Indication

Premedication in patients with MCT, prone to histamine release or gastric ulcers, regurgitation or irritation of the gastrointestinal tract.

B. Dosage

Dogs and cats 0.5–1.0 mg/kg IV, SQ, IM.

C. Duration

Eight to twelve hours.

D. Characteristics

1. Blocks H_2 receptors to help prevent gastric ulcers.
2. Minimizes negative effects of histamine release.
3. Multidose vial contains benzyl alcohol as a preservative.
4. Protect from light.

E. Contraindications

None clinically relevant.

F. Practical notes

May be useful for a patient that has regurgitated under anesthesia or has a history of regurgitation under anesthesia.

XXXV. Fentanyl (see Table 3.12)

XXXVI. Flumazenil (see Table 3.13)

XXXVII. Furosemide: Diuretic

A. Indication

Pulmonary edema, congestive heart failure (CHF).

B. Dosage

0.5–2.0 mg/kg IM or IV.

C. Duration

1–2 hours. (*Note*: In some patients with altered physiology, this drug may last longer.)

D. Characteristics

1. Loop diuretic, which inhibits the reabsorption of sodium and water in the loop of Henle within the kidney
2. Slight vasodilation occurs, which will increase renal perfusion and decrease preload
3. Protect from light.
4. Precipitates in acidic solutions.

E. Contraindications

1. Dehydrated patients
2. Patients with electrolyte imbalances (such as hyponatremia)
3. Do not use in patients that are anuric.
4. High dosages in the feline may result in toxicity.

F. Practical notes

1. Monitor electrolytes when using this drug.
2. Monitor hydration status of the patient when using this drug.

XXXVIII. Gabapentin (see Table 3.9)

XXXIX. Glycopyrrolate (see Table 3.1)

XL. Hydromorphone (see Table 3.12)

XLI. Hydroxyethyl starch "hetastarch" (see Table 3.4)

XLII. Isoflurane (see Table 3.5)

XLIII. Isoproterenol: Beta agonist

A. Indication

Chronotropic; "pharmacological pacemaker" for patients with sick sinus syndrome or third-degree AV block.

B. Dosage

0.0006–0.005 mg/kg/h.

C. Duration

Short-lived if not given as a CRI.

D. Characteristics

1. No alpha agonist effects
2. Sympathomimetic at $beta_1$ and $beta_2$ receptors to increase myocardial contractility, HR, bronchodilate, and reduce bronchial spasms
3. Causes vasodilation
4. May result in tachycardia and tachyarrhythmias
5. Protect from light.

E. Contraindications

Do not use in conjunction with other catecholamines (e.g., epinephrine); effects may be additive.

F. Practical notes

1. When diluted with 5% dextrose, stable for 24 hours
2. Protect dilutions from light.

XLIV. Ketamine (see Table 3.6, 3.9)

XLV. Ketoprofen (see Table 3.10)

XLVI. Lactated ringers solution (LRS) (see Table 3.3)

XLVII. Lidocaine (see Table 3.7, 3.9)

XLVIII. Mannitol: Osmotic diuretic

Chapter 3

A. Indication

Used to reduce ICP following cerebral injury, reduce intraocular pressure (IOP) in cases of glaucoma and for renal support.

B. Dosage

1. Reduction of ICP or IOP: 0.25–2.0 g/kg slow over 20 minutes IV (commonly 0.5 g/kg).
2. For renal support: 6 g/kg/h as a CRI during anesthesia.

C. Duration

Often given once as a single bolus; half-life is likely between 60 and 100 minutes.

D. Characteristics

1. Hyperosmotic diuretic, give slowly IV (generally over 15–20 minutes)
2. Results in increased plasma osmolality
3. In single dose vials, at room temperature, crystals form quickly; keep solution in a warmer or under warm water prior to administration. For this reason, a filter is used when administering this drug.

E. Contraindications

1. Patients with intracranial hemorrhage
2. Dehydrated patients
3. Patient with CHF
4. Anuric renal failure patients
5. Use with caution in hypertensive patients.

F. Practical notes

1. Mannitol is commonly given in neurological patients that present with indications of increased ICP (Cushing's reflex, cerebral edema).

2. When administering this drug, ensuring appropriate fluid therapy and monitoring urine output is necessary.
3. It may be used topically for pharyngeal swelling following brachycephalic surgeries or a traumatic intubation. Place on cotton tip applicators and swab inflamed tissue prior to extubation.

XLIX. Maropitant (see Table 3.9)

L. Meloxicam (see Table 3.10)

LI. Meperedine (see Table 3.12)

LII. Mepivacaine (see Table 3.7)

LIII. Methadone (see Table 3.12)

LIV. Midazolam (see Table 3.11)

LV. Morphine (see Table 3.12)

LVI. Naloxone (see Table 3.13)

LVII. Neostigmine (see Table 3.13)

LVIII. Nitroprusside (see Table 3.2)

LIX. Norepinephrine (see Table 3.2)

LX. Normosol (see Table 3.3)

LXI. Oxymorphone (see Table 3.12)

LXII. Pancuronium (see Table 3.8)

LXIII. Pentobarbital (see Table 3.6)

LXIV. Phenylephrine (see Table 3.2)

LXV. Plasma-lyte 148 (see Table 3.3)

LXVI. Potassium chloride (KCl): Electrolyte supplement

A. Indication

Hypokalemia.

B. Dosage

Rate of administration not to exceed 0.5 mEq/kg/h.

C. Duration

Relatively short-lived if not administered as a part of a CRI.

D. Characteristics

1. Potassium is necessary to prevent muscle weakness, but extreme caution is used when providing supplementation by any route other than oral.
2. Hyperkalemia is fatal in a high enough dosage.

E. Contraindications

Patients with renal insufficiencies.

F. Practical notes

1. Place ECG on patient and monitor for changes if using potassium supplementation.
2. ECG changes associated with hyperkalemia include bradyarrhythmias, spiked T waves, prolonged P–R interval, absent P waves, widened QRS complexes and asystole.
3. Never bolus fluids supplemented with potassium.
4. Monitor serum potassium levels every 30 minutes during supplementation.

LXVII. Procainamide: Class IA antiarrhythmic

A. Indication

Ventricular tachydysrhythmias.

B. Dosage

1. Dogs: 5–10 mg/kg IV followed by an IV CRI 1.5–3.0 mg/kg/h
2. Cats: 1–2 mg/kg IV followed by an IV CRI 0.6–1.2 mg/kg/h.

C. Duration

Effects of the injectable product is short-lived without a CRI.

Chapter 3

D. Characteristic

1. Sodium channel blocker for ventricular ectopic beats and ventricular tachyarrhythmias
2. Metabolized in the liver and excreted by the kidney.

E. Contraindications

1. It is rarely used during anesthesia as this drug may cause cardiovascular depression and hypotension.
2. Reduce dose in patients with hepatic or renal disease.
3. Do not administer in cases of ventricular escape rhythms, sick sinus syndrome, or third-degree AV block.

F. Practical Notes

1. Useful alternative to lidocaine prior to a balloon valvuoplasty to prevent ventricular arrhythmias
2. Useful with ventricular arrhythmias that are refractory to lidocaine.

LXVIII. Propofol (see Table 3.6)

LXIX. Propranolol: Nonselective beta blocker

A. Indication

Tachycardia and supraventricular arrhythmias.

B. Dosage

Dogs and cats: 0.02–0.1 mg/kg IV slowly to effect.

C. Duration

Two to six hours.

D. Characteristics

1. Beta$_1$ and beta$_2$ blocker
2. Class II antiarrhythmic
3. Resultant bradycardia causes a reduction in CO
4. Extensively protein-bound
5. Dependent on liver metabolism
6. Bronchoconstriction may result from beta$_2$ blockade.

E. Contraindications

1. Patients with bradycardia or escape beats
2. Asthmatic patients
3. Use with caution in patients with liver insufficiencies or hypoprotienemia; drug may have profound effect and delayed clearance.

F. Practical notes

In humans, a decrease in local anesthetic and opioid clearance has been reported with administration of propranolol. It is unknown whether this occurs in animals.

LXX. Remifentanil (see Table 3.12)

LXXI. Sevoflurane (see Table 3.5)

LXXII. Sodium bicarbonate: Alkalizing agent

A. Indication

Metabolic acidosis where the underlying cause is low bicarbonate and in the treatment of hyperkalemia.

B. Dosage

1. To correct metabolic acidosis: Give 0.5 dose over slowly over 20 minutes. Reevaluate blood gas; if the patient still exhibits metabolic acidosis, give another 0.5 dose slowly in the same fashion. Target pH correction is no more than 7.2. Equation 3.1 shows calculation of sodium bicarbonate.

$$\text{Body weight (BW)} \times \text{base excess (from blood gas)} \times 0.3 = \text{mEq of sodium bicarbonate} \qquad (3.1)$$

2. For hyperkalemia: 0.5–1.0 mEq/kg slow over 20 minutes

C. Duration

Variable by patient.

D. Characteristics

1. Acts as a base to increase pH
2. Administration will increase CO_2 production (e.g., $EtCO_2$); anesthetist must ensure adequate ventilation
3. Results in alkaline urine
4. Reduction in serum potassium levels may cause hypokalemia

5. Administration leads to hypernatremia
6. Hyperosmolar
7. May result in alkalosis if overdosed.

E. Contraindications

1. Respiratory or metabolic alkalosis
2. Patients with hypocalcemia
3. Patients intolerant of high sodium levels, such as volume overloaded patients or animals with CHF.

F. Practical notes

1. Carefully evaluate patient's acid–base status during bicarbonate administration.
2. Sodium bicarbonate is incompatible with many other drugs, including some opioids and inotropes.

LXXIII. Sodium chloride (see Table 3.3)

LXXIV. Sodium chloride 7.5% (see Table 3.3)

LXXV. Terbutaline: Intermediate-acting beta$_2$-adrenergic agonist

A. Indication

Bronchodilator, helpful in reducing V/Q mismatch.

B. Dosage

0.01 mg/kg SC or IM, or nebulized with 1–2 metered dose from inhaler.

C. Duration

Four hours.

D. Characteristics

1. Increase in HR indicates effect
2. Decrease in potassium (K^+)
3. Tremors can result from beta-receptor stimulation in the muscles
4. Protect from light.

E. Contraindications

1. Patients with cardiac disease (patients with preexisting tachyarrhythmia)
2. Caution in end-stage pregnancy, as beta stimulation can relax the uterine tissue.

F. Practical notes

1. When nebulized, use a chamber that facilitates proper particle dispersion for full effect.
2. When administering this drug to an intubated patient, a significant amount of the drug (50–70%) will reside within the ET tube(1). Therefore, the doses delivered may be increased when administering terbutaline to an intubated patient.

LXXVI. Tiletamine and zolazepam "Telazol" (see Table 3.6)

LXXVII. Tramadol (see Table 3.12)

LXXVIII. Vasopressin (see Table 3.2)

LXXIX. Xylazine (see Table 3.9 and Table 3.11)

LXXX. Yohimbine (see Table 3.13)

References

1. Crogan SJ, Bishop MJ. Delivery efficiency of metered dose aerosols given via endotracheal tubes. Anesthesiology. 1989;70(6):1008–10.
2. Lethagen S, Harris AS, Nilsson IM. Intranasal desmopressin (DDAVP) by spray in mild hemophilia A and von Willebrand's disease type I. Blut. 1990;60(3):187–91.
3. Baxter AL, Ewing PH, Young GB, Ware A, Evans N, Manworren RC. EMLA application exceeding two hours improves pediatric emergency department venipuncture success. Adv Emerg Nurs J. 2013;35(1):67–75.
4. Davis H, Jensen T, Johnson A, Knowles P, Meyer R, Rucinsky R, et al. 2013 AAHA/AAFP fluid therapy guidelines for dogs and cats. J Am Anim Hosp Assoc. 2013;49(3):149–59.
5. Ambros B, Duke-Novakovski T, Pasloske KS. Comparison of the anesthetic efficacy and cardiopulmonary effects of continuous rate infusions of alfaxalone-2-hydroxypropyl-beta-cyclodextrin and propofol in dogs. Am J Vet Res. 2008;69(11):1391–8.
6. Herbert GL, Bowlt KL, Ford-Fennah V, Covey-Crump GL, Murrell JC. Alfaxalone for total intravenous anaesthesia in dogs undergoing ovariohysterectomy: a comparison of premedication with acepromazine or dexmedetomidine. Vet Anaesth Analg. 2013;40(2):124–33.
7. Ferré PJ, Pasloske K, Whittem T, Ranasinghe MG, Li Q, Lefebvre HP. Plasma pharmacokinetics of alfaxalone in dogs after an intravenous bolus of Alfaxan-CD RTU. Vet Anaesth Analg. 2006;33(4):229–36.

Chapter 3

8. Muir W, Lerche P, Wiese A, Nelson L, Pasloske K, Whittem T. Cardiorespiratory and anesthetic effects of clinical and supraclinical doses of alfaxalone in dogs. Vet Anaesth Analg. 2008;35(6): 451–62.

9. Amengual M, Flaherty D, Auckburally A, Bell AM, Scott EM, Pawson P. An evaluation of anaesthetic induction in healthy dogs using rapid intravenous injection of propofol or alfaxalone. Vet Anaesth Analg. 2013;40(2):115–23.

10. Maney JK, Shepard MK, Braun C, Cremer J, Hofmeister EH. A comparison of cardiopulmonary and anesthetic effects of an induction dose of alfaxalone or propofol in dogs. Vet Anaesth Analg. 2013;40(3):237–44.

11. O'Hagan B, Pasloske K, McKinnon C, Perkins N, Whittem T. Clinical evaluation of alfaxalone as an anaesthetic induction agent in dogs less than 12 weeks of age. Aust Vet J. 2012;90(9): 346–50.

12. Michou JN, Leece EA, Brearley JC. Comparison of pain on injection during induction of anaesthesia with alfaxalone and two formulations of propofol in dogs. Vet Anaesth Analg. 2012;39(3):275–81.

13. Kukanich B, Cohen RL. Pharmacokinetics of oral gabapentin in greyhound dogs. Vet J. 2011;187(1):133–5.

14. Pypendop BH, Ilkiw JE. Assessment of the hemodynamic effects of lidocaine administered IV in isoflurane-anesthetized cats. Am J Vet Res. 2005;66(4):661–8.

15. Hickman M, Cox S, Mahabir S, Miskell C, Lin J, Bunger A, et al. Safety, pharmacokinetics and use of the novel NK-1 receptor antagonist maropitant (Cerenia) for the prevention of emesis and motion sickness in cats. J Vet Pharmacol Ther. 2008;31(3):220–9.

16. MacPhail CM, Lappin MR, Meyer DJ, Smith SG, Webster CR, Armstrong PJ. Hepatocellular toxicosis associated with administration of carprofen in 21 dogs. J Am Vet Med Assoc. 1998;212(12):1895–901.

17. Robertson S, Taylor P, Lascelles B, Dixon M. Changes in thermal threshold response in eight cats after administration of buprenorphine, butorphanol and morphine. Vet Rec. 2003;153(15): 462–5.

18. Murphy MR, Hug CC. The anesthetic potency of fentanyl in terms of its reduction of enflurane MAC. Anesthesiology. 1982;57(6):485–8.

19. Steffey EP, Eisele JH, Baggot JD, Woliner MJ, Jarvis KA, Elliott AR. Influence of inhaled anesthetics on the pharmacokinetics and pharmacodynamics of morphine. Anesth Analg. 1993;77(2):346–51.

20. Machado CE, Dyson DH, Grant Maxie M. Effects of oxymorphone and hydromorphone on the minimum alveolar concentration of isoflurane in dogs. Vet Anaesth Analg. 2006;33(1): 70–7.

21. Niedfeldt R, Robertson S. Postanesthetic hyperthermia in cats: a retrospective comparison between hydromorphone and buprenorphine. Vet Anaesth Analg. 2006;33(6):381–9.

22. Posner LP, Pavuk AA, Rokshar JL, Carter JE, Levine JF. Effects of opioids and anesthetic drugs on body temperature in cats. Vet Anaesth Analg. 2010;37(1):35–43.

23. Sturtevant F, Drill V. Tranquilizing drugs and morphine-mania in cats. Nature. 1957; 179(4572):1253.

Chapter 3

Chapter 4

Anesthetic protocols for specific procedures

This chapter gives the reader suggested protocols for specific procedures and is heavily influenced by the authors' opinions; however, the most suitable protocol for any procedure is based on familiarity of the anesthetist with anesthetics available and patient's preanesthetic assessment. Therefore, the user is highly encouraged to try various protocols in healthy patients prior to attempting these protocols for the first time in compromised animals. Also listed are common complications and prevention methods as they relate to anesthesia.

I. Soft tissue surgeries

A. Abdominal exploratory (exploratory laparotomy)

Abdominal exploratory is performed for a variety of reasons such as splenectomy, foreign body removal, septic peritonitis, resection and anastomosis, and gastric dilation and volvulus (GDV). Patient presentation varies substantially. It is important to assess each patient thoroughly with a complete physical examination (PE), complete blood count (CBC), and chemistry. Additional laboratory and diagnostic work is performed as indicated by the differential list. Anesthetic protocols are based on the patient's presentation, PE, blood work (BW), diagnostic test results, and primary differentials. The following information details anesthetic considerations, complications, and suggested protocols for common abdominal surgery procedures.

1. Anesthetic concerns/common complications

(a) Arrhythmias: Arrhythmias (e.g., ventricular premature contractions [VPCs], ventricular tachycardia) are common due to hypoxemia, anemia, metabolic abnormalities, and/or abdominal pain. Often, as in the case of GDV, these may not resolve immediately after the procedure, and continued monitoring of the patient throughout the postoperative period is warranted.

(b) Electrolyte abnormalities and metabolic acid–base disturbances: Vomiting or diarrhea secondary to GI disease results in electrolyte imbalances and altered acid–base balance.

Small Animal Anesthesia Techniques, First Edition. Amanda M. Shelby and Carolyn M. McKune.
© 2014 John Wiley & Sons, Inc. Published 2014 by John Wiley & Sons, Inc.
Companion website: www.wiley.com/go/shelbyanesthesia

(c) Hemorrhage: The abdomen contains highly vascular organs such as the liver, kidneys, and spleen. Blood loss is quantified for an accurate estimation (see Chapter 6, "Blood Loss/Hemorrhage" section).

(d) Hypoproteinemia and/or anemia (loss of protein or bleeding in the gastrointestinal [GI] tract): This contributes to a reduction in effective circulating volume and subsequent hypotension. Additionally, many anesthetic drugs are protein bound. In the hypoproteinemic patient, this results in increased unbound drug, causing a more profound effect.

(e) Hypoventilation: Abdominal distention impedes normal respiration; this is compounded by anesthesia reducing diaphragmatic tone, thus reducing the natural barrier preserving thoracic space. Hypoventilation results (see Chapter 6, "Hypoventilation" section).

(f) Hypovolemia: Animals with GI disease reduce their oral intake of food and water. This leads to dehydration and a resulting decrease in effective circulating volume, which worsens hypotension occurring under anesthesia (see Chapter 6, "Hypotension" section). Volume resuscitation prior to anesthesia is warranted.

(g) Pain (conscious patient)/noxious stimuli (unconscious patient): Pain pathways in the GI tract are triggered by distention. Distention secondary to gas occurs with blockage of the GI tract and results in severe patient discomfort.

(h) Regurgitation: Regurgitation may occur passively secondary to disease or during the procedure from high intra-abdominal pressure (see "Regurgitation").

(i) Sepsis: GI perforations or necrosis of areas of the GI tract result in leakage of bacteria into the abdominal cavity, which induces an inflammatory reaction in the body and bacteria in the blood. This leads to septic shock, a state of profound vasodilation that is exacerbated under anesthesia.

2. Anesthetic protocol

Drug selection depends greatly on the patient's presentation. In American Society of Anesthesiologists (ASA) 1–2 patients requiring an exploratory, IM premedication is acceptable. In ASA 3–5 patients, IV catheters are placed without sedation, and fluids are given prior to anesthesia to correct electrolyte abnormalities and stabilize hemodynamic parameters. In general, reversible drugs are ideal. Opioid and lidocaine constant rate infusions (CRIs) are excellent analgesics in the canine patient and greatly reduce minimum alveolar concentration (MAC) of inhalants intraoperatively (see Table 3.9 and Table 3.12). This also helps balance the anesthetic technique and assists in stabilization of hemodynamic parameters. Postoperatively, a fentanyl CRI 0.002–0.005 mg/kg/h and placement of a lidocaine patch over incision is ideal. Appropriate fluid therapy to correct anemia, electrolyte imbalances, and acid–base disturbances is continued and tailored to the individual patient.

Chapter 4

Table 4.1 Suggested anesthesia protocol for an abdominal exploratory.

Abdominal Explore

Opioid premedication (mg/kg)	Sedative premedication (mg/kg)	Induction (mg/kg)	Maintenance	Intraoperative analgesia (mg/kg/h)	Postoperative analgesia

(a) Methadone 0.5–1 IM, 0.2–0.3 IV
or
(b) Hydromorphone 0.1 IM, 0.05 IV
or
(c) Fentanyl 0.002–0.005 IV
	(a) Acepromazine 0.01–0.02
	or
	(b) Dexmedetomidine 0.003–0.005
	or
	(c) Midazolam 0.2 IM
		(a) Propofol to effect +/– midazolam 0.2 and/or lidocaine 1.0 IV to reduce total dose of propofol
		or
		(b) Fentanyl 0.005–0.01 and midazolam 0.2
			Sevoflurane OR isoflurane + CRI for reduction of inhalant requirement	(a) Opioid CRI
				  i. Fentanyl 0.01–0.042
				  or
				  ii. Hydromorphone 0.03
				  or
				  iii. Remifentanil 0.01–0.042
				(b) Lidocaine CRI 1.5–3
					(a) Opioid CRIs:
					  i. Fentanyl 0.002–0.005 mg/kg/h
					  or
					  ii. Hydromorphone 0.01 mg/kg/h
					(b) Lidocaine 1.5 mg/kg/h
					or
					(c) Intermittent bolus(select one):
					  i. Methadone 0.3 IV q 4–6h
					  or
					  ii. Hydromorphone 0.05–0.1 IV q 4–6h
					and
					(d) Lidocaine patch over incision

Note: Methadone does not cause vomiting. Lidocaine CRI is contraindicated in cats.

Chapter 4

101

3. Key points

(a) Adrenalectomy

(I) CASE SELECTION: An adrenalectomy is indicated in cases of functional (e.g., nonpituitary-dependent hyperadrenocorticism) adrenal tumors or pheochromocytoma. These tumors result in inappropriate hormone secretion and have very different presentations.

(II) COMORBIDITIES: Patients with functional adrenal tumors face several concerning comorbidities, including hypertension, hypercoagulability, and posttumor removal hypoadrenocortisism (e.g., hypotension, electrolyte imbalances).

(III) HEMODYNAMIC CHANGES: Patients with pheochromocytoma face life-threatening conditions intraoperatively. This includes severe and remarkable tachycardia, arrhythmias, and hypertension that fluctuate wildly. The use of phenoxybenzamine prior to surgery significantly reduces mortality from removal of the pheochromocytoma (1). See Chapter 6 for management of tachyarrhythmias and hypertension.

(IV) HEMORRHAGE: Invasiveness of the tumor into surrounding vasculature is associated with the degree of hemorrhage a patient may experience. Cross matching is imperative for these cases as the probability of a transfusion is high.

(b) Gastric dilation and volvulus (GDV)

(I) HYPOVOLEMIA: The first priority for a patient with a GDV is volume resuscitation. At least two large gauge IV catheters are placed; initiate IV fluid shock bolus to prevent circulatory collapse.

(II) INDUCTION: Once the patient is stabilized, induce, intubate, and secure an airway quickly. Inflate the endotracheal (ET) tube cuff to minimize chance of aspiration of stomach contents.

(III) MONITORING: Utilize invasive blood pressure (IBP) monitoring, as rapid changes in hemodynamic variables occur. Central venous pressure (CVP) can be helpful to tailor fluid therapy.

(IV) STOMACH DISTENTION: Passage of a stomach tube to relieve distension of the stomach prior to anesthesia is warranted. Decompression prior to anesthesia improves systemic vascular resistance (SVR), stroke volume (SV), and cardiac output (CO). Often, the surgeon needs a stomach tube passed intraoperatively, so it is warranted for the anesthetist to obtain this piece of equipment and bring it into the OR suite.

(V) VENTRICULAR ARRHYTHMIAS: Arrhythmias are common and may or may not respond to lidocaine (see "Ventricular Arrhythmias").

(VI) VENTILATION: Assist ventilation, as the distended stomach functionally compromises ventilation.

(c) Gastrointestinal obstruction (i.e., foreign body, mass, resection/anastomosis)

(I) VOMITING: Avoid premedication with drugs that results in vomiting, such as morphine or hydromorphone.

(d) Nephrectomy

(I) DRUG ADMINISTRATION: Avoid ketamine especially in the cat, as the cat metabolizes ketamine only to norketamine, an active metabolite reliant on renal excretion.

Additionally, there is much debate in the literature as to pharmacologic support for the kidney with mannitol (2, 3), dopamine in the dog (4), and fenoldopam (5) all having possible utility. It is, however, universally agreed that supporting blood pressure (BP) through the use of inotropes and/or vasopressors as necessary is the best medical practice.

(II) HEMORRHAGE: Massive hemorrhage is possible; the anesthetist confirms the patient is cross-matched and/or blood-typed prior to anesthesia and the compatible products are available to the anesthetist during the procedure.

(III) HYPERTENSION: Patients with disease frequently have hypertension concurrently; obtain a BP prior to anesthesia to determine the patient's "normal" BP range.

(IV) URINE PRODUCTION: Urine output will decrease under anesthesia (6). The option of monitoring urine output with a urinary catheter and collection system is at the discretion of the surgeon. Normal urine output is approximately 0.5–1 mL/kg/hr in the anesthetized patient (6). If one is monitoring urine output and the patient is not producing enough urine, osmotic diuretics such as mannitol and furosemide may be used.

(e) Portosystemic shunt (PSS) (see Chapter 5, "Hepatic Function Disease" section)

(I) DECREASED ONCOTIC PRESSURE: If albumin is less than 2.2 g/dL, give plasma or hetastarch at 2–5 mL/kg/h to provide oncotic support instead of or concurrent with crystalloids. Dextrose is added in cases of hypoglycemia (see later discussion).

(II) HEMORRHAGE (SEE "BLOOD LOSS/HEMORRHAGE"): Prior to the procedure, a patient is cross-matched or blood-typed in case of hemorrhage. Monitor IBP and CVP, if possible, in addition to routine monitoring.

(III) HYPO-COAGULATION: Compared with healthy canines, the activity of clotting factors is decreased in dogs with a PSS; this results in a prolonged PTT (7). This can predispose the patient to increased hemorrhage.

(IV) HYPOGLYCEMIA: Because glycogen storage is one of the liver's primary functions, animals with PSSs (i.e., animals with decreased liver function) often have hypoglycemia. Monitor glucose and supplement fluids with 2.5–5% dextrose as necessary (see Appendix B).

(V) PORTAL HYPERTENSION: Post shunt occlusion, portal hypertension is possible and may contribute to neurological decompensation and seizures postoperatively.

Chapter 4

(VI) DECREASED METABOLISM: The liver's physiologic obligation is metabolism. This is important under anesthesia, as the majority of anesthetic drugs are metabolized hepatically. In a dog with a PSS, reduced liver function results in lower metabolism of anesthetic drugs, leading to relative overdose. Using the low end of drug dosages will reduce this impact.

(f) Splenectomy

(I) DRUG DOSAGES: Often, splenic masses are quite large and have a significant weight before they are surgically addressed. It is prudent to dose the patient at a weight the animal is without the contribution of the mass.

(II) HEMOABDOMEN: In cases of a ruptured splenic mass, hemoabdomen patients are typed and cross-matched; blood products must be readily available. A presurgical packed cell volume/total solid (PCV/TS), as well as intraoperative PCV/TS, will guide blood product and fluid administration (see "Blood Loss/Hemorrhage").

(III) HYPOTENSION: Hypovolemia due to anemia is corrected with appropriate fluid therapy prior to anesthesia, if possible. In case of frank hemorrhage necessitating immediate intervention, the anesthetist does not have the luxury of preemptively volume stabilizing the patient. In this case, the patient is stabilized as best possible in the OR. Positive inotropes (i.e., dobutamine, dopamine) and CRIs to decrease MAC requirements are helpful to maintain normotension.

(V) VENTRICULAR ARRHYTHMIAS: It is common to experience VPCs or even ventricular tachycardia with splenic masses. See "Ventricular Arrhythmias" for instituting therapy.

B. Amputations (hind limb, forelimb, digits, tail)

Amputations are often indicated for certain disease processes (e.g., osteosarcoma) or as a salvage procedure (e.g., financial limitations preventing fracture repair or a failed repair). They do not require specialized expertise or equipment and are performed in a broad range of veterinary hospitals.

1. Anesthetic concerns/common complications

(a) Loss of blood volume: The higher the site of limb removal, the more substantial the risk of blood loss. This is because major arteries branch off the trunk at these regions (e.g., femoral artery or brachial plexus). As arterial branching progresses, arteries become smaller. However, a small artery allowed to hemorrhage still results in significant loss. While the anesthetist may focus on hemorrhage as the major cause of blood loss, it is important to remember that when the limb is removed, all the volume perfusing that limb is removed as well; therefore even in situations of excellent hemostasis, hypovolemia may result.

(b) Pain: During the first year after an amputation, people commonly report phantom limb pain (PLP), with up to 76% of patients experiencing such a phenomena (8). Although the incidence of PLP decreased to only 10% of patients over time in the previous study, our patients are not capable of verbalizing this phenomenon. Therefore, it stands to reason, as humans and animals share the similar pain pathway (see Figure 6.10), our patients experience PLP. To minimize the risk of occurrence, it is important to provide a balanced anesthetic technique with appropriate analgesia (see later discussion).

2. Anesthetic protocol

Drug selection is based on the patient's preanesthetic assessment (see Chapter 1). Analgesia is maximized. This includes regional blocks (see Chapter 8) where appropriate and the use of intraoperative CRIs. Additionally, when the nerve is dissected, local anesthetic is used to provide analgesia when provided sterilely to the surgeon. (*Note*: Direct injection of a nerve with local anesthetic is toxic to the nerve and is avoided (9); the area around the nerve is infused with local anesthetic.) Postoperatively, nonsteroidal anti-inflammatory drugs (NSAIDs) are administered if not contraindicated. Lidocaine patches are applied to the incision for additional analgesia.

3. Key points

(a) Patients undergoing tail or hind limb amputation should receive an epidural if not contraindicated (see Chapter 8, "Epidural" section). For limb amputations, soaker catheters are helpful for providing postoperative analgesia by infusing lidocaine or bupivacaine either as a CRI or, in the case of bupivacaine, every 4–6 hours as an intermittent bolus (see Table 3.7).

(b) Forelimb amputations receive CRI of opioid such as fentanyl or hydromorphone, plus lidocaine and ketamine in an attempt to provide multimodal analgesia (see Appendix D). Soaker catheters are useful in these cases as well (see earlier discussion).

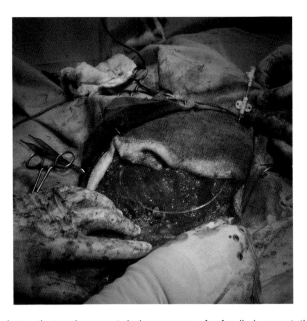

Figure 4.1   Soaker catheter placement during surgery of a forelimb amputation.

(c) Patients with digit amputations are excellent candidates for a Bier block, ring block, or RUMM (radian, ulnar, median, musculocutaneous) nerve block (10) (see Chapter 8).

C. Brachycephalic procedures (laryngeal sacculectomy, stenotic nares correction, and soft palate resection)

Often, these procedures are performed at the same time in a patient with brachycephalic syndrome. The surgeon may request an airway examination during the induction process, to determine which of the procedures are necessary. The goal is to create an airway with less resistance for the patient.

1. Anesthetic considerations/complications

(a) Airway obstruction: The presurgical patient has learned to compensate for his or her inappropriate airway. However, postoperatively, edema from surgical manipulation and correction may worsen the obstruction the patient experiences. This will not manifest itself until extubation. The patient should remain intubated until it has completely recovered from the effects of anesthesia; in the authors' experience, this is sometimes 3–4 hours after the vaporizer is turned off. The dog often tolerates the ET tube because of its misaligned teeth and relief of having a clear airway. Additionally, prior to extubation, the authors find swabbing the inflamed tissue with mannitol applied to cotton tip applicators helps decrease inflammation to the tissues.

(b) Aspiration: The cuff of the ET tube is appropriately inflated at the beginning of the procedure, as blood from the surgical repair is otherwise aspirated. When the ET tube is removed, the cuff is not completely deflated in order to remove accumulated blood or clots.

(c) Desaturation: Desaturation occurs rapidly in a patient after induction, prior to intubation (11). Because the patient is often evaluated by the surgeon prior to intubation, it is best medical practice to preoxygenate all patients prior to and during the induction process.

(d) Equipment selection: In addition to everted laryngeal saccules, stenotic nares, and elongated soft palpate, these dogs also often have a hypoplastic trachea. The anesthetist must select a set of ET tube sizes that are smaller than expected for the average patient of the same weight.

Additionally, because of the risk of postextubation airway obstruction, the anesthetist should have clean tubes available of half a size smaller and enough induction drugs to facilitate re-intubation. Having a tracheostomy kit readily available is wise.

(e) Sedation: Premedication is used to facilitate handling of the patient, provide preemptive analgesia, and reduce the amount of other drugs necessary for induction and maintenance. However, it also worsens the chance of airway obstruction in these patients.

Conservative dosing and drug selection, as well as continuous patient observation post-premedication, is necessary to prevent adverse consequences such as respiratory arrest.

2. Anesthetic protocol

Drug selection is based on the patient's preanesthetic assessment. Propofol is an ideal induction agent because of its titratability and minimal impacts on recovery. If the surgeon elects to pack the back of the laryngeal area with gauze to absorb hemorrhage from the surgical sites, the anesthetist counts the number of gauze pads and ensures they are removed prior to discontinuing anesthesia. The surgical sites are extremely sensitive; it is common for patients to gag or swallow if not at an appropriate surgical plane of anesthesia.

D. External mass removal

A variety of masses of varying size and degree of infiltration may require surgical removal. While it is impossible to present a protocol appropriate for all mass removals, general concepts are listed.

1. Anesthetic concerns/common complications

(a) Analgesia: The size of the mass for removal determines the level of analgesic intervention necessary. If possible (see "Preventing Spread of Disease" later), administration of a local anesthetic as an infiltrative block is incorporated into the mass removal plan, in an attempt to stop pain transmission (see Chapter 8). NSAIDs, if not contraindicated, as well as opioids, are the cornerstone of pain management strategies for these types of procedures.

(b) Preventing spread of disease: If it is unknown whether the tumor is benign or malignant, it is best to avoid using an infiltrative local anesthetic strategy, as there is a hypothetical risk of spreading cancer cells along the needle tract in animals, as has been reported for people (12).

(c) Sedation versus general anesthesia: If a mass is fairly small and the surgeon is comfortable with this technique, the combination of heavy sedation and a local technique (if not contraindicated; see "Preventing Spread of Disease") is often a reasonable alternative to general anesthesia for patients with a truly minor mass removal.

2. Anesthetic protocol

Drug selection is based on the patient's preanesthetic assessment. This will also assist the anesthetist with the choice of general anesthesia or heavy sedation. In a patient with a mellow temperament, heavy sedation is quite useful. In a high-strung patient, general anesthesia (and thus better control over the patient) is often warranted. If procedures are of a short duration, the anesthetist may elect for a "middle of the road" approach and

Chapter 4

Table 4.2 Suggested anesthesia protocol for brachycephalic corrections.

Brachycephalic Procedures

Opioid premedication (mg/kg)	Sedative premedication (mg/kg)	Induction (mg/kg)	Maintenance	Intraoperative analgesia (mg/kg)	Postoperative analgesia (mg/kg)
(a) Methadone 0.5 IM or (b) Hydromorphone 0.05 IM	(a) Acepromazine 0.03 IM	(a) Propofol 2–4 mg/kg IV to effect	(a) Isoflurane or sevoflurane (b) If patient is not intubated: Propofol CRI 12–24 mg/kg/h IV	(a) Intermittent bolus: i. Methadone 0.3 IV q 4–6h or ii. Hydromorphone 0.05–0.1 IV q 4h or iii. Fentanyl, 0.005 IV as needed	(a) Intermittent bolus: i. Methadone 0.5 IM q 4–6h or ii. Hydromorphone 0.05–0.1 IM or IV q 4h

Note: The surgeon may want to evaluate airway/soft pallet during induction. Preoxygenate patient. Because steroids may be necessary to reduce swelling, avoid NSAIDs.

use a TIVA (see Table 1.9). Premedication is ideal in any case to provide preemptive analgesia, facilitate catheter placement, and reduce the amount of other drugs necessary for induction or anesthetic maintenance. Should general anesthesia be deemed necessary, a variety of induction drugs are used; propofol may result in a smooth recovery for short procedures. Maintenance on an inhalant often follows.

3. Key points

(a) Mast cell tumor (MCT)

(I) MAST CELL DEGRANULATION: MCTs are sensitive to manipulation. When aggressively manipulated they can release histamine, serotonin, and heparin. Avoiding aggressive manipulation of the tumor is warranted. While it does not prevent mast cell degranulation, preemptively administering an H_1 blocker (e.g., diphenhydramine 0.5–1 mg/kg) and H_2 blockers (e.g., famotidine 1 mg/kg) will prevent histamine from binding its receptors. If histamine release occurs, it is characterized by vasodilation, hypotension, and tachycardia. Supportive treatment is indicated, and additional diphenhydramine is administered. If the reaction is severe, epinephrine at 0.01 mg/kg may be necessary. Fluid boluses may mitigate the effects of vasodilation in the short term.

(II) ANESTHETIC PROTOCOL MODIFICATIONS: Some opioids are more likely to cause histamine release than others. Avoid opioids such as morphine and meperidine as secondary histamine release may occur. Methadone or hydromorphone are ideal for IM premedication. Acepromazine is the choice sedative if not otherwise contraindicated due to its antihistamine properties. Most induction agents are appropriate. If the mass is large or invasive, appropriate analgesia is required. Lidocaine patches over the incision are ideal postoperatively, along with systemic analgesics.

(b) Mastectomy

(I) PAIN: This procedure is relatively painful, especially when performed bilaterally, due to the stretch of skin for closure. The incision is extensive and inclusion of a lidocaine patch over the site, especially in the cat, provides an excellent option for local analgesia with minimal systemic impacts (13). Additionally, the expected postoperative pain level warrants aggressive preemptive analgesia and a well-balanced analgesic plan.

(II) VENTILATION: Bilateral mastectomy performed in a single surgery may result in a tight skin closure (most common in the cat). While the skin becomes suppler over time, in the immediate postoperative period, the patient may have difficulty ventilating due to this tight closure; while the patient is still intubated, this is evidenced by a high $EtCO_2$ reading. Once the patient is extubated, a venous blood gas is necessary to confirm this. If moderate to severe hypoventilation occurs, the patient must be reanesthetized to allow tension relief of the surgery site. Therefore, it is ideal for the anesthetist to evaluate for this possibility before general anesthesia is discontinued.

(III) ANESTHETIC PROTOCOL MODIFICATIONS: Drug selection is based on the patient's preanesthetic assessment. Intraoperative analgesia targets different pain receptors by use of

Chapter 4

Table 4.3 Suggested protocol for mast cell tumor removal.

Mast Cell Tumor Removal			
Premedication (mg/kg)	Induction (mg/kg)	Maintenance	Intraoperative analgesia (mg/kg)	Postoperative analgesia (mg/kg)
(a) Opioid option (select one): i. Methadone 0.5–1 IM or ii. Hydromorphone 0.1–0.2 IM (b) Diphenhydramine 0.5 (c) Famotidine 1.0 IV (d) Sedative option: i. Acepromazine 0.01–0.03	(a) Propofol 2–4 or (b) Ketamine 5 and diazepam 0.25	Isoflurane or sevoflurane	(a) Intermittent bolus: i. Methadone 0.3 IV q 4–6h or ii. Hydromorphone 0.05–0.1 IV q 4h or iii. Fentanyl, 0.005 IV as needed	(a) Lidocaine patch over incision and (b) Intermittent bolus (select one): i. Methadone 0.3 IV q 4–6h or ii. Hydromorphone 0.05–0.1 IV q 4h and (c) NSAIDs

Note: Patients with MCT require premedication with diphenhydramine and famotidine along with routine opioid and sedative.

multiple agents, including an opioid (morphine, hydromorphone, or fentanyl), ketamine, and lidocaine. (*Note*: Lidocaine CRIs are contraindicated in cats.) Alternatively, a morphine epidural can be performed. Additionally, NSAIDs are a useful adjunctive analgesic postoperatively (see Table 3.10).

E. Head and neck procedures

Head and neck surgeries, as a group, present the anesthetist with some common concerns. Head and neck surgeries include ocular surgeries (which are addressed separately later in this chapter), auricular surgery, airway surgery, and mass removals. However, dental procedures often warrant the same considerations.

1. Anesthesia concerns/common complications

(a) Loss of access: Our most significant anesthetic concern with head and neck procedures is the loss of access to the patient. The anesthetist uses eye signs and jaw tone to assess anesthetic depth (see Table 2.3); now the anesthetist must rely on monitoring equipment to compensate for the loss of ocular and oral signs. Capnography is often a critical piece of monitoring, as disconnections of the ET tube—resulting both in lightening of the patient's anesthetic plane as well as desaturation—is a possible undesirable consequence with loss of access to the head. It is also the habit of most anesthetists to place IV catheters in the cephalic vein (patient's forelimb). Prudence suggests hind limb catheterization for these patients for accessibility.

(b) Trigeminal-vagal response: The trigeminal nerve has three major branches (the ophthalmic, mandibular, and maxillary branches), which ultimately supply feedback into the parasympathetic system. Therefore, stimulation of these nerves (e.g., a surgeon resting his or her hands on a patient's face) may result in a profound bradycardia, potentially proceeding to asystole.

2. Anesthesia protocol

Premedication selection is based on the patient's preanesthetic assessment. The induction agent is chosen based on each patient's profile, but often propofol's titratability makes it the agent of choice. Maintenance on a gas inhalant is used. If the procedure requires the patient to be extubated, TIVA with propofol is utilized.

(a) Laryngeal tie back: Laryngeal paralysis often affects older, large breed dogs, which present in respiratory distress and are commonly given flow-by oxygen and low doses of acepromazine to decrease excitement and prevent hyperthermia. Often, these patients are stabilized sufficiently to undergo surgery during normal business hours. During induction, an airway examination is performed by the surgeon, to determine which of the laryngeal cartilages are affected. Patients are routinely extubated following suture of the affected cartilage to visually ensure sufficient patency of the airway is present.

(I) AIRWAY INFLAMMATION OR EDEMA: Surgical manipulation of the airway may result in swelling or edema. NSAIDs are avoided, so dexamethasone can be administered if necessary.

(II) ASPIRATION PNEUMONIA: Although the true cause of acquired idiopathic laryngeal paralysis is unknown, there is some evidence that it results from a neurologic dysfunction that also effects the esophagus (14). Indeed, many of these dogs develop aspiration pneumonia after the tie back procedure. Avoid drugs that cause regurgitation or vomiting (i.e., hydromorphone, morphine, alpha₂ agonists) postoperatively. If oxygen saturation is inappropriate after extubation, thoracic films are warranted.

(III) HYPERTHERMIA: At presentation, many of these patients present stressed and hyperthermic. In addition to administration of acepromazine, cool fans and oxygen supplementation is often necessary.

(IV) IATROGENIC COMPLICATIONS: The surgeon may accidently suture the cartilage to ET tube; to ensure this has not happened, it is necessary to extubate the patient and assess the integrity of the sutures.

Damage to the recurrent laryngeal nerve either during surgical dissection or subsequently from inflammation may lead to difficulty in swallowing, one of the signs the anesthetist uses to determine when to extubate the patient. In general, the ability to hold the head up also signifies appropriate muscle tone and readiness for extubation.

(V) ANESTHETIC PROTOCOL MODIFICATIONS: Acepromazine produces mild sedation beneficial to patients in respiratory distress. Opioids that cause vomiting are avoided; methadone is the ideal opioid for this patient. Propofol is the induction agent of choice, especially when the surgeon requires an airway examination during induction to check laryngeal function. Propofol is administered slowly so the patient continues spontaneous ventilation for the surgeon to perform a laryngeal examination.

(b) Parathydroidectomy/thyroidectomy: This surgery involves dissection near and around many vital structures, including the major vessels, trachea, esophagus, and recurrent laryngeal nerve.

(I) HORMONAL DYSFUNCTION: The parathyroid gland secretes parathyroid hormone (PTH), which is responsible for the balance of calcium, phosphate, and vitamin D, among other things. After removal, it is necessary to monitor and address fluctuations of calcium, phosphate, and vitamin D. They are often of minimal impact to the anesthetist.

The thyroid gland secretes thyroid hormone and is addressed later.

(II) LARYNGEAL NERVE PARALYSIS: Laryngeal nerve paralysis from damage to the recurrent laryngeal nerve (secondary to inflammation or surgical trauma) results in laryngeal dysfunction. Because this nerve supplies the majority of motor function to the larynx, the patient often has difficulty swallowing and maintaining an open airway upon extubation.

Table 4.4 Suggested anesthesia protocol for a laryngeal tie back.

			Laryngeal Tie Back			
Opioid premedication (mg/kg)	Sedative premedication (mg/kg)	Induction (mg/kg)	Maintenance	Intraoperative analgesia (mg/kg)	Postoperative analgesia (mg/kg)

(a) Methadone 0.5 IM
 	
or
 	
(b) Hydromorphone 0.05 IM
	(a) Acepromazine 0.02
	
	or
	
	(b) Midazolam 0.2
		(a) Propofol 2–4 to effect +/– midazolam 0.2
		
		or
		
		(b) Etomidate 1–2 IV to effect
			Isoflurane or sevoflurane	(a) Intermittent bolus:
				  i. Methadone 0.3 IV q 4–6h
				
				  or
				
				  ii. Hydromorphone 0.05–0.1 IV q 4h
				
				  or
				
				  iii. Fentanyl, 0.005 IV as needed
					(a) Tramadol PO and
					(b) NSAID and
					(c) Methadone 0.2 IV, 0.3–0.5 IM

Note: Preoxygenate.

surgeons request that an epidural with local anesthetic is *not* performed, so an assessment of anal tone following recovery is possible. It is appropriate to discuss this with the surgeon preoperatively.

(b) Noxious stimuli/pain: Due to the level of innervation of this region, surgical stimulation results in a fair amount of noxious stimuli intraoperatively and pain postoperatively. An epidural with 0.1 mg/kg preservative free morphine will provide suitable, long-lasting analgesia. If the surgeon is confident that he or she does not need to assess anal tone following surgery, epidural administration of local anesthetic (such 0.5–1.0 mg/kg bupivacaine), which desensitizes this region, improves the quality of the patient's anesthetic event significantly; this is often combined with preservative-free morphine. When administering an epidural for analgesia in the perianal region, the bevel of the needle is directed caudally, allowing for drug administration delivery to the target dermatomes. An NSAID is warranted postoperatively, if not contraindicated. Tramadol is useful as a send home analgesic.

(c) Patient positioning: For visualization, these patients are often placed on padding to elevate the hind quarters with the head/thorax directed downward. This results in hypoventilation because of the pressure of abdominal contents on the thorax, as well as difficulty in some monitoring placement (such as arterial line). EtCO$_2$ analysis is essential for these patients, and mechanical ventilation (MV) is often necessary. An indirect means for pressure monitoring is used instead of an arterial line or an arterial line is placed in an alternative location (i.e., front limb). Regurgitation also occurs; the patient's esophagus is suctioned postoperatively even if there is no evidence of regurgitation (to address "silent" regurgitation). If there is evidence of regurgitation upon suctioning, the esophagus is appropriately suctioned and lavaged (see "Regurgitation").

2. Anesthetic protocol

Premedication and induction drugs are based on the patient's preanesthetic assessment. Opioid (hydromorphone or fentanyl) with or without lidocaine CRIs are ideal intraoperatively. A&D ointment over the incision postoperatively helps soothe the wound as well as assist in keeping fecal matter from contacting the incision. Often, these patients had a purse string suture placed preoperatively to close the anus; the anesthetist ensures this suture is removed before discontinuing anesthesia.

G. Reproductive

Castrations and ovariohysterectomies are common procedures in a veterinary setting. While general anesthesia is used for most reproductive procedures, appropriate pain management has gained significant attention for these cases (15) (rightly so). Pain is addressed for any animal undergoing a surgical procedure; however, it is important to recognize that an ovariohysterectomy is an open abdominal procedure; that is, the level of pain for all reproductive procedures is not equal.

1. Anesthesia concerns/common complications

(a) Pain: A balanced analgesic plan is warranted for all patients undergoing reproductive procedures. This includes appropriate premedication, induction agents such as ketamine when not contraindicated to provide preemptive analgesia, and local blocks where applicable to reduce noxious stimulus transmission. Postoperatively, NSAIDs are administered when not contraindicated, and send home medication (e.g., tramadol) is prescribed.

(b) Hemorrhage: Major arteries perfuse the reproductive organs; inappropriate hemostasis from a slipped ligation or tearing of a pedicle requires aggressive volume support while the surgeon locates the hemorrhaging vessel.

2. Anesthesia protocol

(a) Cat castration: Castration of the cat is a quick procedure that rarely requires intubation. If the cat is a young healthy patient, a cat total injectable combination is administered. While several varieties of this cocktail exist, it usually involves the combination of an opioid (e.g., butorphanaol), sedative (e.g., dexmedetomidine), and dissociative (i.e., ketamine). While most drug doses are calculated based on the patient's ideal body weight, cat total injectable combinations are commonly administered as a volume per cat. Table 4.6 shows some common cat total injectable combinations. Postoperatively, meloxicam is given SQ.

(b) Dog castration: Dogs for castration are premedicated, catheterized, intubated, and placed on maintenance anesthetic. It is common for premedication to include an opioid and sedative. Testicular block with lidocaine attempts to provide a balanced technique (see Table 4.7). The opioid premedication is usually sufficient for intraoperative and

Table 4.6 Cat total injectable combinations.

Option 1: Drug dosage	Option 2: Volume (for every 4 kg of cat)
Butorphanol 0.4 mg/kg or buprenorphine 0.03 mg/kg Dexmedetomidine 0.01–0.015 mg/kg Ketamine 7.5–10 mg/kg	Butorphanol [10 mg/mL] 0.16 mL or buprenorphine [0.3 mg/mL] 0.4 mL Dexmedetomidine [0.5 mg/mL] 0.08–0.12 mL Ketamine 0.3–0.4 mL

Table 4.7 Testicular block.

Materials: 22 gauge needle, syringe, aseptic scrub, lidocaine
Method: 1. Calculate 2 mg/kg of lidocaine. Stay under this dose. No more than 2 mL per testicle is required for block. 2. Clip and aseptically prepare for castration. 3. Holding testicle in one hand, insert needle and aspirate. If no blood is present, inject half of calculated dose or 2 mL. Repeat for second testicle.

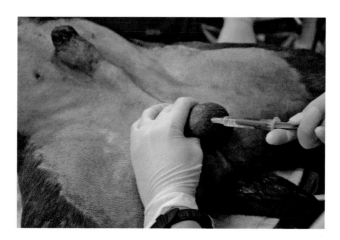

Figure 4.2 Testicular block in canine patient. Courtesy of Patricia Queiroz-Williams.

postoperative analgesia. An injectable dose of a NSAID is administered postoperatively in the healthy patient. If necessary, tramadol is dispensed for postoperative pain relief as well.

(c) Ovariohysterectomy (OHE): For both cat and dog spays, it is common to combine an opioid and sedative for premedication. Mu agonist opioids, such as morphine, hydromorphone, methadone, or buprenorphine are appropriate opioid selections. Sedation with an alpha$_2$ agonist also provides analgesia; however, drug selection is based on the patient's preanesthetic assessment. Postoperative analgesia includes repeating a dose of opioid for postoperative pain and at minimum a single dose of NSAIDs, with possibly additional NSAIDs for administration at home. A lidocaine patch over the incision also provides additional analgesia. Tramadol is ideal for sending home with the patient.

3. Key points

(a) Cesarean section (C-section)/dystocia: C-sections, either as emergencies or as scheduled procedures, are performed when fetal survival is prioritized (even if the owner elects to spay the animal after the neonates are removed). Certain breeds, such as the Bulldog, Boston Terrier, and French Bulldog, have a high incidence of C-section (16). Nonurgent surgery, nonbrachycephalic dams, and smaller litters are associated with live puppies at delivery. Radiographs provide a fetal head count, so the number of puppies for removal is quantified. An ultrasound is performed to see if any of the fetuses are viable in an emergency C-section. Viable fetuses will influence drug selection in the anesthetic protocol. The anesthetist takes into consideration drugs that will pass to the fetus and how these drugs impact the fetus. It is important to obtain preoperative BW in the mother (especially electrolytes and hydration status). If the surgeon elects to perform an OHE where fetal survival is not intended, the anesthetic plan follows a similar protocol for an OHE (see "Ovariohysterectomy").

(I) DELAYED GI MOTILITY: Decreased GI motility in the bitch and queen means that although the mother may not have eaten for a prolonged period of time, there may still be food in the stomach. In humans, Mendelson's syndrome is one cause of maternal death; this syndrome is characterized by aspiration of GI contents during anesthesia. It is prudent to promptly inflate the cuff on the ET tube after the patient is intubated and prepare for suctioning of GI contents in these patients. If aspiration is suspected postoperatively, appropriate therapy for aspiration pneumonia is instituted.

(II) EFFECTIVE CIRCULATING VOLUME: As noted earlier, these patients present often after having gone off food and water in preparation for the delivery of the young. If the patient appears dehydrated, preoperative volume loading with 10–30 mL/kg of crystalloids is warranted. Otherwise, placing the mother on twice maintenance fluid therapy (5 mL/kg/h) until the team is ready for induction is appropriate.

(III) FETUS: The fetus is completely dependent on maternal support for survival, so it is not surprising that almost everything the mother receives will also pass to the neonate. Fetal and neonatal metabolism of drugs is inferior to that of an adult, due in large part to the immaturity of the liver and kidneys, where the majority of drugs are broken down and excreted, respectively. Therefore, minimizing the drugs administered to the mother by conservative dosing or the use of nonsystemic drug routes (i.e., epidural) is the best way to minimize the impact of the drugs on the young. Using drugs such as propofol, which has some extrahepatic metabolism, gives the young another alternative to hepatic metabolism. Conversely, agents such as ketamine and thiopental are associated with decreased puppy vigor at birth (17). Xylazine is also contraindicated (18). Minimizing the time between induction and delivery of the neonates reduces the impacts of inhaled anesthetics on the neonates. In the case of compromised neonates, neonatal resuscitation is begun immediately (see Table 4.8).

Table 4.8 Neonatal resuscitation supplies.

Supplies	Use
Small ET tubes (2.5 mm ID) or 18–16 G catheter with stylete removed	Intubate if neonate not breathing
Bulb syringe	Suction mouth and nares
Warming units (circulating hot water blankets, air warming units, incubators, etc.)	Keep neonates warm until mother recovers
Small oxygen mask or large enough mask to fit pup inside	Provide supplemental oxygen
Flow by oxygen source	Provide supplemental oxygen
Reversal agents for any drugs used in mom (i.e., naloxone, flumazenil)	Increase neonate vigor by reversing drugs exposed to *in utero*
Glucose supplement	Hypoglycemia
Warm towels	For rubbing neonates to stimulate breathing

(IV) HYPOCALCEMIA: An ionized calcium level is assessed in the mother prior to beginning the procedure; supplementation with calcium in the fluids is used as needed (see Chapter 3, "Calcium Gluconate" section).

(V) HYPOVENTILATION: As the bitch or queen nears term, hypoventilation becomes a more significant problem due to the functional obstruction of diaphragmatic tone secondary to abdominal filling. Assisted ventilation is often necessary in these cases.

(VI) PAIN: A bitch or queen that is in pain may reject or even become aggressive toward young attempting to nurse. Therefore, it is recommended to manage the mother's pain appropriately. If an epidural is not preemptively administered in an attempt to minimize time from induction to delivery, it is common to administer the epidural postoperatively before discontinuing general anesthesia. If a conservative dose of preoperative opioids was administered, additional opioid is given once the neonates are removed and/or when the mother recovers; morphine is hydrophilic, making it less likely to pass through the milk to the neonates, and thus a suitable choice. A single dose of NSAIDs is warranted.

(VII) RECOVERY TO NURSE NEONATES: As soon as possible after closure and cleaning of the surgery site, the neonates are encouraged to nurse to prevent hypoglycemia.

(VIII) ANESTHETIC MODIFICATIONS:

Step 1: Obtain IV access. This is usually accomplished without sedation, as high progesterone levels present in the pregnant animal facilitate handling. If IM sedation is required to obtain IV access, opioids are preferred, as they are reversible. Crystalloid fluids, ideally containing calcium (e.g., lactated Ringer's solution [LRS]), are started.

Step 2: Minimize time between induction and the OR suite. The patient is provided supplemental oxygen via oxygen mask during preoperative preparation. Preparation includes clipping surgical area and epidural area, as well as a dirty scrub before induction (try to allow patient to remain in sternal/standing position). The surgeon is scrubbed and has table opened and ready.

Step 3: Induce with propofol IV to effect (ideally, in the OR). If no IM sedation was necessary, 4–8 mg/kg may be needed to intubate patient. Including a low dose of fentanyl (2–5 mcg/kg) as an IV premedication or a low dose of morphine (0.5 mg/kg) IM immediately prior to induction provides some analgesia. Opioids will cross the placental barrier.

Step 4: Gas inhalants are routinely used for maintenance. Without premedication, inhalant requirements are high. Regional anesthetic techniques (i.e., line blocks) are helpful to minimize inhalant requirement. Epidurals (morphine 0.1 mg/kg and bupivacaine 0.5–1 mg/kg) are administered if the anesthetist is experienced and administration is quick. Incisional line block with 1–2 mg/kg of bupivacaine is placed. Intraoperatively, pedicle blocks with bupivacaine 1 mg/kg can be performed. Once the last fetus is removed, a full mu agonist opioid is given IV to mother. Crystalloid fluids are continued at 10–15 mL/kg/h intraoperatively.

Table 4.9   C-section with fetal survival.

Step 1: Obtain IV catheter without sedation; use EMLA cream on clipped skin to facilitate placement. Clip and scrub abdomen and lumbosacral area for procedure and epidural, respectively. Morphine, 0.5 mg/kg, IM is administered to the patient.
Step 2: Fluid bolus 30 mL/kg over 10 min. Continue fluids at 15 mL/kg/h.
Step 3: Preoxygenate, maintain patient in sternal recumbency (avoid dorsal recumbency). Place monitoring equipment on patient.
Step 4: Propofol 4–6 mg/kg IV to effect. Epidural if expedient.
Step 5: Gas inhalant
Step 6: Incisional line block with bupivacaine 1 mg/kg and lidocaine 1 mg/kg.
Step 7: Sterile prep. When puppies are out, give full mu opioid (methadone 0.3 mg/kg or hydromoprhone 0.1 mg/kg IV) and turn down vaporizer.
Step 8: Administer epidural postoperatively, if it not given before.
Step 9: Recover, postoperative pain control with an opioid and NSAID.

Chapter 4

Step 5: Fetal resuscitation: If sedatives or opioids were used in the mother, place drop of reversal agent under the newborns tongue. For opioids, naloxone is a common reversal; for benzodiazepines, flumazenil is used. A bulb syringe is used to clear mucous from mouth and nares. Flow by oxygen is used via mask to provide supplemental oxygen. Vigorous rubbing from caudal to cranial along the neonate's dorsum helps stimulate breathing and clearing of airway. A warm area should be dedicated for the neonates until the mother is recovered from anesthesia. Circulating water blankets and/or air warming units are helpful in providing appropriate warmth.

Step 6: Recovering the mother involves providing adequate analgesia without significant sedation so the mother is capable of cleaning and nursing the newborns.

(b) Pyometra (open vs. closed): Pyometra is a uterine infection in an unspayed female dog or cat (although it occurs in the uterine stump of patients where an ovarian remnant is left at the time of the animal's OHE). Patients with an open pyometra are usually less systemically affected. In a closed pyometra, patients are often severely septic before they are diagnosed, making them a higher anesthetic risk.

(i) ENDOTOXEMIA AND SEPTICEMIA: (See also Chapter 5, "Shock" section.) One of the most common pathogens in pyometra is *Escherichia coli*, which releases endotoxins into the bloodstream (endotoxemia). As the disease progresses, the pathogens risk infecting the bloodstream (septicemia) as well as the primary organ. While both conditions sicken a patient significantly, septicemia is life-threatening. The animal presents in shock with significant vasodilation. While IV antibiotics may improve the situation, the patient is at significant risk because surgery is required to remove the primary source of infection (i.e., the uterus). Inhalant anesthetics exacerbate vasodilation. Vasopressor support (epinephrine, ephedrine, or phenylephrine) is often necessary in addition to standard management for hypotension. Additionally, as sepsis worsens, diseases such as acute respiratory distress (ARD), systemic inflammatory response (SIR), secondary multiorgan failure, and disseminated intravascular coagulation (DIC) develop.

(II) ANESTHETIC PROTOCOL MODIFICATIONS: The anesthetic protocol for an open pyometra is based on the patient's preanesthetic assessment. For a closed pyometra, one carefully examines the patient for signs of shock (begins addressing this prior to induction, if possible) as well as the patient's BW to see if other organs are damaged. These cases are often an ASA 4-5; owners are informed there is a real risk the patient may die with anesthesia and consulted regarding cardiopulmonary resuscitation (CPR) status. The severity of this disease means a cautious approach to anesthesia. Often a neuroleptic induction with an opioid such as fentanyl and a benzodiazepine is used to facilitate intubation followed by a CRI such as fentanyl to keep the vaporizer at the lowest possible setting to prevent consciousness. Heavy BP support is required to keep the patient stable and a short surgical time is a must. All emergency drugs are drawn up prior to induction.

H. Thoracotomy

Respiration is important both for oxygenation of the body as well as removal of CO_2. Gas exchange is based on normal lung anatomy and shape, which is maintained by negative pressure in the thorax. When the thorax is entered, intrathoracic pressure equalizes with atmospheric pressure (i.e., negative pressure is lost). This results in the lung collapsing to its residual volume, which is not compatible with adequate gas exchange.

1. Anesthetic concerns/common complications

(a) Hypoxemia: When alveoli have collapsed, there is no longer adequate surface area for normal gas exchange (see Chapter 6, "Hypoxemia" section). A patient will have significant ventilation to perfusion (V/Q) mismatch. Coupled with the concurrent hypoventilation, there is profound risk for severe and prolonged hypoxemia if appropriate interventional steps are not taken. One such step is the use of a peak end-expiratory pressure (PEEP) valve; a PEEP valve maintains a residual amount of pressure in the airway, preventing the alveoli from collapsing completely. Not only does this allow for continued gas exchange, it also helps with re-expanding alveoli once negative pressure is restored. These patients are always maintained on 100% oxygen. Monitoring with a pulse oximeter (see Chapter 2) is essential both intraoperatively and postoperatively. Additionally, arterial blood gas analysis is key to evaluation of hypoxemia and ventilation.

(b) Hypoventilation: Because adequate gas exchange is compromised when the lungs equalize with atmospheric pressure, CO_2 is not effectively removed. This results in hypercapnia (hypoventilation). Respiration is assisted (manually or with a mechanical ventilator, often based on the needs of the surgeon); see Chapter 2 for instructions on how to use a mechanical ventilator. $EtCO_2$ monitoring is critical for moment-to-moment information on hypoventilation, as well as determining the effectiveness of assisted ventilation. $EtCO_2$ compared to $PaCO_2$ is beneficial to assess ventilation.

(c) Iatrogenic pneumothorax: It is understood that a thoracotomy will result in a pneumothorax; while this is managed during the procedure, the majority of concern for this iatrogenic pneumothorax occurs postoperatively. Chest tubes are a vital part of the post-operative plan. Staff working with these patients postoperatively need appropriate instruction on how to manually evacuate the chest. If at any time there is concern the patient is "not right," the chest is evacuated! It takes very little time for respiratory collapse to occur if there is build up of air or fluid in the thorax. Continued monitoring with pulse oximetry is warranted postoperatively; rectal probes are available for patients with a significant amount of pigment or that resist a pulse oximeter around their face.

(d) Pain: The median sternotomy approach for a thoracotomy is particularly painful, both intraoperatively as well as postoperatively. A 0.2 mL/kg total volume epidural with morphine and saline assists with pain management in some of these patients, with this maximal volume intended to move the drug closer to its target site. In a lateral thoracotomy, if the surgeon is provided with sterile local anesthetic, a local block (e.g., intercostal block) is administered. Because of the way the nerve fibers branch, it is important to block at least two intercostal spaces cranial and caudal to the surgical approach site. Additionally, intraoperative multimodal CRIs (such as opioid, lidocaine, and ketamine) and postoperative NSAIDs (if not contraindicated) help balance an analgesic plan. There is some debate about intrapleural drug administration via the chest tube postoperatively (19). It is the opinion of the author (CM) that other options be employed first. A lidocaine patch over the incision site may also help postoperatively.

2. Anesthetic protocol

If catheterization is not possible without sedation, premedication includes a full agonist opioid IM. Hydromorphone may cause the patient to pant when given IM so this drug is avoided, if possible. Methadone (0.5–1 mg/kg IM) is a nice alternative. Selecting a sedative will depend on the patient's preanesthetic assessment (PE, BW, and disposition) and is avoided if unnecessary. If an IV catheter is placed without sedation, an opioid with/without a benzodiazepine is ideal IV. Once the patient is induced, an arterial line (see Chapter 2) is placed to monitor IBP as well as to allow sampling for blood gas analysis. ECG, capnography, Doppler, temperature, and SpO_2 are also monitored. Upon recovery, chest tubes are left in place until negative pressure is consecutively obtained (usually for the first 24 hours after a procedure). Supplemental oxygen (see Table 6.8) is available and used for any patient that cannot maintain a pulse oximeter reading greater than 94%. Patients are placed in a setting where they are closely monitored for respiratory distress. It may be helpful to maintain the arterial catheter during the first 12–24 hours of recovery.

3. Key points

(a) Diaphragmatic hernia: Diaphragmatic hernias present either acutely (secondary to trauma, for example) in respiratory distress, or chronically (secondary to a congenital malformation; the patient usually presents for unrelated reasons). A recent, traumatically

Chapter 4

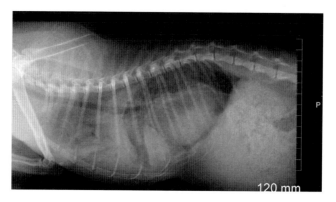

Figure 4.3 Radiographic image of cat with DH.

induced diaphragmatic hernia is a suitable candidate for immediate surgical correction. A patient with a congenital diaphragmatic hernia has often compensated quite well over time for this abnormality; a thorough abdominal palpation, presence of a "heave" line (hypertrophied abdominal musculature to assist with breathing), and thoracic radiographs may confirm its presence. However, the choice of surgical repair for these chronic cases necessitates excellent anesthesia support; indeed, of the two, the congenital diaphragmatic hernia is the more difficult case to manage.

(I) HYPOVENTILATION: In addition to the preceding reasons, hypoventilation occurs in these patients because of an actual functional obstruction to respiration. Time under anesthesia is minimized between induction and when a patient is placed in dorsal recumbency, at which point the patient may acutely decompensate. The patient is clipped if possible prior to the procedure. Elevate the patient's thorax and head above the abdomen when transporting the patient (even once anesthetized). Assisted ventilation (manual or mechanical) is instituted immediately following intubation.

(II) RE-EXPANSION PULMONARY EDEMA: Once a patient's abdominal contents are replaced, the real work begins for the anesthetist. In the case of acute traumatic diaphragmatic hernias, the patient may tolerate lung re-expansion without any adverse consequence. This is not so for the patient that has compensated for a chronic diaphragmatic hernia. In this case, re-expansion, especially if it is done quickly, results in re-expansion pulmonary edema, which progresses in severity and results in hypoxemia. It is the goal of the anesthetist in the case of a chronic diaphragmatic hernia to minimally expand the lungs and not exceed pressures that generated sufficient breaths preoperatively (usually 5–10 cmH₂0). A chest tube is usually placed, but in an ideal situation, the animal is allowed to re-expand its own lungs over the course of time. In the face of hypoxemia (see previous concerns for thoracotomies), it is necessary to assist ventilation. Ideally, this assistance is strictly manual and begun by increasing respiratory frequency (breaths per minute), not tidal volume, if hypoxemia is present.

Table 4.10 Suggested anesthesia protocol for a median sternotomy.

	Median Sternotomy				
Opioid premedication (mg/kg)	Sedative premedication (mg/kg)	Induction (mg/kg)	Maintenance	Intraoperative analgesia (mg/kg/h)	Postoperative analgesia (mg/kg/h)
Full agonist opioid: (a) Methadone 0.5 IM or (b) Hydromorphone 0.2 IM or 0.1 IV	(a) Dexmedetomidine 0.003–0.005 IM or (b) Midazolam 0.1–0.2 IV or IM	(a) Ketamine 5 + diazepam 0.25 or (b) Ketamine 0.5 + lidocaine 1 + propofol 2–4 IV to effect	Isoflurane or Sevoflurane	(a) HLK CRI (Hydromorphone 0.03, ketamine 1.2 and lidocaine 3) or (b) FLK CRI (Fentanyl 0.01–0.042, ketamine 1.2, lidocaine 3) or (b) Morphine 0.1 mg/kg epidural to 0.2 mL/kg total volume (dilute with sterile 0.9% NaCl)	(a) Lidocaine patch over incision site and (b) Continue HLK CRI (hydromorphone 0.01, ketamine 0.3, lidocaine 1.5) and (c) NSAID

Note: Lidocaine CRI is contraindicated in cats.

Table 4.11 Suggested anesthesia protocol for a lateral sternotomy.

Lateral Sternotomy					
Opioid premedication (mg/kg)	Sedative premedication (mg/kg)	Induction (mg/kg)	Maintenance	Intraoperative analgesia	Postoperative analgesia
Full agonist opioid (a) Methadone 0.5 IM, 0.3 IV or (b) Hydromorphone 0.2 IM, 0.1 IV	(a) Dexmedetomidine 0.003–0.005 IM or IV (b) Midazolam 0.2 IM or IV	(a) Ketamine 5 + diazepam 0.25 or (b) Ketamine 0.5 + lidocaine 1 + propofol 2–4 IV to effect	Isoflurane or sevoflurane	(a) Fentanyl CRI 0.01–0.042 mg/kg/h and (b) Intercostal nerve block and (c) Morphine 0.1 mg/kg epidural to 0.2 ml/ kg total volume (dilute with sterile 0.9% NaCl)	(a) Fentanyl CRI 0.002–0.005 mg/ kg/h and (b) NSAID and (c) Lidocaine patch over incision site

Note: Lidocaine CRI is contraindicated in cats.

I. Urological (cystotomy, perineal urethrostomy [PU])

A cystotomy is a simple procedure often used to remove urinary calculi or masses. Caudal abdominal radiographs are performed to evaluate for the presence/number count of uroliths in patients where the calculi are radiopaque. A PU is commonly performed due to urethra obstruction in neutered male cats. Abdominal ultrasound assists with the evaluation of free fluid in the abdomen; if this free fluid is urine, intervention for a bladder rupture is warranted as soon as possible (see Appendix H, "Abdominal Tap"). BW is performed to evaluate kidney function and electrolyte values (especially serum potassium). A preoperative ECG is monitored to evaluate for any bradyarrhythmias associated with elevated serum potassium.

1. Anesthetic concerns/common complications

(a) Hyperkalemia (see also Chapter 6, "Hyperkalemia" section): One of the greatest concerns with a ruptured bladder or a blocked cat is the presence of hyperkalemia. This is life-threatening as serum potassium values elevate above 7.5 mEq/L, resulting in severe bradycardia that may progress to asystole.

(b) Urinary diuresis or retention: For surgeries involving the urological system, avoid large fluid boluses or drugs that cause diuresis (e.g., alpha$_2$ agonists) until the procedure is completed. Systemic and epidural morphine has been demonstrated to result in an increase in antidiuretic hormone (ADH) and thus increases urinary retention. Because these cases of urinary retention receive more notoriety when they receive an epidural as opposed to routine premedication, a morphine epidural is often avoided. An epidural with local anesthetic is acceptable, as it should not affect ADH release.

Postobstructive diuresis occurs following the unblocking of an obstructed cat. The patient requires a higher fluid rate or risks becoming dehydrated if urologic surgery follows the unblocking of the animal.

2. Anesthetic protocol

The protocol is targeted at avoiding or reducing the dosage for drugs excreted by the kidney (e.g., ketamine). Otherwise, drugs are selected based on the patient's preanesthetic assessment. Aggressive fluid therapy is only used once the bladder has been incised or a patent urinary catheter is in place.

II. Orthopedic/neurology procedures

A. Dorsal hemilaminectomy

Patients requiring a dorsal hemilaminectomy have a herniated disk with spinal cord compression in the thoracic or lumbar spine. While some animals (e.g., dachshunds) exhibit an inherent tendency toward a ruptured disk (Type I disk disease), a slow protrusion of the disk over time causes compression (Type II disk disease) generally of older,

128

Table 4.12 Suggested anesthesia protocol for cystotomy and PU.

Cystotomy and PU				
Opioid premedication (mg/kg)	Sedative premedication (mg/kg)	Induction (mg/kg)	Maintenance	Intraoperative analgesia (mg/kg)	Postoperative analgesia (mg/kg)
(a) Methadone 0.5–1 IM or (b) Hydromorphone 0.1–0.2 IM or (c) Morphine 0.5 IM	(a) Acepromazine 0.02 mg/kg or (b) Midazolam 0.2 mg/kg	(a) Propofol 2–4 or (b) Ketamine 5 and diazepam 0.25	Isoflurane or sevoflurane	(a) Epidural with local anesthetic (e.g., bupivacaine) only. (b) Opioid options: i. Intermittent bolus: (Methadone 0.3 IV q 4–6 h or Hydromorphone 0.05–0.1 IV q 4 h or Fentanyl, 0.005 IV as needed) ii. Fentanyl CRI 0.01– 0.042 mg/kg/h IV	(a) Intermittent bolus: i. Methadone 0.3 IV q 4–6 h or ii. Hydromorphone 0.05–0.1 IV q 4 h

Note: Avoid alpha$_2$ agonists especially if urinary obstruction causes diuresis and may increase chance of rupture. Avoid ketamine in cats with renal insufficiency.

large breed dogs. Diagnosing the location of the protrusion requires a neurological examination, +/− spinal radiographs, computed tomography (CT), and/or magneric resonance imaging (MRI) depending on the surgeon's preference or experience.

1. Anesthesia concerns/common complications

(a) Dehydration: Immobile patients commonly present slightly dehydrated with an increased PCV and total protein (TP). It is helpful to restore volume by placing a catheter and administering maintenance fluids to the patient while the anesthetist prepares for anesthesia. Care is taken to make sure the animal does not have a distended bladder (palpate and express, if necessary).

(b) Noxious stimuli/pain: Manipulation of tissues around the spinal cord is intensely stimulating, and pain management for these patients is key. Premedication includes a full mu agonist and an alpha$_2$ agonist if not contraindicated. (*Note*: If surgeon preference is a CT for imaging confirmation of disk site, this premedication may provide heavy enough sedation where general anesthesia is unnecessary for CT.) Intraoperatively, opioid, ketamine, and lidocaine CRIs work nicely to manage noxious stimuli. Before the use of steroids or NSAIDs, the anesthetist must ensure these drugs have not been previously administered. A lidocaine patch over the incision site and a postoperative analgesic CRI is warranted.

(c) Progressive spinal cord degeneration: The animal will gradually and progressively lose neurologic function. Initially, the animal may lack conscious proprioception, in which case the patient is often managed medically. As the disease worsens to include loss of motor function and ability to urinate, the supervising clinician may decide to proceed to surgery. It is important for the anesthetist to help with bladder expression (to avoid bladder atony), as this is often easily performed once the patient is asleep. When deep pain is lost, the decision to proceed to surgery is often an urgent attempt to remove compression and restore motor function, although prognosis is at best guarded. These patients are considered true emergencies and anesthesia is prioritized for them.

2. Anesthetic protocol

The anesthetic protocol is based on patient presentation. No drugs are specifically contraindicated. The classic "back dog" is usually healthy otherwise; however, it is always important to do a complete PE and routine BW.

B. Ventral slot

When disk herniation occurs in the cervical spine, the surgical approach is performed ventrally. This requires the surgeon to work around many delicate and important structures, including the trachea, esophagus, carotid arteries, and the jugular vessels to access the spinal cord.

Chapter 4

1. Anesthetic concerns/complications

(a) Hemorrhage due to venous sinus proximity as well as vascular disruption may be profound. Intraoperative blood loss should be watched closely. A preoperative cross-match and blood typing is recommended.

(b) Nonambulatory

(c) Noxious stimuli/pain: A full agonist opioid (morphine, hydromorphone, or fentanyl), ketamine, and lidocaine CRI is ideal intraoperatively and continued postoperatively. Avoid extending or flexing the neck especially during restraint and intubation.

(d) Occlusion of the ET tube is common: $EtCO_2$ is essential. The anesthetist must measure the ET tube to beyond thoracic inlet to avoid the surgeon possibly occluding the ET tube during the surgical approach. Some anesthetists prefer the use of wire-guarded ET tubes to prevent occlusion.

2. Anesthetic protocol

The drug protocol is tailored to the patient's preanesthetic assessment. Premedication includes a full mu agonist opioid. Drugs that cause vomiting are avoided (i.e., hydro-morphone or morphine IM). It is ideal to avoid hyperextension of the neck during intuba-tion. Multimodal intraoperative and postoperative analgesia is required (see comments earlier).

C. Orthopedic surgeries

Patients may require an orthopedic procedure secondary to trauma, malignancy, malfor-mation or degeneration, or rupture of joints and ligaments. These surgeries involve manipulation of bone and produce a significant degree of somatic pain. Examples of these procedures include fracture repairs, cranial cruciate repairs (lateral suture, tibial plateau leveling osteotomy [TPLO], and tibial tuberosity advancement [TTA]), total hip replacement, angular limb deformity corrections, mandibulectomy, maxillectomy, and arthroscopies.

1. Anesthesia concerns/complications

(a) Aspiration: When an orthopedic procedure is performed in the mouth, such as with a maxillectomy or mandibulectomy, there is risk of aspirating blood or surgical flush. If the surgeon chooses to pack the pharyngeal region with gauze, the number of gauze is counted and a prominent reminder note is placed to ensure removal of the packing mate-rial. Extubating with the cuff partially inflated helps minimize aspiration.

(b) Hemorrhage: Major arteries course through many of the approaches for orthopedic procedures. While every surgeon strives for adequate hemostasis, occasionally, this is not achieved. The anesthetist notes if significant quantities of blood are present in the suction canister or there is a fair amount of soaked 4×4 gauze sponges. This is unusual during an orthopedic procedure, and if hemorrhage becomes visually significant, it is quantified to see if intervention (i.e., a blood transfusion) is required.

(a) Noxious stimuli/pain: These procedures warrant aggressive pain management from the start of the case. Preemptive, multimodal analgesia is important as well as appropriate intraoperative analgesia to avoid "wind-up" (see Table 4.13). Multimodal analgesia involves the use of regional techniques (see Chapter 8) where possible, as well as oral and injectable drugs. See "Anesthesia Protocol" that follows for a suggested plan with a focus on pain management. Frequent (q 4 h) reassessment of pain with a suitable pain scale (see Appendix A) is necessary for the first 24 hours, so adjustments tailored to each patient are implemented.

2. Anesthetic protocol

No drugs are specifically contraindicated in most orthopedic procedures. It is important to create a protocol based on the patient's preanesthetic assessment. The following plan optimizes analgesia.

Premedication includes a mu opioid agonist and alpha$_2$ agonists, if not contraindicated, as both of these drug families possess analgesic properties. Induction with ketamine (if not contraindicated) provides a loading dose as a CRI is indicated (see later discussion); diazepam facilitates muscle relaxation if ketamine is used as induction agent. If one chooses to use an alternative induction drug, a subanesthetic dose of ketamine (0.5 mg/kg) is included to help decrease wind-up and provide the loading dose for the CRI if desired. Maintenance with inhalant anesthetic plus a local block (see Chapter 8) is desirable. A local block will not simply modify pain transmission; it will prevent transmission from occurring. If a local block for the surgery site is not available or successful, a multimodal CRI such as an opioid, ketamine, and lidocaine (avoid lidocaine CRI in felines) is a suitable alternative. If hypotension was not a prevalent comorbidity during the procedure, postoperative administration of a NSAID is warranted, as well as continued administration of a full mu agonist opioid for at least the next 24 hours. When recovering patients that underwent an orthopedic procedure involving the facial bones near or around the mouth, one should ensure the patient swallows and suction the back of mouth before extubating.

III. Ocular procedures

These procedures are categorized into procedures involving the globe (i.e., enucleation, lens luxation, phacoemulsification) and those involving tissues surrounding the globe (i.e., cherry eye, entropion repair).

A. Anesthesia concerns/common complications

See "Anesthesia Concerns/Common Complications" under "Head and Neck Procedures," as loss of access and trigeminal vagal responses are applicable for ophthalmologic procedures as well.

Chapter 4

Table 4.13 Analgesia for orthopedic procedures.

Orthopedic Procedure	Analgesia Options
Facial bones (maxillectomy and mandibulectomy)	Regional techniques (nerve blocks; see Ch. 8) Opioid, lidocaine, and ketamine CRI NSAIDs post-op Tramadol post-op Opioid bolus post-op
Forelimbs below elbow	Brachial plexus block Opioid, lidocaine, and ketamine CRI NSAIDs post-op Tramadol post-op Opioid bolus post-op
Forelimbs above elbow	Paravertebral nerve block Opioid, lidocaine, and ketamine CRI NSAIDs post-op Tramadol post-op Opioid bolus post-op
Hind limb	Epidural/epidural catheter Femoral and sciatic nerve block Opioid, lidocaine, and ketamine CRI NSAID post-op Tramadol post-op Opioid bolus post-op
Pelvis/hips	Epidural/epidural catheter Opioid, lidocaine, and ketamine CRI NSAID post-op Tramadol post-op Opioid bolus post-op

1. Noxious stimuli/pain

Because vision and thus the eye are key to survival, it is heavily innervated and procedures involving the eye are very painful. Fortunately, local anesthetic delivered either topically or as a local block (see Chapter 8), when appropriately applied, prevents pain transmission from occurring. Indeed, when topical proparacaine is given as two drops, 1 minute apart, the cornea is anesthetized for up to 55 minutes (20) in dogs, although the duration is much shorter in cats (21). Combined with adequate premedication (i.e., a full mu agonist) and analgesic medication postoperatively (NSAIDs if not contraindicated), effective pain management is feasible.

B. Anesthesia protocol

Full mu agonist opioids cause miosis in dogs and mydriasis in cats. Atropine, administered topically or systemically, will result in mydriasis and is often combined into the premedication protocol for the dog. Alternatively, phenylephrine is used topically to dilate the pupil; systemic effects may be noticeable following topical application (i.e., profound hypertension secondary to vasoconstriction). Drugs causing vomiting (hydromorphone, morphine, and dexmedetomidine) are avoided in patients where IOP is a concern. Ketamine increases IOP via muscle contracture around the globe, so it is only used in a patient that has effective muscle relaxation from premedication or general anesthesia. There is debate about increases in IOP from the use of propofol (22, 23). In studies demonstrating an increase in IOP, the increase was 3–5 mmHg as compared with dogs induced with thiopental, which is a small although statistically significant increase. However, these studies were also performed in clinically normal dogs (as opposed to dogs with glaucoma). Unfortunately, as thiopental is no longer commercially available in some parts of the world, propofol is still preferable to etomidate in cases where pupillary diameter is of concern (24). It is the authors' recommendation to use thiopental, when available, as the induction agent of choice (unless contraindicated) in patients with glaucoma requiring anesthesia and propofol after significant muscle relaxation when thiopental is not available. Concurrent diseases may influence anesthetic protocol (see "Key Points" that follows). In addition to applicable local blocks, intraoperative analgesia with lidocaine or opioid CRIs as well as intermittent opioid boluses is warranted. Eye ointment/lubricant is not placed in the eye undergoing surgery, unless specifically requested by the ophthalmologist (usually after completion of procedure). If the ophthalmologist requires the eye to remain central, a neuromuscular blocking (NMB) is included (see Table 3.8).

No specific drugs are contraindicated for ocular procedures involving the tissues surrounding the eye. The protocol is selected based on the patient's preanesthetic assessment.

C. Key points

1. Ophthalmology procedures involving the globe (e.g., enucleation, lens luxation, cataract phacoemulsification, corneal conjunctiva graft)

(a) Concurrent disease: While not all patients with ocular disease have concurrent disease, there is a high prevalence of dogs presenting for phacoemulsification secondary to cataract disease that are diabetic. Appropriate anesthetic management of the diabetic patient (see Chapter 5, "Diabetes Mellitus" section) is necessary.

(b) Concurrent medications: In addition to routine screening for concurring medications as is done for any patient undergoing anesthesia, these patients are often receiving medication from the ophthalmologist to promote pupillary dilation (especially important in patients with a lens luxation or cataract) or reduce IOP. These drugs (such as phenylephrine) manifest their presence during anesthesia, so it is good practice for the anesthetist to confirm what medications the patient is receiving, both from the owner and from the ophthalmologist.

(c) Increased IOP: Vision is the ultimate result most owners desire for their pets. Glaucoma compromises vision and therefore is a medical emergency. The anesthetist's goal is not worsening glaucoma through his or her actions. Drugs that worsen glaucoma are avoided (including atropine and ketamine). Anything that will cause vomiting

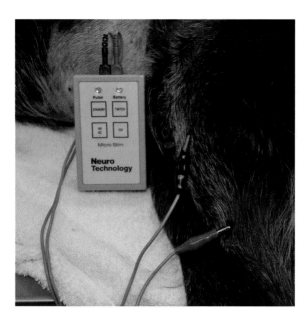

Figure 4.4   Patient with a PNS over the peroneal nerve (line). Courtesy of Patricia Queiroz-Williams.

(as vomiting increase IOP) is avoided. Coughing significantly increases IOP. The patient is intubated *only* at an adequate plane of anesthesia. Glaucoma is a very painful disease, and appropriate analgesia (opioids such as methadone) is incorporated into the analgesic plan.

(d) Ocular positioning: For certain procedures, such as phacoemulsification, a centrally located eye is necessary. In these cases, where a surgeon prefers not to use a stay suture for placement, an NMB is incorporated into the protocol. Prior to use of an NMB, a nerve stimulator is placed on the patient, usually over the common peroneal nerve.

A train of four is observed, comparing visually the first twitch to the fourth twitch. While it is possible to provide neuromuscular blockade to only the eye, for safety reasons, the anesthetist must assume it will paralyze the respiratory muscles as well. Therefore, before administration of NMB, mechanical ventilation is begun (see Chapter 2, "Mechanical Ventilation" section).

Once NMB is administered (see Chapter 3), the twitches will diminish from fourth to first before disappearing altogether. Ultimately, the appropriate effect of NMB, regardless of how many twitches are present, is the ocular position for the ophthalmologist. Because the eye is very sensitive to the effect of neuromuscular blockade, even when four twitches are present post drug administration, the eye may still remain central. Re-administration of the NMB is at the discretion of the ophthalmologist.

The next challenge is reversal of the blockade near the end of the procedure. See Table 3.13 for more information on reversing NMB. The anesthetist's greatest concern with the use of NMB is continued paralysis in recovery, which may go unnoticed. This iatrogenic respiratory arrest will proceed rapidly to cardiac arrest. Therefore, it is incumbent upon the anesthetist to ensure the patient is adequately ventilating before leaving the OR, regardless of when the procedure was completed (i.e., if timing is not optimized, the anesthetist may spend another hour in the OR after the procedure is completed, ensuring the patient is fit for recovery).

IV. Scoping procedures

Scoping procedures are minimally invasive means to visualize internal structures and obtain cultures or biopsies. A scope is also useful to assist with therapeutic interventions, such as the placement of feeding tubes or removal of a foreign body, in order to avoid more invasive approaches.

A. Anesthesia concerns/common complications

Minimal; see "Key Points."

B. Anesthesia protocol

The anesthetic protocol is tailored to the patient's preanesthetic assessment and underlying diseases. Premedication includes an opioid and sedative combination. Whatever induction combination is chosen, additional induction drug is available, as one of the hallmarks characteristic of these procedures is periods of intense stimulation (e.g., distention of the stomach or biopsy of the nasal sinus) intermittently in an otherwise minimally stimulated patient, resulting in an abrupt change of the anesthetic plane. For this reason, adequate analgesia is maintained with intermittent boluses of opioids (such as fentanyl) as opposed to CRIs. Recovery is a concern because the procedure has often disrupted a patient that was previously stable; that is, there is now gas in the stomach, fluid in the lungs, or hemorrhage in the nasal cavity that was iatrogenically caused. These patients warrant close postanesthetic monitoring although not for sole purposes of ensuring adequate analgesia, as they often are only mild to moderately painful.

C. Key points

1. Bronchial alveolar lavage (BAL)

(a) Airway: This procedure performed in small patients is a challenge to the anesthetist because the diameter of the scope may exceed the internal diameter of the ET tube (which is not the case for larger patients). In small patients, this means it is not possible to have the patient intubated while performing the bronchoscopy. This is problematic both because it compromises the patient's gas exchange and it requires an alternative to gas inhalant for maintaining anesthesia. Without connection to an anesthesia circuit, the anesthetist cannot manually ventilate for the patient and thus, hypoventilation will ensue. Additionally, without supplemental oxygenation delivered through the circuit, the patient may rapidly desaturate and become hypoxemic. Respiratory, and subsequently, cardiac

Chapter 4

arrest, may occur in these cases. Maintenance of anesthesia is often accomplished with TIVA. See "Head and Neck Procedures" for additional information concerning loss of access and trigeminal vagal response.

(b) Anesthetic protocol modification: This procedure is not painful. The anesthetic protocol is selected based on drugs that result in minimal respiratory depression, are reversible, and have a short duration. IV access is an absolute necessity. Stress is minimized to avoid respiratory distress. Placement of monitoring equipment is completed in the cooperative patient before induction. While this procedure is not painful, it is often helpful to select a full mu agonist for premedication in case an opioid CRI is necessary to reduce the amount of maintenance drug necessary for anesthesia. Propofol is the induction agent of choice and is suitable for maintaining anesthesia when administered as a CRI. Additionally, administering midazolam during induction will reduce the amount of propofol required. If available, jet ventilation is ideal for these patients; however, many institutions do not have a jet ventilator. This means the patient is extubated before the procedure begins; however, it is wise to begin with induction and intubation of the patient to allow the anesthetist to get all monitoring in order. If the clinician wishes to collect cultures, a sterile ET tube is required for intubation. Once the anesthetist is comfortable that the patient's monitoring equipment is functional and the patient is stable, then the patient is extubated and the scoping procedure begins. Obviously, it is ideal to intubate and secure an airway; prior to the procedure, the anesthetist confirms with the clinician which scope is necessary and will physically see if the scope fits through the proposed ET tube for the patient (this must be done prior to scope sterilization). If the scope will fit through the ET tube, there is an adapter available with a port that has a diaphragm, through which the scope enters (see Figure 4.5). The diaphragm allows maintenance of the anesthesia circuit so the anesthetist can ventilate the patient. In a patient that is not intubated, supplemental oxygen is administered through the scope or by red rubber catheter attached to the fresh gas outlet on the anesthesia machine. In these patients, re-intubation occurs

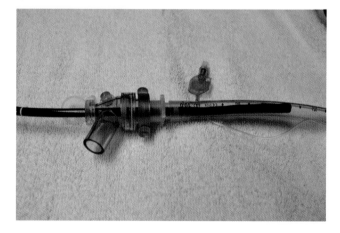

Figure 4.5   Supplies for oxygen insufflation during a BAL. Courtesy of Patricia Queiroz-Williams.

when the patient desaturates, and immediately following the bronchial lavage. The patient is allowed to recover with supplemental oxygen, before reintroducing the scope. Special attention is paid to the pulse oximetry reading, and the procedure is transiently aborted when the SpO_2 drops below 93%. In recovery, it is ideal to have available supplemental oxygen following extubation. Albuterol is available to assist in bronchodilation.

2. Gastroscopy (upper/lower GI)

(a) Distension of the stomach: Pain fiber upregulation occurs in the GI tract with visceral organ distension; therefore, insufflating the stomach significantly leads to discomfort for the patient. Fortunately, visualization for the individual performing the endoscopy is usually adequate without hyperinflating the stomach. The anesthetist palpates the stomach at the edge of the ribs prior to beginning the procedure; this allows for a comparison as the stomach is inflated. Hyper-distending the stomach also leads to hypoventilation by compression on the thorax and negatively impacts venous return (and thus BP). If hyper-inflation is suspected or confirmed by palpation, the anesthetist communicates this to the individual performing the endoscopy with the request to desufflate the abdomen margin-ally. At the end of the procedure it is necessary to desufflate the entire stomach to prevent problems in recovery.

(b) Anesthetic protocol modifications: The premedication choice of atropine and morphine may make passage of the endoscope through the pyloric sphincter more difficult (25). These drugs are avoided.

3. Rhinoscopy and biopsy

(a) Hemorrhage: The nasal passage is well perfused and thus rhinoscopy may result in hemorrhage; a small number of these cases will have marked and significant hemorrhage (26). Coagulation panels are assessed preoperatively to ensure that a patient will ade-quately clot if biopsies are performed. Nasal phenylephrine and ice packing are common therapies to control continued hemorrhage. In case of profound hemorrhage, the patient may need diagnostic tests for blood compatibility and a transfusion. (Even if hemorrhage is not remarkable, aspiration of blood is always a risk.)

(b) Noxious stimulation/pain: Rhinoscopy and biopsies are very stimulating procedures, often necessitating rapid changes in anesthetic plane. There is evidence that inclusion of a local block, particularly a maxillary nerve block (see Chapter 8, "Maxillary Nerve Block" section), may reduce the level of responsiveness for patients undergoing these procedures (27).

(c) See "Head and Neck Procedures" for additional information concerning loss of access and trigeminal vagal response.

(d) Anesthetic protocol: In some cases, the stimulation from the procedure is so intense, the surgeon may require a single bolus of NMB be given, as long as ventilation is supported

Chapter 4

(see "Ocular Positioning"). A quiet recovery is desirable to avoid dislodging any clots following biopsies. A low dose of acepromazine, if not given as a premedication, may be administered IV following extubation. The ET tube cuff is left partially inflated for extubation to help minimize chances of aspiration of blood surrounding the ET tube.

V. Miscellaneous procedures

A. Deep ear flush/myringotomy

Deep ear flushes are performed in patients with chronic ear infections, to clear debris and gross infection from the ear. Often these patients have painful ears and may or may not have an intact tympanic membrane. In cases where middle or inner ear infection is suspected, a myringotomy (incision into the tympanic membrane) is used to reduce pressure and pain.

1. Anesthesia considerations/common complications

(a) Acute on chronic pain: Patients that present for a deep ear flush often have chronic ear infections, which are a source of chronic pain. When the flush is performed in these patients, it adds an element of acute pain. This results in an "acute on chronic" noxious or painful event, which adversely affects quality of life. Every attempt to optimize analgesia is done for these animals.

(b) Unintentional myringotomy: This is possible during a deep ear flush. The complications from this are usually minimal, but may include vestibular disease present at recovery. Additionally, a myringotomy will create communication between the ear canal and trachea, possibly increasing chances for aspiration of fluid from ear flush.

2. Protocol

Anesthetic protocol is based on the patient's preanesthetic assessment. Often these are short procedures (less than 20 minutes). Short acting or reversible drugs are preferred (i.e., fentanyl and dexmedetomidine), bearing in mind that reversal of the sedative effects of the drug will reverse their analgesic benefits as well. The inclusion of alpha$_2$ agonists, if not contraindicated, and an opioid, are suitable for premedication if warranted. Induction with ketamine, if not contraindicated, will serve both as a loading dose should a ketamine CRI be instituted. Maintenance anesthesia includes a ketamine CRI to address the chronic pain issue, as well as either intermittent boluses or a CRI of opioids. Patients are intubated, and the ET tube cuff is properly inflated. Caution is suggested with inclusion of NSAIDs for these dogs, as they may already be receiving steroids as part of their ear disease management. However, sending home tramadol is warranted.

B. Dentals with extractions

Routine dental cleanings have very few complications when one takes the proper precautions securing the patient's airway; however, many patients requiring extensive dental work are older with concurrent disease. Preanesthetic assessment with full BW and a complete PE is very important to ensure a suitable anesthetic plan.

1. Anesthesia considerations/common complications

(a) Aspiration of fluid: Copious amounts of fluid are present in the mouth during dental procedures, including fluid to keep the drill from overheating as well as blood from working in such a vascular area. To reduce the possibility of the patient aspirating these fluids, ensure ET tube cuff is well inflated. Place sponge or gauze 4 × 4 with string secured to ET tube (dental floss works well) in the back of the mouth to prevent aspiration; however, one must take extreme care to ensure pack removal at the end of the procedure. It is recommended to record on the anesthesia record if a pack is placed and when pack is removed. Simple positioning helps as well; elevating the neck with towels and trying to keep nose down facilitates drainage of fluid from the mouth. The anesthetist may choose to remove the ET tube with the cuff partially inflated if there is concern about fluid compromising the airway.

(b) Noxious stimuli/pain: Dental extractions are painful both because of the innervation to the tooth as well as the sensitivity of the oral mucosa. Whenever possible, incorporation of a local block (see Chapter 8), is warranted, as this will prevent pain transmission.

(c) See "Head and Neck Procedures" for additional information concerning loss of access and trigeminal vagal response.

2. Anesthesia protocol

Drug selection is based on the patient's preanesthetic assessment. As eluded to previously, many dental cases have a myriad of diseases in addition to requiring extensive dental work. These patients may require alterations in the anesthetic protocol to accommodate their concurrent diseases (see Chapter 5). Premedication involves an opioid appropriate for the extent of dental work intended (e.g., if several extractions are involved a full agonist opioid is indicated) and a sedative. Induction and maintenance of anesthesia is accomplished by an agent appropriate for the patient. Dental nerve blocks are indicated for any patient with extractions (see Chapter 8). An opioid CRI may be required to reduce MAC and provide additional analgesia in patients with extremely painful mouths. Patients are not extubated until they are capable of swallowing and lifting their head. Remember to include appropriate analgesia in the postoperative period, such as NSIADs, if not contraindicated.

References

1. Herrera MA, Mehl ML, Kass PH, Pascoe PJ, Feldman EC, Nelson RW. Predictive factors and the effect of phenoxybenzamine on outcome in dogs undergoing adrenalectomy for pheochromocytoma. J Vet Intern Med. 2008;22(6):1333–9.

2. Goksin I, Adali F, Enli Y, Akbulut M, Teke Z, Sackan G, et al. The effect of phlebotomy and mannitol on acute renal injury induced by ischemia/reperfusion of lower limbs in rats. Ann Vasc Surg. 2011;25(8):1118–28.

3. Lewis RM, Rice JH, Patton MK, Barnes JL, Nickel AE, Osgood RW, et al. Renal ischemic injury in the dog: characterization and effect of various pharmacologic agents. J Lab Clin Med. 1984;104(4):470–9.

4. Yatsu T, Arai Y, Takizawa K, Kasai-Nakagawa C, Takanashi M, Uchida W, et al. Effect of YM435, a dopamine DA1 receptor agonist, in a canine model of ischemic acute renal failure. Gen Pharmacol. 1998;31(5):803–7.

5. Halpenny M, Markos F, Snow HM, Duggan PF, Gaffney E, O'Connell DP, et al. Effects of prophylactic fenoldopam infusion on renal blood flow and renal tubular function during acute hypovolemia in anesthetized dogs. Crit Care Med. 2001;29(4):855–60.

6. Boscan P, Pypendop BH, Siao KT, Francey T, Dowers K, Cowgill L, et al. Fluid balance, glomerular filtration rate, and urine output in dogs anesthetized for an orthopedic surgical procedure. Am J Vet Res. 2010;71(5):501–7.

7. Kummeling A, Teske E, Rothuizen J, Van Sluijs FJ. Coagulation profiles in dogs with congenital portosystemic shunts before and after surgical attenuation. J Vet Intern Med. 2006; 20(6):1319–26.

8. Burgoyne LL, Billups CA, Jirón JL, Kaddoum RN, Wright BB, Bikhazi GB, et al. Phantom limb pain in young cancer-related amputees: recent experience at St Jude children's research hospital. Clin J Pain. 2012;28(3):222–5.

9. Nouette-Gaulain K, Capdevila X, Rossignol R. Local anesthetic 'in-situ' toxicity during peripheral nerve blocks: update on mechanisms and prevention. Curr Opin Anaesthesiol. 2012;25(5):589–95.

10. Trumpatori BJ, Carter JE, Hash J, Davidson GS, Mathews KG, Roe SC, et al. Evaluation of a midhumeral block of the radial, ulnar, musculocutaneous and median (RUMM block) nerves for analgesia of the distal aspect of the thoracic limb in dogs. Vet Surg. 2010;39(7): 785–96.

11. McNally E, Robertson S, Pablo L. Comparison of time to desaturation between preoxygenated and nonpreoxygenated dogs following sedation with acepromazine maleate and morphine and induction of anesthesia with propofol. Am J Vet Res. 2009;70(11):1333–8.

12. Yamauchi Y, Izumi Y, Hashimoto K, Inoue M, Nakatsuka S, Kawamura M, et al. Needle-tract seeding after percutaneous cryoablation for lung metastasis of colorectal cancer. Ann Thorac Surg. 2011;92(4):e69–71.

13. Ko JC, Maxwell LK, Abbo LA, Weil AB. Pharmacokinetics of lidocaine following the application of 5% lidocaine patches to cats. J Vet Pharmacol Ther. 2008;31(4):359–67.

14. Jeffery ND, Talbot CE, Smith PM, Bacon NJ. Acquired idiopathic laryngeal paralysis as a prominent feature of generalised neuromuscular disease in 39 dogs. Vet Rec. 2006;158(1):17.

15. Williams VM, Lascelles BD, Robson MC. Current attitudes to, and use of, peri-operative analgesia in dogs and cats by veterinarians in New Zealand. N Z Vet J. 2005;53(3):193–202.

16. Evans KM, Adams VJ. Proportion of litters of purebred dogs born by caesarean section. J Small Anim Pract. 2010;51(2):113–8.

17. Moon-Massat P, Erb H. Perioperative factors associated with puppy vigor after delivery by cesarean section. J Am Anim Hosp Assoc. 2002;38(1):90–6.

18. Moon P, Erb H, Ludders J, Gleed R, Pascoe P. Perioperative risk factors for puppies delivered by cesarean section in the United States and Canada. J Am Anim Hosp Assoc. 2000;36(4): 359–68.

19. Dabir S, Parsa T, Radpay B, Padyab M. Interpleural morphine vs bupivacaine for postthoracotomy pain relief. Asian Cardiovasc Thorac Ann. 2008;16(5):370–4.

20. Herring IP, Bobofchak MA, Landry MP, Ward DL. Duration of effect and effect of multiple doses of topical ophthalmic 0.5% proparacaine hydrochloride in clinically normal dogs. Am J Vet Res. 2005;66(1):77–80.

21. Binder DR, Herring IP. Duration of corneal anesthesia following topical administration of 0.5% proparacaine hydrochloride solution in clinically normal cats. Am J Vet Res. 2006;67(10):1780–2.

22. Hofmeister EH, Williams CO, Braun C, Moore PA. Propofol versus thiopental: effects on peri-induction intraocular pressures in normal dogs. Vet Anaesth Analg. 2008;35(4):275–81.

23. Batista CM, Laus JL, Nunes N, Patto Dos Santos PS, Costa JL. Evaluation of intraocular and partial CO2 pressure in dogs anesthetized with propofol. Vet Ophthalmol. 2000;3(1):17–9.

24. Gunderson EG, Lukasik VM, Ashton MM, Merideth RE, Madsen R. Effects of anesthetic induction with midazolam-propofol and midazolam-etomidate on selected ocular and cardio-respiratory variables in clinically normal dogs. Am J Vet Res. 2013;74(4):629–35.

25. Donaldson LL, Leib MS, Boyd C, Burkholder W, Sheridan M. Effect of preanesthetic medication on ease of endoscopic intubation of the duodenum in anesthetized dogs. Am J Vet Res. 1993;54(9):1489–95.

26. Lent SE, Hawkins EC. Evaluation of rhinoscopy and rhinoscopy-assisted mucosal biopsy in diagnosis of nasal disease in dogs: 119 cases (1985–1989). J Am Vet Med Assoc. 1992;201(9): 1425–9.

27. Cremer J, Sum SO, Braun C, Figueiredo J, Rodriguez-Guarin C. Assessment of maxillary and infraorbital nerve blockade for rhinoscopy in sevoflurane anesthetized dogs. Vet Anaesth Analg. 2013; 40(4):432–9.

Chapter 4

1. Anesthesia concerns/common complications

(a) Bradyarrhythmias: Because CO is equal to heart rate (HR) multiplied by stroke volume (SV), a slow HR will decrease CO. In light of decreased CO secondary to the use of general anesthesia, there is a risk of severely compromising perfusion to vital tissues including the brain, kidney, and liver.

(b) Tachyarrhythmias: Perfusion to the heart occurs during diastole. When a tachyarrhythmia occurs, the heart spends very little time in diastole, which results in compromised myocardial perfusion, significantly worsening ventricular arrhythmias in particular (as the ventricle is the largest cardiac muscle body to perfuse).

2. Anesthesia protocol

A patient that is scheduled for an elective procedure but has an arrhythmia on PE must have at minimum an ECG analyzed before anesthesia proceeds. In cases where the procedure is urgent and anesthesia is unavoidable, goals are to stabilize and/or reduce the impact of the arrhythmia. This means using cardiac friendly drugs for premedication (i.e., opioids and benzodiazepines), induction (i.e., etomidate or neuroleptic anesthesia [fentanyl and a benzodiazepine]), and reducing the amount of inhalant administered (i.e., through the use of opioids for their minimum alveolar concentration (MAC) sparing effect). Additionally, in bradyarrhythmias, it is necessary to increase HR, either through the use of anticholinergics, isoproterenol, or a temporary pacemaker. In cases of tachycardia, it is essential to know whether the tachycardia is ventricular or preventricular in origin. Ventricular arrhythmias may slow in response to lidocaine; see Chapter 6 for treatment of arrhythmias.

3. Key points

Wolff–Parkinson–White syndrome is a syndrome where there is an additional conduction pathway between the atria and ventricle (i.e., the AV node is the normal conduction path). The AV node slows conduction between the atria and the ventricles, which this additional pathway does not. Thus, tachycardia results. This disease uncommonly occurs in the dog, and when it does happen, often the patient may not displace any abnormal conduction because of it. However, if tachycardia does develop, treatment with procainamide (5 mg/kg IV over 2–3 minutes) is indicated.

B. Structural abnormalities

1. Systolic dysfunction

Systolic dysfunction includes diseases such as valvular insufficiencies (mitral regurgitation [MR] or tricuspid regurgitation [TR]) and dilated cardiomyopathy (DCM). Under anesthesia, hypotension is common. In patients with DCM, arrhythmias are common and some may necessitate treatment.

Chapter 5

(a) Anesthesia concerns/common complications

(i) Maintain HR within 25% of resting HR; if the anesthetist must choose between slightly below or slightly above resting HR, these cases often benefit from a slightly elevated HR.

(ii) Avoid peripheral vasoconstriction as this will increase after load and decrease SV, both of which compromise CO.

(iii) Maintain myocardial contractility by using inotropic agents, such as dopamine or dobutamine (see Table 3.2).

(iv) Avoid volume overload by using a conservative fluid therapy plan (usually 2–5 mL/ kg/h).

(v) Minimize stress.

(b) Anesthetic protocol (see Table 5.1): Premedication facilitates IV catheterization with minimal stress and reduces drug requirements, but the anesthetist is careful to use drugs that are reversible in the cardiac patient. Opioids, given in higher doses, will reduce the need for sedatives that impact the cardiovascular system. Patients with mild MR might benefit from a low dose of acepromazine (0.01 mg/kg) to reduce afterload; benzodiazepines are also suitable based on the patient's temperament. However, dexmedetomidine is contraindicated in these patients. Preoxygenation is done for a minimum of 5 minutes prior to induction and up to the point of intubation. Monitoring equipment is placed on the patient prior to induction if possible. Etomidate is an ideal induction agent for these cases, as it minimally affects HR and blood pressure (BP). If a benzodiazepine is not administered at the time of premedication, it is useful to combine it with etomidate at induction. Gas inhalants are routinely used to maintain anesthesia; however, constant rate infusions (CRIs) such as fentanyl are used to reduce the MAC requirement of inhalant, thus minimizing negative cardiovascular side effects. Positive inotropes such as dopamine or dobutamine are used to support BP. Monitoring includes an ECG, Doppler, and ideally invasive blood pressure (IBP) if obtainable. In extremely critical cardiovascular patients, central venous pressure (CVP) is performed to closely monitor preload. Fluid therapy is conservative (2–5 mL/kg/h). In recovery, patients may require supplemental oxygen depending on the procedure and severity of cardiovascular disease. Often, patients with mild to moderate cardiovascular disease tolerate anesthesia with minimal complications, provided the protocol is appropriate for them.

Chapter 5

(c) Key points

(i) DCM is one of the most difficult cardiac diseases to manage for the anesthetist. Knowing the patient's ejection fraction (i.e., how severely the patient's ability to provide forward flow is impacted) will give the anesthetist an idea of how seriously the patient is compromised. In addition to the above goals, the best possible management of these patients is to keep anesthesia time to a bare minimum, and only undergo elective procedures when they are "stable," which often includes management of any concurrent arrhythmias as well as the use of drugs such as pimobedan (a positive inotrope).

146

Table 5.1 Suggested anesthesia protocol for patients with systolic dysfunction.

Opioid premedication (mg/kg)	Sedative premedication (mg/kg)	Induction (mg/kg)	Maintenance	Intraoperative analgesia (mg/kg/h)	Postoperative analgesia (mg/kg)
(a) Methadone 0.3–0.5 IM, 0.2–0.3 IV or (b) Hydromorphone 0.1 IM, 0.05 IV or (c) Fentanyl 0.002–0.005 IV	(a) Midazolam 0.2 IM	(a) Etomidate 1–2 IV +/– midazolam 0.1–0.2 IV or (b) Propofol to effect +/– midazolam 0.2 and/or lidocaine 1.0 IV to reduce total dose of propofol or (c) Fentanyl 0.01 and midazolam 0.2	Sevoflurane or isoflurane + CRI for reduction of inhalant requirement	(a) Opioid CRI i. Fentanyl 0.012–0.042 or ii. Hydromorphone 0.03 or iii. Remifentanil 0.012–0.042	(c) Intermittent bolus: i. Methadone 0.3 IV q 4–6 h or ii. Hydromorphone 0.05–0.1 IV q 4-6 h

Note: An anticholinergic IM is ideal if HR is low following premedication, prior to induction. Lidocaine is avoided in cats.

2. Diastolic dysfunction

This includes diseases such as hypertrophic cardiomyopathy (HCM) and pericardial disease, where there is limited filling of the ventricle due to small chamber size.

(a) Anesthesia concerns/common complications:

(i)   Avoid excessive peripheral vasodilation or constriction.

(ii) Maintain HR within 25% of baseline; if the anesthetist must choose between slightly below or slightly above resting HR, these cases often benefit from a slightly decreased HR to allow more filling time.

(iii) Avoid increases in myocardial contractility and myocardial oxygen consumption. This includes avoiding drugs such as ketamine and positive inotropes.

(iv) Maintain adequate circulating volume without causing fluid overload (conservative fluid rates of 2–5 mL/kg/h and monitor CVP in critical cardiac patient).

(v)   If BP is compromised, the first step is reducing the MAC of inhalant through the use of CRIs (i.e., opioids). If this is not enough, phenylephrine is used to tighten vascular tone. The goal is to return vascular tone back to its baseline before the impact of inhalant anesthesia (which reduces systemic vascular resistance [SVR]). It is difficult to know in cases of routine monitoring, however, if vasoconstriction is too profound. Invasive cardiovascular monitoring equipment and measuring of lactate levels (which should remain below 2.0 mmol/L), provides general information on adverse effects due to the use of phenylephrine. If lactate levels increase, it is possible there is compromised perfusion secondary to vasoconstriction. If this occurs, phenylephrine is decreased or discontinued.

(b) Anesthetic protocol (see Table 5.2): If sedation is needed in patients with HCM, low doses of dexmedetomidine facilitate the goal of decreasing HR to allow more time in diastole as well as reducing MAC of inhalant. In general for cardiac patients, it is good practice to administer drugs that are reversible and have minimal cardiovascular effects. Patients are preoxygenated before induction and up to the point of intubation. Induction with etomidate and midazolam is ideal. If the patient is cooperative, monitoring equipment is placed before induction. Isoflurane or sevoflurane at low concentrations are used routinely for maintenance. Fentanyl or lidocaine CRIs are used to reduce MAC of inhalant as well as provide analgesia if needed. Recovery should occur in a stress free environment. Supplemental oxygen is available if necessary.

3. Obstructive dysfunction

Obstructive dysfunction includes diseases such as fulminant heartworm disease or valvular stenosis (pulmonic or aortic). Cardiac diseases with obstructive dysfunction have reduced CO and limited cardiac reserve. In addition, the ventricular chambers begin to hypertrophy in response to pushing volume against an obstruction. As with other types of cardiovascular disease, these patients often compensate with their disease until heart failure develops. Anesthetizing these animals carries the risk, therefore, of decompensation.

Table 5.2 Suggested anesthesia protocol for patients with diastolic dysfunction.

Opioid premedication (mg/kg)	Sedative premedication (mg/kg)	Induction (mg/kg)	Maintenance	Intraoperative analgesia (mg/kg/h)	Postoperative analgesia (mg/kg)
(a) Methadone 0.3–0.5 IM, 0.2–0.3 IV or (b) Hydromorphone 0.1 IM, 0.05 IV or (c) Fentanyl 0.002–0.005 IV	(a) Midazolam 0.2 IM or (b) Dexmedetomidine 0.003–0.005	(a) Etomidate 1–2 IV +/– midazolam 0.1–0.2 IV or (b) Propofol to effect +/– midazolam 0.2 and/or lidocaine 1.0 IV to reduce total dose of propofol	Sevoflurane or isoflurane + CRI for reduction of inhalant requirement	(a) Opioid CRI i. Fentanyl 0.012–0.042 or ii. Hydromorphone 0.03 or iii. Remifentanil 0.012–0.042 b. +/– Lidocaine 1.5	(c) Intermittent bolus: i. Methadone 0.3 IV q 4–6 h ii. Hydromorphone 0.05–0.1 IV q 4–6 h

Note: Lidocaine is contraindicated in cats.

(a) Anesthesia concerns/common complications:

(i)   Maintain HR within 25% of resting HR; if the anesthetist must choose between slightly below or slightly above resting HR, these cases often benefit from a decreased HR, allowing hypertrophied cardiac muscles time in diastole to perfuse.

(ii) Avoid peripheral vasoconstriction, which adds additional resistance to forward flow (increasing afterload).

(iii) Avoid volume overload by using a conservative fluid therapy (usually 2–5 mL/kg/h).

(iv) Avoid increases in myocardial contractility and oxygen consumption by avoiding drugs like ketamine and positive inotropes.

(v)   Minimize stress.

(b) Anesthetic protocol (see Table 5.3): In general for cardiac patients, it is good practice to administer drugs that are reversible and have minimal cardiovascular effects (i.e., an opioid and benzodiazepine). The goal of premedication is to provide sufficient sedation to minimize stress, facilitate IV catheterization, and reduce the amount of drugs necessary for induction and maintenance. If the patient is cooperative, IV catheterization is performed with the assistance of eutectic mixture of local anesthetic (EMLA) cream in the nonsedated patient. It is important to preoxygenate these patients. Placement of monitoring equipment prior to induction is ideal (Doppler, ECG, noninvasive blood pressure [NIBP], and, when obtainable, IBP). Rapid access to the airway is important to minimize oxygen desaturation. Neuroleptic anesthesia (opioid + benzodiazepine) or etomidate is ideal for induction. Low doses of propofol may be used following bolus of opioid, benzodiazepine, and/or lidocaine.

MAC sparing CRIs are indicated to reduce inhalants; extremely critical patients may require minimal to no gas inhalant when placed on high doses of fentanyl or remifentanil CRIs. Monitoring includes at least IBP, CVP when time allows, ECG, Doppler, SpO_2, and capnography. In recovery, be prepared to provide oxygen supplementation. Recovery should occur in a stress free environment where the patient is closely monitored.

II. Endocrine diseases

A. Diabetes insipidus

Diabetes insipidus (DI) is rare in veterinary patients. This disease occurs either centrally or at the level of the kidney (nephrogenically); the patient either does not secrete or does not respond to (respectively) antidiuretic hormone (ADH). The lack of ADH effect results in an animal that urinates large volumes and thus must drink large volumes to accommodate its polyuria. It is important to stabilize these patients prior to anesthesia. Animals with confirmed DI are not anesthetized for elective procedures until their DI is managed, through the use of desmopressin. For nonelective procedures, volume status is of critical importance prior to anesthesia. Generally speaking, these patients have a free water deficit that is corrected as best as possible prior to anesthesia.

Table 5.3 Suggested anesthesia protocol for patients with obstructive heart disease.

Opioid premedication (mg/kg)	Sedative premedication (mg/kg)	Induction (mg/kg)	Maintenance	Intraoperative analgesia (mg/kg/h)	Postoperative analgesia (mg/kg)
(a) Methadone 0.3–0.5 IM, 0.2–0.3 IV or (b) Hydromorphone 0.1 IM, 0.05 IV or (c) Fentanyl 0.002–0.005 IV	(a) Midazolam 0.2 IM	(a) Etomidate 1–2 IV +/− midazolam 0.1–0.2 IV or (b) Fentanyl 0.005–0.01 and midazolam 0.2	Sevoflurane or isoflurane + CRI for reduction of inhalant requirement	(a) Opioid CRI i. Fentanyl 0.012–0.042 or ii. Hydromorphone 0.03 or iii. Remifentanil 0.012–0.042	(c) Intermittent bolus: i. Methadone 0.3 IV q 4–6h or ii. Hydromorphone 0.05–0.1 IV q 4–6h or iii. Burprenorphine 0.01–0.03 IV q 6–8h

1. Anesthesia concerns/common complications

(a) Water is not restricted at any point for these patients. These patients are considered dehydrated, both systemically and cerebrally.

(b) Monitor electrolytes (especially sodium) throughout anesthesia and into recovery; use of fluid therapy assists with keeping sodium in the patient's target range (150–160 mEq/L). See Chapter 6 for management of hypernatremic patients, as rapid changes in sodium have severe neurologic consequences.

(c) Fluid of choice is 5% dextrose in water (D5W) or 2.5% dextrose in 0.45% NaCl.

2. Anesthetic protocol

No anesthetic is specifically contraindicated for patients with diabetes insipidus; however, it is important to select drugs based on patient presentation and preanesthetic assessment. Judicious fluid therapy is warranted. In order to minimize the time it takes the patient to return to full function (and thus drinking on its own), it is wise to use reversible drugs whenever possible. Premedication is tailored to level of invasiveness of the procedure, with invasive procedures warranting full mu agonist opioids and minimally invasive procedures warranting mildly depressive drugs such as butorphanol. Induction with propofol is smooth, and the drug is metabolized quickly. Maintenance anesthesia with gas inhalants also includes the use of an opioid CRI, such as remifentanil, which reduces MAC of inhalant but is rapidly metabolized systemically. Postoperative analgesia is tailored to the level of invasiveness of the procedure.

Chapter 5

B. Diabetes mellitus

Diabetes mellitus is characterized by either relative or absolute insulin deficiency. Most commonly, the patient is insulin dependent. The cat, unsurprisingly, is a possible exception, and may have transient diabetes, noninsulin dependent diabetes, or traditional insulin-dependent diabetes. Ultimately, the body's inability to regulate glucose with insulin leads to osmotic diuresis and excessive urination. If insulin is not exogenously administered, the body will attempt to utilize other energy sources, which results in ketone formation and, especially with any perpetuating factors (such as stress), ketoacidosis. Ketoacidosis is a life-threatening emergency that is addressed before anything else but the most crucial of surgeries. Therefore, the anesthetist is typically confronted with the managed diabetic, although how well managed the diabetes is varies considerably. Routine BW including a complete blood count (CBC) and chemistry is performed; knowing electrolytes are essential. A urinalysis to assess for ketonuria is warranted. During the PE, pay special attention to hydration. Diabetic patients may have an enlarged liver and weakened muscles, which will contribute to inadequate ventilation during anesthesia.

1. Anesthesia concerns/common complications

(a) The focus of the anesthetic protocol is minimizing time out of the patient's routine feeding schedule. Elective procedures are scheduled in the morning so the patient recovers by the evening. Additionally, short-acting, reversible drugs are used where appropriate to minimize the "hangover" effects.

(b) In managed diabetics, patients are fasted for 8 hours (overnight), with 0.5 dose of their regular insulin given in the morning. Blood glucose (BG) is measured at admission to ensure the patient is not hypoglycemic.

(c) Monitor BG every 45–60 minutes, beginning immediately after induction. A sampling line (either an arterial line or a large bore catheter) is convenient for this purpose. Normal glucose is 80–120 mg/dL, but knowing a diabetic patient's level of regulation will tell the anesthetist how realistic this is. Typical diabetic patients have a BG of 200–250 mg/dL; a glucose drop below 200 mg/dL may prompt intervention. If glucose is less than 120 mg/dL in any diabetic patient, give dextrose 2.5–5% at 5–10 mL/kg/h. This is often accomplished with a buretrol or smaller bag of fluids, as the patient's requirements for dextrose may fluctuate over the anesthetic period.

If glucose levels exceed the patient's "normal blood glucose" based on BW, regular insulin at 0.1–0.2 IU/kg is administered. Alternatively, a CRI of regular insulin at 0.05 IU/kg/h, if continually monitored, may assist in regulation. It is prudent for the anesthetist to remember, however, that the patient is better off "sweet than sour," and therefore, aggressively lowering BG is inappropriate.

(d) Dehydration is common in these patients; this is corrected prior to anesthesia if possible.

2. Anesthetic protocol (see Table 5.4)

Dexmedetomidine results in a transient hyperglycemia and is avoided when possible. Selection of premedication and induction drugs are based on patient presentation with a preference given to titratable drugs (i.e., propofol or etomidate). Most induction agents are relatively short acting and will be metabolized quickly. Gas inhalants are routinely used. CRIs are used to provide analgesia as well as reduce inhalant requirements. The patient receives continued glucose checks at 45- to 60-minute intervals until it resumes eating, including time spent in recovery. Glucose supplementation (2.5–5%) in crystalloid fluids may be required throughout the recovery phase at 2–5 mL/kg/h. Appropriate and balanced postoperative analgesia is necessary in cases of invasive procedures so the patient resumes normal function as quickly as possible.

C. Hyperadrenocorticism (Cushing's disease)

Hyperadrenocorticism is an increase in corticosteroids, either exogenously due to supplementation or from the adrenal glands themselves (as a result of a primary adrenal mass or secondary to a pituitary gland tumor causing stimulation of the adrenal gland). While the term "Cushing's disease" indicates the pituitary form of hyperadrenocorticism, it is often used interchangeably for all forms of hyperadrenocorticism. Hyperadrenocorticism is confirmed or suggested based on a variety of test methods, including adrenocorticotropic hormone (ACTH) stimulation, low-dose dexamethasone suppression test, high-dose dexamethasone suppression test, and urine cortisol to creatinine ratio.

Table 5.4 Suggested anesthesia protocol for patients with diabetes mellitus.

Opioid premedication (mg/kg)	Sedative premedication (mg/kg)	Induction (mg/kg)	Maintenance	Intraoperative analgesia (mg/kg/h)	Postoperative analgesia
(a) Methadone 0.3–0.5 IM, 0.2–0.3 IV (*Note:* Methadone does not cause vomiting.) or (b) Hydromorphone 0.1 IM, 0.05 IV	(a) Acepromazine 0.01–0.02 or (b) Midazolam 0.2 IM	(a) Propofol to effect +/− midazolam 0.2 or (b) Etomidate 1–2 IV +/− midazolam 0.1–0.2 IV	Sevoflurane or isoflurane + CRI for reduction of inhalant requirement	(a) Opioid CRI i. Fentanyl 0.012–0.042 or ii. Hydromorphone 0.03 or iii. Remifentanil 0.012–0.042 (b) Lidocaine CRI 1.5–3	(a) Opioid CRIs: i. Fentanyl 0.002– 0.005 mg/kg/h or ii. Hydromorphone 0.01 mg/kg/h (b) Lidocaine 1.5mg/ kg/h (c) Intermittent bolus: i. Methadone 0.3 IV q 4–6h or ii. Hydromorphone 0.05–0.1 IV q 4–6h

Note: Lidocaine is contraindicated in cats; alternatively, lidocaine patches are an option alongside incision for both the cat and dog.

Chapter 5

153

CS of this disease include polyuria and polydipsia (PU/PD), polyphagia, thin hair and skin especially on the flank and abdomen along with pyoderma, a "pot belly" appearance, panting, muscle weakness, and lethargy. On PE, hepatomegaly is present. Concurrent disease processes may include hypertension, hypercoagulability, renal disease, diabetes mellitus, congestive heart failure (CHF), and neurologic disease. All of these diseases merit investigation when the anesthetist is presented with the hyperadrenocortical patient. Characteristic BW abnormalities include a stress leukogram, increases in RBC counts, BG, ALP, ALT, and cholesterol, and a decrease in phosphate. Urinalysis reveals a decreased urine specific gravity (USG), proteinuria, and possibly bacterial infection.

1. Anesthesia concerns/common complications

(a) Fragile skin: Care is taken when clipping these patients. Their skin is prone to bruising and lacerations. The hair that is clipped does not grow back as quickly or aesthetically as the hair of a normal patient, so minimizing the clipped areas is indicated.

(b) Concurrent medications: As with all patients, a thorough understanding of all medications or supplements a hyperadrenocortical patient receives is important for the anesthetist. A patient that has iatrogenic adrenocortical disease (i.e., is on glucocorticoid supplementation) is *not* abruptly taken off glucocorticoids prior to anesthesia, as an Addisonian crisis may result (see "Hypoadrenocorticism (Addison's Disease)" later).

Some patients with the pituitary form of Cushing's disease are treated with Anipryl. This drug is an irreversible monoamine oxidase inhibitor (MAOI), meaning that until new MAOs are formed, monoamines are not oxidized and therefore increase in circulation. While this is useful in certain disease states, too much monoamine may result in a serotonergic crisis. This is characterized by hyperthermia, tachycardia, hypertension, and muscle tremors, which range in severity from mild to fatal. Additional drugs that increase the availability of monoamines are contraindicated (e.g., tramadol). During the anesthetic period, meperidine is avoided, as are fentanyl and pentazocine. It appears morphine is the most suitable opioid, although neurologic depression may accompany administration of morphine in a patient on Anipryl. Some authors suggest avoiding ketamine as it may exacerbate the symptoms of a seretonergic crisis, but there is little, if any, nonanecdotal information for this recommendation.

(c) Hypoventilation: This results from muscle weakness and abdominal distension secondary to hepatomegaly and fat redistribution; mechanical ventilation (MV) is warranted.

(d) Management of concurrent diseases: The possibility of a pulmonary thromboembolism (PTE) secondary to hypercoagulability is something the anesthetist is vigilant to monitor for; this is suggested by a large difference between $EtCO_2$ and arterial CO_2 (see Chapter 6, "PTE" section).

2. Anesthetic protocol (see Table 5.5)

Premedication reduces stress and facilitates IV catheterization; often a sedative is unnecessary, but the anesthetist includes acepromazine in low doses or midazolam as necessary.

Table 5.5 Suggested anesthesia protocol for patients with hyperadrenocorticism.

Opioid premedication (mg/kg)	Sedative premedication (mg/kg)	Induction (mg/kg)	Maintenance	Intraoperative analgesia (mg/kg/h)	Postoperative analgesia
(a) Methadone 0.3–0.5 IM, 0.2–0.3 IV or (b) Hydromorphone 0.1 IM, 0.05 IV or (c) Morphine 0.5 IM	(a) Acepromazine 0.01–0.02 or (b) Midazolam 0.2 IM	(a) Propofol to effect +/− midazolam 0.2 or (b) Etomidate 1–2 IV +/− midazolam 0.1–0.2 IV or (c) Fentanyl 0.005–0.01 and midazolam 0.2	Sevoflurane or isoflurane + CRI for reduction of inhalant requirement	(a) Opioid CRI 　i. Fentanyl 0.012–0.042 　or 　ii. Hydromorphone 0.03 　or 　iii. Remifentanil 0.012–0.042 (b) Lidocaine CRI 1.5–3	(a) Opioid CRIs: 　i. Fentanyl 0.002–0.005 mg/kg/h 　or 　ii. Hydromorphone 0.01 mg/kg/h (b) Lidocaine 1.5 mg/kg/h (c) Intermittent bolus: 　i. Methadone 0.3 IV q 4–6h 　or 　ii. Hydromorphone 0.05–0.1 IV q 4–6h

Note: Lidocaine is contraindicated in cats; alternatively, lidocaine patch can be placed alongside incisions in cats and dogs. Preoxygenate patients. In patients on Anipryl, meperidine is avoided, as are fentanyl and remifentanil.

Morphine is a safe choice that provides appropriate analgesia for invasive procedures. Longer lasting opioids (i.e., hydromorphone or methadone) are used to provide intraoperative analgesia as well. Following IM premedication, patients are watched for respiratory depression. Preoxygenation is recommended. If the patient is cooperative, monitoring equipment such as the Doppler and ECG are placed prior to induction. Induction is accomplished with many options depending on the patient's anesthetic assessment and drug availability. Etomidate results in adrenocortical suppression, although whether this is beneficial is unknown. Inclusion of a benzodiazepine helps reduce the amount of etomidate necessary; however, even small amounts of etomidate will result in adrenocortical suppression (1). Neuroleptic induction may work well for extremely critical patients. Gas inhalants are used to maintain anesthesia. A CRI of opioids (i.e., remifentanil or hydromorphone) and/or lidocaine helps provide analgesia and reduce MAC requirements of the inhalant. Diligent monitoring of ventilation, IBP, acid–base status, and electrolyte analysis are performed throughout the procedure, and possibly into recovery. Patients are extubated only when they are able to adequately ventilate themselves and monitored after extubation for trouble ventilating. Supplemental oxygen is provided to patients that need it.

D. Hypoadrenocorticism (Addison's disease)

A deficiency of glucocorticoid and/or mineralocorticoid from the adrenal glands is called hypoadrenocorticism (Addison's disease). While Addison's disease in most patients is idiopathic, high ACTH levels or adrenal damage secondary to drug therapy (i.e., lysodren) are causes as well. The adrenal gland's outermost layer, the zona glomerulosa, is responsible for secreting mineralocorticoids (aldosterone is one of the most important); when the zona glomerulosa no longer secretes aldosterone, sodium, potassium, chloride, and water regulation becomes dysfunctional. The subsequent layer, the zona fasciculata, is responsible for cortisol production, and when this is impaired, many normal functions of the body (such as metabolism, cardiovascular stability, and response to stress) are compromised.

Addison's disease is often referred to as "the great pretender" because the CS of this disease are vague; they include weakness, lethargy, inappetence, chronic vomiting and diarrhea, pre-renal azotemia (sometimes mistaken for renal failure), and occasionally PU/PD. The patient may be hypotensive with abnormalities related to hyperkalemia (bradycardia and ECG changes including loss of P waves, wide and bizarre QRS waves, and tall, tented T waves). Suspected Addison's disease is confirmed by testing the adrenocortical reserve with ACTH stimulation. Elective procedures in an unmanaged Addisonian patient are postponed until the patient is stabilized.

Even in the managed Addisonian patient, it is recommended that a CBC and chemistry is performed. Common abnormalities on the CBC include absence of stress leukogram—this is unusual for an animal presenting as ill or "not doing right." Anemia is likely present but may be masked by hypovolemia resulting in a relatively normal packed cell volume (PCV). Abnormalities on the chemistry include a host of electrolyte abnormalities, such as hypoglycemia, hyperkalemia with hyponatremia (ratio Na : K <27), hypochloremia, and hypercalcemia, as well as azotemia and acidosis (which are secondary to hypovolemia). A urinalysis may reveal a low USG.

1. Anesthesia concerns/common complications

(a) Addisonian crisis: An Addisonian crisis manifests as life-threatening hypovolemic shock in patients acutely removed from glucocorticoids. Patients must receive large volumes of 0.9% NaCl for resuscitation.

(b) Effective circulating volume: This is the most relevant concern in these patients. Fluid stabilization with 0.9% NaCl is necessary prior to any procedure; aggressiveness of stabilization is based on how well managed the Addisonian patient is. Unstable cases may require up to 90 mL/kg of 0.9% NaCl for the first hour.

(c) Hyperkalemia: Pre-instrumentation, especially an ECG, is warranted if the patient allows. Arrhythmias associated with hyperkalemia are discussed in Chapter 6, as is the treatment.

(d) Hypoglycemia: Hypoglycemic patients may require a 2.5–5% dextrose supplementation.

(e) Hypotension: Obtain a BP measurement prior to induction, as well as a CVP in any unstablized case (a central venous catheter serves many purposes in these patients, including a sampling line, means for measuring CVP, and a port for fluid administration). Hypotension is difficult to manage in these cases, but heavily relies on volume support. IBP measurement is optimal.

(f) Stress: These patients compensate poorly for stress; of all patients, minimizing stress is a top priority in the Addisonian.

(g) Supplementation: Ensure any managed Addisonian has received its corticoid supplementation for the day. Unmanaged cases receive hydrocortisone 2–4 mg/kg IV prior to induction.

2. Anesthetic protocol (see Table 5.6)

These patients usually require lower drug dosages than the standard patient; when possible, use reversible, short-acting drugs. Premedication with an opioid and application of EMLA cream will reduce the stress associated with IV catheterization. A neuroleptic anesthesia premedication/induction will often facilitate intubation. Propofol to effect, with midazolam 0.2 mg/kg to reduce the amount of propofol necessary, is used as well. Etomidate is contraindicated in these patients due to its inhibition of steroidicogenisis. Gas anesthetics are routinely used for anesthesia maintenance. Opioid CRIs are used to reduce the MAC requirement of inhalant anesthetics. Provide MV if necessary; however,

Chapter 5

(d) Hypoventilation: If respiratory muscles are weak, hypoventilation is evident under anesthesia.

(e) Multiorgan involvement: Given the number of organ systems impacted by hyperthyroidism, minimizing time under anesthesia and maintaining adequate tissue perfusion (i.e., preventing hypotension) is critical to success in these patients.

(f) Tachycardia: Patients that are severely hypertensive and tachycardic are stabilized on beta blockers prior to anesthesia; this may also decrease the incidence of arrhythmias.

(g) Hypothermia: In an underweight patient, thermoregulation is difficult due to increased body surface area and use of a non-rebreathing (NRB) system.

(h) Thyroid storm: This complication is life-threatening and is characterized by a rapid release of thyroid hormones into systemic circulation (usually in response to stress). CS include tachycardia and hyperthermia; a patient that experiences this can develop pulmonary edema and decompensate rapidly. While this occurs most commonly postoperatively, it can occur intraoperatively. Treatment involves controlling the symptoms. Cool patient with cool IV fluids and use abdominal lavage for open abdominal procedure. Short-acting beta blockers will control tachycardia (see Chapter 3, "Esmolol" section). Provide supplemental oxygen.

(i) If a subtotal thyroidectomy is performed, damage to the recurrent laryngeal nerves and swelling can contribute to airway obstruction at extubation.

2. Anesthetic protocol

It is important the anesthetist thoroughly understands all systems affected and the level of involvement of each system; all of these conditions are managed. It is the opinion of the author (CM) that premedication with an opioid tends to make most cats euphoric; this may or may not alleviate enough agitation to facilitate IV catheterization, although inclusion of EMLA cream may help in this regard (2). High doses of opioids will result in dysphoria (3, 4). In the case of significantly unmanageable patients, inclusion of dexmedetomidine may render the patient more manageable as well as decrease the HR. Smooth, short-acting induction agents such as propofol given slowly to effect are warranted. The anesthetist includes a benzodiazepine to reduce the amount of propofol. Cats that show cardiac changes are induced with etomidate and a benzodiazepine combination. Anesthetics causing sympathetic stimulation are avoided (i.e., ketamine). Unfortunately, there are very few options to allow for a reduction in MAC in cats, but an opioid CRI will provide analgesia even in light of a vaporizer setting that is not reduced. An ECG is vital to detect arrhythmias, and an arterial line gives continuous information on BP. It is also important to monitor body temperature closely.

F. Hypothyroidism

Hypothyroidism, manifested as a deficiency in thyroid hormone, is one of the most common diseases seen in older dogs. The disease commonly occurs secondary to idiopathic thyroid atrophy, but is also secondary to a lymphocytic thyroiditis. The function of the thyroid gland is to maintain a normal metabolic state, and therefore hypothyroidism results in a decreased metabolic state. Common CS include lethargy, depression, intolerance of cold, and obesity. Cardiovascular changes secondary to hypothyroidism include bradycardia and decreased CO due to decreased myocardial contractility. Decreased metabolic rate makes patients more sensitive to anesthetics, as the drugs are not metabolized as quickly. Common BW abnormalities include a nonregenerative anemia, elevation in cholesterol, and a decrease in total T4. For a full discussion on diagnosis of hypothyroidism utilizing thyroid assays, the reader is referred to other texts.

1. Anesthesia concerns/common complications

(a) Delayed gastric emptying: With the overall slow down in metabolism, the GI tract does not empty in a timely manner. Even with fasting, the anesthetist is prepared for regurgitation.

(b) Drug dosages: Use lower drug doses, drugs "to effect" or reversible, short-acting drugs when possible.

(c) Hypotension: Patients that have not returned to normal T4 levels have multiple cardiovascular issues, but hypotension frequently manifests itself under anesthesia, due to the increased drug sensitivity coupled with an already decreased CO and decrease in intravascular volume. These patients are minimally responsive to traditional management of hypotension with positive inotropes.

(d) Hypothermia: Core temperature is poorly maintained in these patients due to a decrease in metabolism.

(e) Prolonged recovery: Slow drug metabolism and hypothermia both prolong recovery in these patients.

2. Anesthetic protocol

The modifications to a routine anesthesia protocol are dependent on how well a patient's hypothyroid disease is controlled; in patients that are fully stabilized, minimal changes are necessary. However, patients with a degree of unmanaged hypothyroidism will present the anesthetist with some challenges. Lower drug doses are generally given due to the decrease in metabolic rate. Preferentially, the anesthetist selects drugs that are short acting and reversible. Often, only a low dose of an opioid (no sedative) is required for premedication, although this is often combined with anticholinergic to increase HR. Preoxygenation and pre-instrumentation are important for these patients. Ketamine is considered the induction agent of choice, if not otherwise contraindicated, to increase HR and stimulate release of catecholamines. This agent is combined with a benzodiazepine for muscle relaxation. A CRI of ketamine will balance the anesthesia technique.

Chapter 5

Gas inhalants are used but kept as low as possible due to the patient's sensitivity to anesthetic drugs; a short-acting opioid CRI such as remifentanil allows the anesthetist to keep the inhalant levels low. Ephedrine is useful in management of intraoperative hypotension. Close monitoring of the patient is warranted throughout the prolonged recovery period.

G. Pheochromocytoma

Pheochromocytomas are catecholamine-producing adrenal tumors. Often these tumors are found incidentally. Patients frequently have indistinct signs, and it is not until a patient is anesthetized that the ramifications of these tumors come to light. CS include lethargy and weakness, inappetence and weight loss, vomiting, and PU/PD. On PE, panting, pale mucus membranes (secondary to vasoconstriction), tachycardia, and a possibly a fever are present. BW changes include anemia, a stress leukogram, increased liver enzymes (ALP, ALT, AST), azotemia, and electrolyte alterations. If there is a suspicion of an adrenal tumor, a complete workup before anesthesia is indicated.

1. Anesthesia concerns

(a) Hemorrhage: This tumor is highly invasive, and any attempts to remove it may result in massive hemorrhage. It is prudent to cross-match these patients and to ensure that blood products are available.

(b) Hypertension and tachycardia: The secretion of epinephrine (canine) or norepinephrine (feline) results in profound vasoconstriction (via stimulation of the alpha adrenergic receptors), as well as tachycardia. The body compensates for this unrelenting increase in vascular tone by decreasing circulating volume. The only relief is stimulation of the beta receptors by catecholamine release, which results in some small degree of vasodilation. When this patient is anesthetized, the ensuing vasodilation in light of the decreased effective circulating volume may result in cardiovascular collapse. To reduce this possibility, a patient with a pheochromocytoma is administered alpha adrenergic blocking drugs such as phenoxybenzamine prior to its anticipated anesthesia, with the intention of allowing the patient relief of vasoconstriction in order to restore effective circulating volume. This has significantly improved outcome (5); ideally, this is done for 14 days prior to anesthesia. It is inappropriate to administer a beta blocker (i.e., esmolol) to reduce tachycardia if the patient is not alpha blockaded, as the beta blockade may worsen hypertension by blocking the beta smooth muscle effects.

(c) Impaired venous return: This tumor is very invasive into surrounding vasculature, including the vena cava. In addition to possible intraoperative blood loss, there is also concern regarding the degree of impairment on venous return to the heart and compounding compromise to CO.

2. Anesthesia protocol

Premedication with a full mu agonist opioid will provide sedation, preoperative analgesia, and a reduction in the drugs necessary for induction and maintenance of anesthesia.

If a sedative is necessary, benzodiazepines have the least amount of cardiovascular side effects. As much monitoring and support equipment as possible is pre-placed in the awake patient; use things such as EMLA to facilitate arterial line placement and large bore second catheter (central jugular catheter ideal). Minimizing time under anesthesia is critical. The only induction agent contraindicated is ketamine. Due to its very safe profile, a neuroleptic induction with fentanyl and a benzodiazepine is often chosen in these cases. Maintenance with inhalant and a balanced technique with an opioid and lidocaine CRI are suitable. Intraoperatively, in a patient that has received phenoxybenzamine, esmolol is used to address tachycardia, and nitroprusside is administered to reduce hypertension. Blood for transfusion is available if necessary. The patient will continue to have high levels of circulating catecholamines for several days, so the postoperative period is a critical time for these patients; as much monitoring as possible is carried over (i.e., arterial line is left in the patient).

III. Hepatic function diseases

Hepatic function is of critical importance to the anesthetist. The liver is responsible for protein synthesis, drug metabolism, glycogen storage, and production of clotting factors. Certain disease states will alter hepatic leakage enzymes; these disease states must be very advanced to alter hepatic function, however. Therefore, the focus of this section is on disease that impairs hepatic function. Portosystemic shunts (PSS) are prototypical examples of such alteration, but things like end-stage cirrhosis or liver damage secondary to drug (i.e., NSAID) overdose result in similar changes. On PE, the patient with PSS is dull, small in size, and may have a history of seizures. Dullness is often due to hepatic encephalopathy; medical management is warranted prior to anesthesia to resolve the hepatic encephalopathy. On BW, anemia, an increase in ammonia and bile acids, and a decreased blood urea nitrogen (BUN), BG, albumin, and coagulation factors are present. Urinalysis may reveal ammonium biurate crystals, which result in calculi.

A. Anesthetic concerns/common complications

1. Congenital abnormalities

In any animal presenting with a congenital abnormality such as a PSS, a particularly thorough PE is warranted to ensure there are no congenital abnormalities of other body systems, such as the cardiovascular, respiratory, and renal systems.

2. Drug metabolism

Select drugs that are extrahepatically metabolized or short acting/reversible. Drugs dependent on the liver for metabolism have a more profound effect for a longer duration in patients with insufficiencies. Barbiturates are contraindicated. If the patient has neurological hepatic encephalopathy due to a PSS, benzodiazepines are controversial as well. Lidocaine may rapidly accumulate in patients with extreme liver insufficiencies.

3. Hemorrhage (see also Chapter 6, "Hemorrhage" section)

The liver is extremely vascular. Liver biopsies and PSS ligations all have the potential for significant hemorrhage. This is compounded by the concurrent coagulation disorders of PSS. Two IV catheters (one large gauge) are recommended; the patient is blood-typed or cross-matched before surgery.

4. Hypoglycemia

Monitor BG every 45–60 minutes. Supplement fluids with 2.5–5% dextrose as necessary.

5. Hypotension

Maintain hepatic perfusion (i.e., BP). These patients are commonly hypotensive when maintained under general anesthesia. Monitoring IBP is ideal. Hypotension from the anesthetics is compounded by the reduction in oncotic pressure secondary to the decrease in protein production; often, plasma is the fluid of choice for patients where albumin is low (give plasma if albumin is less than 2.2 g/dL). Alternatively, a hetastarch bolus of 2–5 mL/kg is an option. However, hetastarch may worsen coagulopathies. Positive inotropes as well as reducing MAC requirements with fentanyl or remifentanil CRIs will help reduce the hypotension the patient faces.

6. Hypothermia

The small size of these patients and the use of an NRB circuit make thermoregulation very difficult for the anesthetist. Circulating warm water blankets, forced air warming devices, and plastic wrap may reduce the degree of hypothermia, but the patient is unlikely to be normothermic if anesthetized for a procedure involving an open abdomen.

7. Mentation

Patients that present clinically with hepatic encephalopathy are medically managed prior to anesthesia. If the patient is not medically managed, recovery in these patients is markedly prolonged (i.e., >24 hours) and may require MV.

B. Anesthetic protocol (see Table 5.7)

Agents metabolized by the liver (e.g., barbiturates and phenothiazine tranquilizers), highly protein-bound agents (e.g., diazepam and barbiturates), and hepatotoxic agents (e.g., halothane) are avoided because of poor hepatic function and hypoalbuminemia. Use reversible, short-acting, extrahepatically metabolized drugs when possible. An opioid such as morphine +/− an anticholinergic (as necessary) is administered as a premedication. Induction with propofol is smooth and has extrahepatic metabolism. Although isoflurane is considered the inhalant of choice in patients with liver disease, in

Table 5.7 Suggested anesthesia protocol for patients with hepatic disease.

Opioid premedication (mg/kg)	Sedative premedication (mg/kg)	Induction (mg/kg)	Maintenance	Intraoperative analgesia (mg/kg/h)	Postoperative analgesia

(a) Methadone 0.3 IM, 0.2 IV
 	
or
 	
(b) Morphine 0.5 IM +/−
(c) Glycopyrrolate 0.01 IM
	Avoid if possible.	(a) Propofol 2–4 mg/kg IV to effect	Isofluane + CRI for reduction of inhalant requirement	(a) Opioid CRI
				  i. Fentanyl 0.012–0.042
				  or
				  ii. Remifentanil 0.012–0.042
					(a) Fentanyl CRI 0.002–0.005 mg/kg/h or
					(b) Intermittent bolus: Methadone 0.5 IM q 4–6 h

Note: Use of benzodiazepines such as midazolam or diazepam is controversial in patients with hepatic encephalopathy. Preoxygenate patient.

Chapter 5

165

reality, sevoflurane is only marginally more metabolized by the liver and the two are likely comparable (6). Remifentanil, if available, is metabolized by plasma esterases and therefore is not dependent on the liver for termination of effect, making it a suitable choice to reduce inhalant levels and provide analgesia. Check BG periodically throughout surgery and supplement with dextrose as needed. Keeping anesthetic time to a minimum may improve outcome in PSS cases. The patient's mentation and degree of hypothermia will impact recovery, which is likely to be prolonged.

IV. Neurological disorders: Intracranial disease

The calvarium is a fixed space, and as such, there is a balance of tissue and fluid (i.e., blood and cerebral spinal fluid [CSF]) within that space. If one of the proceeding components increases, another must decrease, or an increase in ICP will result. The concern for patients with intracranial disease is the increase of ICP causing herniation of brain tissue, resulting in death. Unfortunately, anesthetizing these patients disrupts the cerebral blood flow (CBF), one of the three major components in the calvarium, and this becomes critical in patients that already have a disrupted balance (i.e., intracranial disease). History helps to identify presence, frequency, and duration of seizures, trauma, or a neurotoxin in cases of intracranial disease of unknown cause. A thorough neurologic exam as part of a complete PE is important in these patients. The following are signs of increased intracranial pressure (ICP): altered levels of consciousness, miosis, mydriasis, differing pupillary sizes, decreased pupillary reflex, papilledema, bradycardia with hypertension (Cushing's reflex), and breathing disturbances. CBC, chemistry and urinalysis may be normal but will help to identify any contributing comorbidities.

A. Anesthetic goal/special considerations

1. Autoregulation

Inhalant anesthesia will disrupt the brain's normal ability to autoregulate its own perfusion pressure; inhalants allow for a dose-dependent increase in CBF, which is detrimental to these patients.

2. Cerebral metabolic rate (CMRO$_2$)

One of the anesthetist's goals for these patients is to reduce CMRO$_2$. In general, anesthesia does this. The anesthetist, however, is careful to avoid dissociatives (ketamine) which may increase the CMRO$_2$. Allowing the patient to become mildly hypothermic (95–96.8° F) will also reduce CMRO$_2$.

3. Glycemic control

Hyperglycemia worsens neurologic outcomes in people, but hypoglycemia was not beneficial either (7). Little information on animals is available in this regard. It is best for the anesthetist to monitor BG, with a target goal of maintaining euglycemia through the use of regular insulin if necessary.

Chapter 5

4. Hypoxemia

PaO_2 below 60 mmHg will trigger more blood flow to the brain in order to maintain perfusion of this tissue. If hypoxemia is present, careful steps are taken to determine the underlying cause and begin treatment (see Chapter 6, "Hypoxemia" section).

5. Cushing's reflex

This reflex occurs in response to significant increases in ICP, and heralds impending brain herniation; as such, it is a life-threatening emergency. It is easily recognized by profound bradycardia and significant hypertension. Any anesthetic utilized is immediately discontinued. Treatment involves reducing ICP by giving 4 mL/kg hypertonic saline over 2–5 minutes or mannitol 0.5–1.5 g/kg over 10–20 minutes. The patient is repositioned with the head raised, and the head is packed with ice packs. Ventilation targets an $EtCO_2$ of 30 mmHg. Any compression around the neck (e.g., positioning devices) is removed. Anticholinergic are avoided as the decrease in HR is the physiologic response to the massive increase in BP. A neurologist may also choose to include corticosteroids in the treatment plan as well and is consulted in this regard.

6. ICP

The target goal of maintaining as normal ICP as possible is achieved through several practical steps:

(a) Avoid vomiting (hydromorphone or morphine IM, $alpha_2$ agonists)
(b) Avoid jugular compression
(c) Avoid coughing or gagging
(d) Avoid fluid overload
(e) Position patient with the head elevated
(f) Seizures: Seizures are detrimental in that they increase $CMRO_2$. Seizures occur at any time during anesthesia and will go unnoticed in the adequately anesthetized patient. In the conscious patient, diazepam 0.5–1 mg/kg IV is used as treatment. Supplemental oxygen is given to seizing patients due to increased cerebral oxygen demands.
(g) Ventilation: Changes in $EtCO_2$ will also impact CBF. As CO_2 increases, so does CBF. Unfortunately, CO_2 too low may result in cerebral ischemia. Maintain $PaCO_2$ between 32 and 38 mmHg and $EtCO_2$ between 30 and 35 mmHg. MV is often necessary for this maneuver.

B. Anesthetic protocol (see Table 5.8)

Sedation is often unnecessary for IV catheterization; however, if IM premedication is needed, avoid drugs that cause vomiting and extreme respiratory depression. Methadone 0.3 mg/kg IM or IV with midazolam 0.2 mg/kg is the authors' preferred premedication (Table 5.8). Preoxygenate all patients prior to induction. The induction drug of choice is propofol given slowly IV to effect, but etomidate will reduce CBF as well. Anesthesia is maintained with a propofol CRI with or without lidocaine CRI. If MV is utilized, an

Table 5.8 Suggested anesthesia protocol for patients with intracranial disease.

Opioid premedication (mg/kg)	Sedative premedication (mg/kg)	Induction (mg/kg)	Maintenance (mg/kg/h)	Intraoperative analgesia (mg/kg)	Postoperative analgesia (mg/kg)
(a) Methadone 0.3 IM, 0.2 IV or (b) Butorphanol 0.3	(a) Midazolam 0.2 IM	(a) Propofol 2–4 mg/kg IV to effect or (b) Etomidate 1–2 IV +/– midazolam 0.1–0.2 IV	Propofol CRI 12–24 + Fentanyl or remifentanil CRI 0.01–0.02 +/–Lidocaine CRI 1.5–3	(a) Intermittent bolus: i. Methadone 0.3 IV q 4–6 h or ii. Fentanyl, 0.005 IV as needed	(a) Intermittent bolus: i. Methadone 0.5 IM q 4–6 h

Note: Continuously observe patient after premedication. Because steroids may be necessary to reduce swelling, avoid NSAIDs. Preoxygenate patients. Lidocaine CRI is contraindicated in cats.

opioid CRI such as remifentanil will reduce the amount of drug necessary to maintain immobility. If it is not possible to maintain the patient solely on an opioid and propofol CRI, inhalants are added but kept at less than 1 MAC. It is ideal to monitor blood gas analysis to ensure $PaCO_2$ is within optimal range (32–38 mmHg); however, it is often more practical to monitor $EtCO_2$. IBP is preferred so a Cushing's reflex is detected early and reliably.

C. Key points

1. Traumatic brain injury

In cases of traumatic brain injury, complications arise both from the direct injury itself and the brain's response to this injury (swelling and inflammation, vasospasm, etc.). These cases are not anesthetized unless absolutely necessary; indeed, a large portion of things that would normally require anesthesia are performed without anesthesia due to the degree of obtundation of the patient. Mannitol is avoided in these patients as they often have a disrupted blood–brain barrier and therefore mannitol may worsen cerebral edema. Oxygen support is provided to these patients.

V. Renal insufficiencies

To the anesthetist, the kidney serves to eliminate fluids and drugs after they are metabolized by the liver; however, the kidney's role physiologically is much broader, and the reader is referred to other texts for a more thorough discussion on the many functions of the kidney. Renal disease is a broad term indicating dysfunction of the kidney; the scope of this dysfunction ranges from renal insufficiency to true renal failure. Indeed, CS and BW changes are slow to manifest because of the kidney's incredible reserve. By the time renal failure is diagnosed, over 75% of the kidney's functional capacity has been lost (when BUN and creatinine begins to elevate). Renal failure results from a number of causes, including toxins, parathyroid disease and concurrent hypercalcemia, infectious disease and sepsis, and idiopathic renal failure. Renal failure is acute or chronic. It is unusual that the anesthetist is presented with a patient in acute renal failure, as this condition is possibly reversible and thus anesthesia (which will worsen renal perfusion) is contraindicated in these patients. This section will focus on chronic renal failure, a permanent and ultimately fatal disease. CS of chronic renal failure includes depression, weight loss, vomiting, and PU/PD. As uremia (a systemic disease resulting from the accumulation of toxins) develops, mentation becomes dull (uremic encephalopathy), and there is an odor to the pet's breath. On PE, kidneys are palpably small, and oral ulcerations are present. On auscultation, cardiac arrhythmias are present in some of these patients. BP is evaluated as well, as hypertension is incredibly common. BW reveals an anemia, elevations in BUN and creatinine, acidosis, hypoproteinemia, hyperamylasemia, electrolyte changes including hypokalemia, hyperphosphatemia, hypocalcemia, hypermagnesemia, and a possible hyperglycemia.

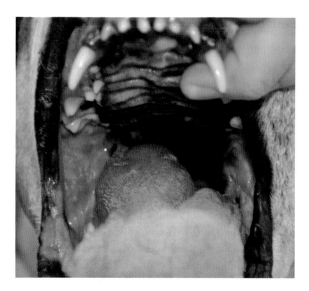

Figure 5.1   Airway obstruction. Courtesy of Anderson da Cuhna.

(b) Obstruction: An obstruction of the airway may manifest preoperatively or postoperatively. In certain patients (i.e., brachycephalic patients), the animal may live its life with an obstruction. However, premedication and sedation worsens this obstruction. Postoperatively, while these patients are recovering, sedation contributes to their inability to maintain a patent airway. Obstruction increases work of breathing, which will eventually exhaust respiratory muscles. Hypoxemia also results from airway obstruction. Preoxygenation is always warranted in these cases.

(c) Securing an airway: Depending on what type of upper airway disease is present, routine intubation is a challenge for the anesthetist (i.e., in the patient with a tumor of the pharyngeal region). If this is suspected prior to anesthesia (usually based on stridorus noises), having a variety of endotracheal (ET) tube sizes, stylets, retrograde intubation equipment (see Table 5.9), and possibly an endoscope may assist the anesthetist in obtaining a difficult airway.

Once the ET tube is placed, presence of $EtCO_2$ is used to verify accurate placement.

2. Anesthesia protocol

The objective of the premedication is to provide enough sedation to minimize restraint for IV catheterization, while avoiding excessive relaxation that may predispose the patient to airway obstruction. Alpha$_2$ agonists are avoided for this reason (e.g., sedation is too profound). An opioid without a sedative is a suitable option in manageable patients. Low doses of acepromazine are beneficial to facilitate IV catheterization. Hydromorphone may increase panting, so alternatively, methadone is often used. Preoxygenate

Table 5.9 Retrograde intubation.

Materials: Clippers, scrub, sterile gloves, 18 g needle, guide wire, ET tubes, laryngoscope

Technique:
1. Clip and prep an area of the skin over the trachea, approximately halfway between the mandible and thoracic inlet. Once the anesthetist is appropriately gloved, ensure the guide wire will fit through the 18-g needle. Another assistant positions the patient and opens its mouth appropriately.
2. Induce the patient.
3. Insert an 18-g needle between tracheal cartilages, directing the needle cranially.
4. Advance the guide wire through the needle; the wire should course cranially and exit between the arytenoids.
5. Advance the wire out of the mouth and place an ET tube on the wire; the anesthetist will need enough length protruding from the mouth so the guide wire exits the connection on the ET tube.
6. Advance the ET tube down the guide wire. When the ET tube is successfully placed, remove the needle and guide wire. Place a light wrap if desired.

---

the patient prior to induction for at least 3 minutes. Apply ECG and other monitoring equipment if patient will allow prior to induction. The goal of induction is rapid airway access. Proper use of a laryngoscope and having several sizes of ET tubes readily available assists with this. Gas inhalants (isoflurane or sevoflurane) are routinely used, although a propofol CRI is suitable in cases where extubation is anticipated. Opioid, ketamine, and lidocaine CRIs decrease MAC and provide analgesia where appropriate. These animals may require MV. Recovery takes place in a quiet location where the patient is continuously monitored for respiratory distress. Respiratory distress is more likely to occur in brachycephalic breeds due to bronchospasm, laryngospasm, airway obstruction by soft palate or swelling laryngeal tissue from traumatic intubation. Corticosteroids are beneficial in treating postoperative complications due to swelling and edema, so NSAIDs are often withheld. Patients are placed in sternal recumbency with head and neck comfortably supported and extended. Leave ET tube in place as long as possible—this may take hours. Only after the patient is strongly protesting, able to lift and support the head independently, and swallow is the ET tube removed. Continue to monitor SpO₂ and respiratory effort. Be prepared with laryngoscope, small ET tube, propofol, and 100% oxygen to re-intubate. In some cases, supplemental oxygen via mask is all that is needed. For extremely prolonged recoveries, reversal of drugs (i.e., opioids) given during procedure is required. Usually, patience and time are the best methods of recovery for brachycephalic breeds.

3. Key points

(a) Brachycephalic syndrome (see Chapter 4): Figure 5.2 shows a brachycephalic patient.

(I) COMPONENTS: Stenosis (narrowing) of the nares, elongated soft palate, hypoplastic trachea, and everted saccules. In addition, these breeds tend to be overweight (making adequate ventilation difficult) and have high vagal tone.

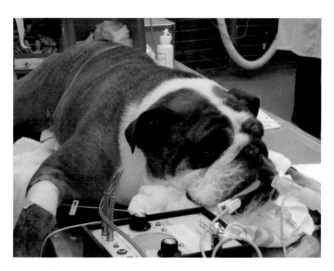

Figure 5.2 Brachycephalic patient. Courtesy of Anderson da Cuhna.

B. Lower airway disease

Lower airway disease encompasses structures below the level of the larynx (i.e., trachea, bronchi and the lungs). Trachea and large bronchial disease compromise the delivery of oxygen to the lungs; this includes diseases such as tracheal collapse or trauma, foreign bodies, and tumors. Gas exchange takes place in the lungs; diseases resulting in V/Q mismatch or diffusion barrier impairment (e.g., pulmonary edema, pneumonia, and asthma) are lower airway diseases that concern the anesthetist, as hypoxemia and increased work of breathing result. As is true for most patients with compromising disease, a complete PE and diagnostic workup are recommended. Diagnostic workup involves radiographs, pulse oximetry, and possible blood gas analysis. Depending on the severity of the disease, the patient may need supplemental oxygen even to complete a PE.

1. Anesthesia concerns/common complications

(a) Bronchodilation: Anticholinergics are simple bronchodilators the anesthetist already has at his or her disposal. Anticholinergics result in smooth muscle relaxation and therefore a degree of bronchodilation. Additionally, bronchodilation is achieved with beta$_2$ agonists, which are administered either aerosolized or intravenously. Albuterol or terbutaline are two routinely used bronchodilators.

(b) Minimize stress: Although this is ideal for all patients, patients with respiratory disease are maximally compensating. Additional stress may result in decompensation and respiratory arrest.

(c) NSAIDs: NSAIDs are avoided (unless directly indicated) in patients with airway disease, as steroids may be necessary to address inflammation that is present or iatrogenically induced.

(d) Elective procedures: All elective procedures are postponed until the lower airway disease is managed, if not cured.

(e) MV: MV reduces the work of breathing, which reduces the respiratory fatigue these animals are experiencing. When setting up the ventilator, it is important to allow for adequate duration of inspiration to maximize time for gas exchange.

(f) Recovery: The patient is allowed to recover where continuous monitoring is possible, and in a quiet, stress-free environment. Sadly, these two requirements are often mutually exclusive. Supplemental oxygen is provided, and the pulse oximeter is continually monitored until the patient maintains a reading of 94–96% or greater without oxygen support.

2. Anesthesia protocol

Premedication includes an opioid and an anticholinergic. While it is prudent to avoid opioids that result in histamine release, opioids as a class decrease tracheal sensitivity, reduce stress, and are antitussive. All patients with respiratory disease are continually observed after administration of premedication. If the animal is tolerant, begin preoxygenation at least 3–5 minutes prior to induction, and throughout the course of induction. If the patient is cooperative, instrumentation is placed prior to induction (i.e., ECG, NIBP, and Doppler). Propofol is the induction agent of choice for a smooth, controlled induction; however, there are no injectable induction drugs specifically contraindicated in these cases. The addition of a benzodiazepine will reduce the amount of propofol necessary. Additional induction agent is kept available to the anesthetist, as is the laryngoscope and spare ET tubes of appropriate size, in case the patient requires re-intubation during recovery. Maintenance of the patient on gas inhalant, $+/-$ opioid CRIs, is common. These patients are not extubated unless absolutely required, and if so, are rapidly re-intubated if pulse oximeter drops below 92%. Specialized monitoring equipment includes spirometry loops for volume loop assessment. Otherwise, monitoring for these patients includes monitoring ventilation and oxygenation closely with SpO_2 and $EtCO_2$ as well as arterial blood gases if possible. Monitoring equipment is left on the patient until the patient is completely recovered and oxygenating well on its own.

Chapter 5

3. Key points

(a) Pulmonary edema: Pulmonary edema in small animal patients is often secondary to cardiovascular disease (i.e., CHF); these patients must have their cardiac disease thoroughly worked up, as well as CHF managed, prior to anesthesia for any elective procedure.

(I) DIURETICS: Diuretics, such as furosemide, reduce circulating volume and therefore reduce the amount of pulmonary edema present. Although the patient may already receive diuretics as part of its maintenance therapy, additional diuretics are occasionally necessary intraoperatively due to changes in volume status subsequent to anesthesia. If the patient is on diuretics such as furosemide already, a blood gas to assess electrolytes (particularly potassium) is warranted prior to anesthesia.

(ii) FLUID THERAPY: Fluid therapy is kept to no more than 5 mL/kg/h, to prevent volume overload from worsening this disease.

(iii) VENTILATION: Intermittent positive pressure ventilation (IPPV) is indicated in these patients, as it might help move fluid out of the tracheobronchial tree as well as recruit compromised alveoli, ultimately increasing lung volume and the area for gas exchange. Sigh breathes (manually administered supramaximal pressures of 25–30 cmH$_2$0 every 4 to 6 breaths) also assist with this recruitment.

(b) Tracheal rupture: Tracheal rupture appears more common in the cat than in the dog, and is often associated with previous intubations with a high pressure, low-volume cuffed ET tube. This, coupled with negligent handling (rotating the cat without disconnecting the animal from the circuit, etc.), may result in a tracheal tear (11). These patients often present with subcutaneous emphysema after an anesthetic procedure. Further diagnostics to rule out a pneumothorax or pneumomediastinum is warranted; in case of pneumothorax, a chest tap is warranted (see Table 6.10).

Often, these patients are medically managed, but if the case is surgical, there are several management steps.

(i) INTUBATION: The level of the tear is important for the anesthetist, who will preferentially intubate past this tear. Unfortunately, this is sometimes difficult in cases of intrathoracic tracheal rupture. The key lesson here is to never intubate beyond the thoracic inlet in your own patients (see Chapter 1).

(ii) MV: Leakage of air from the tracheal rupture will alter respiratory compliance, significantly increasing work of breathing and chance of hypoxemia for these patients. MV reduces the work of breathing for these patients, and offers recruitment options for compromised alveoli.

C. Space-occupying respiratory disease

Air, fluid (e.g., chyle, blood, pus, or transudates) or tissue (see Chapter 4, "Diaphragmatic Hernia" section) accumulation affects the ability of the lungs to expand within the thoracic cavity. Underlying causes include a traumatic event (e.g., hit by car [HBC]), pathology (e.g., cancer or infectious agents), or idiopathic disease. This is also iatrogenically induced in procedures such as thoracoscopy or a thoracotomy (see Chapter 4, "Thoracotomy" section). A thorough PE includes evaluation of respiratory effort and auscultation of the chest for lung sounds; however, in the case of acute respiratory disease, such as HBC, there may not be time to perform such an exam before respiratory arrest ensues. In the case of trauma, if an animal appears to have difficulty oxygenating (pale MMC, increased RR, and obtunded mentation), a thoracentesis ("chest tap") is warranted as the first step with a simple butterfly catheter and large volume syringe (see Table 6.10). It is far better to attempt to tap air off the chest and find none than to try to run diagnostic tests in a patient with a pneumothorax. The chest tap itself will give valuable information (i.e., whether or not a pneumothorax is present). A more thorough auscultation is performed after the tap. A small amount of air may be introduced into the thorax in the event of negative tap; while this is clinically of little consequence, radiographs may reveal this air, and the primary clinician is mislead if he or she is not informed about a tap. BW including a CBC and chemistry, arterial blood gas (when possible), chest/abdominal radiographs, and a thoracic ultrasound are performed to work up the disease in stabilized patients. These diagnostics indicate the type of space-occupying disease present, help rule out possible causes, and quantify the degree of severity. When air or fluid is the cause of the space-occupying disease (e.g., pneumothorax or pyothorax), thoracentesis is performed immediately following diagnosis. Supplemental oxygen is available to the patient at all times.

1. Anesthesia concerns/common complications

(a) Atelectasis: Space occupation results in lung atelectasis and subsequent hypoxemia. Monitoring at minimum includes frequent blood gas analysis (q 30–60 minutes), $EtCO_2$, and SpO_2. IBP, a Doppler and ECG are recommended.

(b) Elective procedures: As with all respiratory diseases, elective procedures are not performed until the underlying disease is addressed and stabilized.

(c) Hypoventilation: Hypoventilation, defined by an increase in CO_2, results from space occupation. Respiratory acidosis is evident as well. In the stable patient prior to anesthesia with gas or fluid present in the chest, a thoracentesis is performed prior to induction of anesthesia (see Table 6.10). Because hypoventilation results from most anesthetics, it is imperative that any gas or fluid is removed. The anesthetist must not allow residual volume to compound anesthetic hypoventilation.

(d) Hypovolemia: Hemothorax will result in hypovolemia and a decrease in effective circulating volume as well as space occupation. In cases of hemothorax, a cross-match or blood type is performed and blood is available.

(e) MV: Defining the underlying etiology in cases of pneumothorax is necessary before MV is safely started. For example, in case of trauma, MV may rupture bullae that are currently stable. Therefore, in cases of trauma, it is best to manually assist ventilation with a second set of hands rather than place the patient on a ventilator. In other cases of space occupation, MV is safe and often necessary. $EtCO_2$ target range is 30–35 mmHg. High peak inspiratory pressure (PIP) (20–25 cmH$_2$O) provides effective ventilation due to the space-occupying disease (i.e., increased resistance).

2. Anesthesia protocol

IV catheterization is usually accomplished without sedation in compromised patients. However, a premedication involving an opioid with minimal respiratory effects (i.e.,

Chapter 5

methadone) in combination with a sedative (i.e., midazolam or low dose of aceproma-zine) is administered IM to facilitate catheterization and reduce stress when necessary, or IV after catheter placement to reduce the amount of induction drug necessary as well as provide preemptive analgesia. The patient is continuously monitored after premedica-tion when respiratory disease exists. All patients are preoxygenated. When possible, prior to the administration of drugs, place monitoring equipment (i.e., ECG, Doppler, NIBP) on the patient. A smooth induction allows quick access to the airway, so assisted manual ventilation is started immediately. Drug selection will depend greatly on the degree of compromise of the patient. In severely compromised patients, the premedication IV may allow intubation (neuroleptic induction). Propofol is the induction agent of choice. Main-tenance with inhalant anesthetics is routine. Often, CRIs are necessary in critical patients to reduce MAC of inhalant as well as provide other benefits (i.e., analgesia). Supporting ventilation is important in these cases. If chest tubes are not present prior to induction, the anesthetist has all equipment needed to tap the chest (see Table 6.9 and Table 6.10) readily available if suspect pneumothorax occurs. Chest tubes, if placed, are left in place for recovery. Check for negative pressure with patient in two positions (i.e., a lateral and sternal recumbency). If negative pressure is not achieved, a vacuum system for continual drainage is necessary. The arterial line is maintained (if possible) for continued blood gas analysis. The patient remains intubated as long as possible; the anesthetist must have the supplies on hand to re-intubate, if necessary. Supplemental oxygen is provided either in an oxygen cage with 40–60% O_2 or via nasal cannulas or face mask (see Chapter 6, "Hypoxemia" section). Try to create a quiet, calm environment during recovery. Provide adequate analgesia.

VII. Other conditions that influence anesthesia

A. Age

Patients that are young or old have different physiology than the average adult patient.

1. Anesthesia concerns/common complications

(a) Anesthetic risk: When assessing a large number of patients, studies indicate age does not increase anesthetic risk in a patient 11 years or younger (12). Breed is likely to play some roll in this, as a Great Dane is unlikely to ever reach 11 years of age, and a toy poodle may live well beyond that.

(b) Inhalant requirement: Inhalant requirement (i.e., MAC) is highest at puberty and steadily declines after that in humans (13). If this is true in dogs, it is likely the geriatric patient has the lowest MAC requirement.

(c) Altered drug disposition: Reduced liver and renal function, due to organ immaturity in the very young and decrease in organ mass in the aged, will result in a reduction in the amount of drug that is metabolized and excreted. In addition to drug metabolism, the liver is responsible for many other important functions, including production of proteins. Hypoalbuminemia is present in both the young and the elderly. Because many of our anesthetic drugs are highly protein-bound, this means there is a higher free fraction of circulating drug, resulting in a greater effect than intended. These factors combine to result in the possibility of relatively overdosing a patient. Reduce drug dosage and use short-acting, reversible drugs (i.e., opioids or benzodiazepines) when possible.

2. Anesthesia protocol

See "Key Points."

3. Key points

(a) Geriatrics: These animals are characterized by those patients that have reached 75% of their expected life span. As patients age, physiologic changes (as listed in Table 5.10) may affect general anesthesia; additionally, concurrent systemic diseases may manifest over time. A thorough preanesthetic exam and history (with a focus on systemic disease and current medications) is evaluated and addressed prior to anesthesia. This includes CBC, chemistry, urinalysis, and ECG.

Table 5.10   Geriatric changes.

Cardiovascular system	Decreased arterial compliance Decreased myocardial compliance Decreased maximal HR Decreased maximal CO Blunted beta adrenergic receptor activity
Respiratory system	Reduced gas exchange efficiency Reduced vital capacity Increased work of breathing Decreased thoracic compliance Decreased lung elasticity Increased closing volume
Nervous system	Altered sympathetic activity and outflow Downregulation of beta adrenergic receptors Decreased parasympathetic activity Decreased central neurotransmitter activity
Renal and hepatic systems	Decreased drug clearance Decreased glomerular filtration rate Decreased capability to handle water and sodium loads
Body composition	Decreased skeletal muscle mass Increased lipid fraction Decreased perfusion and organ blood flow Decreased tissue mass

Chapter 5

2. Anesthetic goals/considerations

(a) Hypothermia: As animals age and become geriatric, unless they have underlying disease (i.e., hypothyroidism), they tend to lose both fat and muscle mass. This decrease in weight often leads to difficulty thermoregulating when anesthetized. Circulating warm water blankets, forced air-warming units, fluid warmers, and warm water bottles are necessary to reduce hypothermia these patients experience under anesthesia.

(b) Patient positioning: Osteoarthritis is an insidious disease occurring in our geriatric patients that, because of its slow progression, owners may not notice in their pets. Tension on joints and pressure points on muscles during anesthesia result in considerable pain postoperatively, so care is taken to pad the patient and position it appropriately.

(c) Physiologic reserve: Physiologic parameters are important due to geriatrics' limited functional reserve of organ systems.

(I) CARDIOVASCULAR: As a patient ages, in addition to decreased organ mass, there is also stiffening of cardiac and vascular tissues, which increases afterload and may manifest as hypertension. A patient's response to catecholamines decreases as well. Age-related cardiovascular structural changes (e.g., mitral and tricuspid regurgitation) occur and progress over time.

(II) NEUROLOGIC: A generalized cerebral atrophy occurs as a patient ages; this manifests itself as an increase in anxiety and possible cognitive dysfunction. Anesthetic drugs (e.g., sedatives) may enhance these behaviors.

(III) RESPIRATORY: As thoracic wall compliance and lung capacity decreases, a decrease in functional lung capacity occurs. These patients are at increased risk for hypoxemia and hypoventilation especially when administered anesthetics.

(IV) RENAL: Renal function is decreased over time due to a decrease in functioning glomeruli and decreased tubular function. This is present in some patients in spite of laboratory changes (see "Renal Disease"); anesthesia goals for geriatric patients include supporting BP to maintain perfusion to the kidney.

(d) Anesthetic protocol (see Table 5.11): Premedication with an opioid, without a sedative, is suitable for many geriatric patients. If a sedative is required and the patient's temperament is appropriate, a benzodiazepine such as midazolam is included in the premedication. While multiple induction agents are suitable in the elderly, titrating the drug to effect is appropriate, as much less drug is necessary in this class of patient. Inclusion of a benzodiazepine, if not administered as part of the premedication, is appropriate to reduce the amount of induction drug. Maintenance with gas anesthesia is suitable, but an opioid CRI is almost always included in an effort to reduce the amount of inhalant necessary. Maintain HR within 25% of baseline rate, and manage hypotension as necessary (see Chapter 6, "Hypotension" section).

Chapter 5

Table 5.11 Suggested anesthesia protocol for patients that are geriatric.

Opioid premedication (mg/kg)	Sedative premedication (mg/kg)	Induction (mg/kg)	Maintenance	Intraoperative analgesia (mg/kg/h)	Postoperative analgesia (mg/kg)

(a) Methadone 0.3IM, 0.2IV
or
(b) Hydromorphone 0.05IM, IV
	(a) Midazolam 0.1IM	(a) Propofol to effect +/– midazolam 0.2
		or
		(b) Etomidate 1–2IV +/– midazolam 0.1–0.2IV
		or
		(c) Fentanyl 0.005–0.01 and midazolam 0.1
			Sevoflurane or Isoflurane + CRI for reduction of inhalant requirement	(a) Opioid CRI
				  i. Fentanyl 0.012–0.042
				  or
				  ii. Remifentanil 0.012–0.042
				(b) Lidocaine CRI 1.5
					(a) Intermittent bolus:
					  i. Methadone 0.3IV q 4–6 h
					  or
					  ii. Hydromorphone 0.05–0.11V q 4–6h

Note: Opioid selection is appropriate for the degree of pain the procedure will involve. See Table 3.12. Preoxygenate patient.

Chapter 5

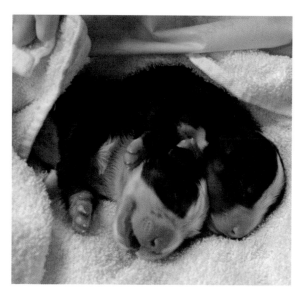

Figure 5.3   Neonate patients. Courtesy of Anderson da Cuhna.

Table 5.12   Neonatal pediatric patients.

Cardiovascular system	Low myocardial contractility
	Low ventricular compliance
	Low cardiac reserve
	CO dependent on HR
	Increased cardiac index
	Poor vasomotor control
Respiratory system	High oxygen consumption
	High minute volume (higher RR)
	Low pulmonary reserve
Renal and hepatic system	Immature glomerular filtration rate
	Inability to metabolize drugs due to immature liver
Body composition	Limited thermoregulation
	Low body fat and muscle ratio
	Hypoalbuminemia
	Low hematocrit
	High total body water content
	Large extracellular fluid compartment
	Fixed and centralized circulating fluid volume
Nervous system	Increased permeability of blood–brain barrier
	Immature sympathetic nervous system

(e) Neonatal and pediatric patient: A dog or cat is considered a neonate in the first six weeks of life. A pediatric patient is 16–20 weeks (4–5 months) of life. Differences impacting neonatal and pediatric anesthesia are listed in Table 5.12. Minimal laboratory tests include PCV, total protein (TP), and BG. Neonates are not fasted. Pediatrics are not fasted longer than 2–4 hours. Do not withhold water.

2. Anesthetic goals/considerations

(a) Blood–brain barrier: The blood–brain barrier is more permeable in young patients, and therefore drugs that cross into the CNS have a more profound effect.

(b) Cardiovascular: CO is highly dependent on HR, as SV is relatively fixed in the young (reminder: CO is equal to HR $\times$ SV). Because SVR is naturally low due to the immature sympathetic system of the young, it is imperative the HR is maintained at or above resting rate. This is usually achieved by the avoidance of drugs such as alpha$_2$ agonists and with the use of anticholinergics.

(c) Hypoglycemia: If a patient's liver has not fully matured, glycogen storage is imperfect. Young patients may have hypoglycemia during an anesthesia procedure. Monitoring of BG and/or supplementation with 2.5–5% dextrose in crystalloid solution is warranted.

(d) Hypothermia: Because these patients have very large body surface area to body mass ratio, they often become hypothermic during a procedure. Minimizing heat loss through the use of bubble wrap over the animal, fluid warmers, circulating warm water blankets, and forced air warming devices is warranted.

(e) Respiratory: Until the bones further calcify, the thorax of these young patients remains very compliant, and at least in the first 6 weeks of life, lungs are still relatively stiff. While this overall results in normal ventilation, anesthesia disrupts this balance. MV is not often warranted in these patients, but the anesthetist may need to hand-ventilate the patient in periods of relatively minimal stimulation.

(f) Venous access: In small patients, IV access is difficult to obtain. Intraosseous (IO) catheters are useful in emergency situations. An 18G or 20G needle works nicely as an IO catheter but require more advanced experience to place and may be difficult to stabilize in place.

4. Anesthetic protocol (see Table 5.13)

Neonates and pediatric patients present challenges to the anesthetist due to their size. Premedication with an opioid, without a sedative, is suitable for most young patients. If a sedative is required and the patient's temperament is appropriate, a benzodiazepine such as midazolam is included in the premedication. Reversal drugs for the premedication are at least calculated if not drawn up. Oxygen is administered for at least 3–5 minutes before induction occurs. Drug dose volumes are often so small that dilutions are necessary to ensure adequate dose delivery. Propofol is carefully titrated to minimize the cardiopulmonary side effects, using the smallest volume syringe suitable (e.g., 1 mL of propofol is drawn up in a 1-mL syringe, *not* a 3-mL syringe). One should pay attention to how much heparinized saline (flush) is given to the patient. Small volumes of just a several milliliters are often the patient's hourly fluid dose. Crystalloid fluid therapy with 2.5–5% dextrose at 10–15 mL/kg/h is recommended. Use a syringe pump for accurate

Table 5.13 Suggested anesthesia protocol for patients that are neonatal or pediatric.

Opioid premedication (mg/kg)	Sedative premedication (mg/kg)	Induction (mg/kg)	Maintenance	Intraoperative analgesia (mg/kg/h)	Postoperative analgesia (mg/kg)
(a) Methadone 0.5 IM or (b) Hydromorphone 0.1 IM	(a) Midazolam 0.2 IM	(a) Propofol 2–4 to effect or (b) Ketamine 5–7	Sevoflurane or isoflurane	(a) Opioid CRI: Remifentanil 0.012–0.042 (b) Local blocks as necessary	(a) Intermittent bolus: i. Methadone 0.3 IV q 4–6 h or ii. Hydromorphone 0.05–0.1 IV q 4–6 h

Note: Glycopyrrolate is included in premedication at 0.01 mg/kg IM.

Table 5.14 Normal vital parameters for neonates and pediatrics.

Vital parameter	Low	High
HR	140 bpm	240 bpm
RR	24 breaths	40 breaths/min
MAP	50–60 mmHg	–
Temperature	100°F	103°F
Glucose	70 mg/dL	160 mg/dL

hourly delivery and monitor BG every 45–60 minutes. Inhalant anesthesia is recommended for procedures of more than 15 minutes. Intubate immediately and use an NRB system. Monitoring of cardiopulmonary function is mandatory. Normal vital parameters for neonates and pediatrics are shown in Table 5.14. Shivering postoperatively increases oxygen consumption requiring supplemental O_2 during the recovery period. Avoid NSAIDs in patients less than 12 weeks of age.

B. Body condition

An animal's body condition score is assigned as part of a routine PE. Body condition score reflects overall health and is also related to anesthetic risk.

1. Anesthesia concerns/common complications

(a) Anesthesia risk: In a recent study examining factors associated with increased anesthetic morbidity and mortality, it was found that underweight canine patients had an increase in anesthetic mortality as compared with their normal weight counterparts (14). Interestingly, both under- *and* overweight felines had an increase in anesthesia-related mortality (15).

(b) Drug dosage: Because fat serves as a depot for our lipid-soluble anesthetic drugs, it is appropriate to calculate a patient's drug dosage based on ideal body weight in obese animals, and actual body weight in underweight animals.

(c) Thermoregulation: Patients at either extreme of body conditions will thermoregulate differently than their normal weight counterparts because of changes in body surface area to mass ratios. Underweight patients will experience a worsened degree of hypothermia. Obese patients are hard to rewarm once hypothermic but are also prone to hyperthermia.

2. Anesthesia protocol

No drugs are specifically contraindicated or indicated; a protocol is selected based on the patient's temperament, signalment, disease process, and anticipated procedure. Temperature is diligently monitored.

Chapter 5

D. Shock/trauma patient

Shock refers to inadequate delivery of oxygen to tissues. There are several forms of shock: hemorrhagic shock, anaphylactic shock, cardiogenic shock, and septic shock, among others. Ultimately, shock is a life-threatening condition requiring immediate intervention, and therefore the anesthetist commonly sees the patient after stabilization. However, in some cases, such as septic shock and hemorrhagic shock, surgical intervention is necessary to address the nidus of the disease. This section will focus on these two forms of shock.

1. Anesthesia concerns/common complications

(a) Decreased effective circulating volume (ECV): A decrease in ECV is due to either true volume loss (hemorrhagic shock) or ineffective circulating volume due to vasodilation (septic shock). In either case, improving ECV is critical. Aggressive volume resuscitation with crystalloids, colloids, and other blood products are indicated to improve BP and perfusion. CRI of positive inotropic agents such as dopamine or dobutamine also improve BP and support myocardial function. Vasopressive agents such as epinephrine, norepinephrine, and phenylephrine are often necessary as well.

(b) Management of underlying disease: Shock is a symptom of a severe underlying disease, rather than a disease itself. In order to resolve, and not just manage shock, the underlying disease is addressed.

(c) Tissue hypoxemia: Tissue hypoxemia results in lactic acidosis (see Chapter 6, "Metabolic Acidosis"); supplemental oxygen may not restore the delivery of oxygenation, but it will improve the concentration of oxygen available.

(d) Circulatory collapse/cardiac arrest: As multiple-organ systems become starved for oxygen and appropriate perfusion, circulatory collapse and cardiac arrest become evident (see Chapter 6, "Cardiac Arrest" section or Appendix C for CPR).

2. Anesthesia protocol

Multiple large gauge IV catheters are placed; no premedication is necessary. Preoxygenate the patient for as long as possible. IV drug administration is preferred as IM injections are compromised due to poor peripheral blood flow. Stabilization with appropriate fluid therapy is ideal before anesthesia. Large volume replacement is indicated (shock doses 50–60 mL/kg in cats, 90 mL/kg in dogs). When patients require anesthesia, drugs are selected based on short duration and reversibility. This makes fentanyl and midazolam the ideal combination as a neuroleptic induction. Prompt placement of the ET tube and inflation of cuff is recommended to guard against aspiration. Either isoflurane or sevoflurane are used; the most important factor is using low vaporizer settings. Supplement with opioid or lidocaine CRIs to maintain a suitable depth and analgesia level. The patient is kept as light as possible to optimize the hemodynamic function. Monitoring is critical and pre-placed to the fullest extent possible. IBP measurement, CVP measurement, and blood gas analysis are indicated, beginning preoperatively and continued into recovery. The patient must recover where 24-hour care and oxygen supplementation is available.

References

1. Preda VA, Sen J, Karavitaki N, Grossman AB. Etomidate in the management of hypercortisolaemia in Cushing's syndrome: a review. Eur J Endocrinol. 2012;167(2):137–43.
2. Wagner KA, Gibbon KJ, Strom TL, Kurian JR, Trepanier LA. Adverse effects of EMLA (lidocaine/prilocaine) cream and efficacy for the placement of jugular catheters in hospitalized cats. J Feline Med Surg. 2006;8(2):141–4.
3. Brosnan R, Pypendop B, Siao K, Stanley S. Effects of remifentanil on measures of anesthetic immobility and analgesia in cats. Am J Vet Res. 2009;70(9):1065–71.
4. Sturtevant F, Drill V. Tranquilizing drugs and morphine-mania in cats. Nature. 1957; 179(4572):1253.
5. Herrera MA, Mehl ML, Kass PH, Pascoe PJ, Feldman EC, Nelson RW. Predictive factors and the effect of phenoxybenzamine on outcome in dogs undergoing adrenalectomy for pheochromocytoma. J Vet Intern Med. 2008;22(6):1333–9.
6. Yuan Z, Liu J, Liang X, Lin D. Serum biochemical indicators of hepatobiliary function in dogs following prolonged anaesthesia with sevoflurane or isoflurane. Vet Anaesth Analg. 2012;39(3):296–300.
7. Atkins JH, Smith DS. A review of perioperative glucose control in the neurosurgical population. J Diabetes Sci Technol. 2009;3(6):1352–64.
8. Muir WW, Gadawski J. Cardiorespiratory effects of low-flow and closed circuit inhalation anesthesia, using sevoflurane delivered with an in-circuit vaporizer and concentrations of compound A. Am J Vet Res. 1998;59(5):603–8.
9. Halpenny M, Markos F, Snow HM, Duggan PF, Gaffney E, O'Connell DP, et al. Effects of prophylactic fenoldopam infusion on renal blood flow and renal tubular function during acute hypovolemia in anesthetized dogs. Crit Care Med. 2001;29(4):855–60.
10. Flournoy W, Wohl J, Albrecht-Schmitt T, Schwartz D. Pharmacologic identification of putative D1 dopamine receptors in feline kidneys. J Vet Pharmacol Ther. 2003;26(4):283–90.
11. Mitchell SL, McCarthy R, Rudloff E, Pernell RT. Tracheal rupture associated with intubation in cats: 20 cases (1996–1998). J Am Vet Med Assoc. 2000;216(10):1592–5.
12. Brodbelt D. Perioperative mortality in small animal anaesthesia. Vet J. 2009;182(2):152–61.
13. Eger EI. Age, minimum alveolar anesthetic concentration, and minimum alveolar anesthetic concentration-awake. Anesth Analg. 2001;93(4):947–53.
14. Brodbelt D, Pfeiffer D, Young L, Wood J. Results of the confidential enquiry into perioperative small animal fatalities regarding risk factors for anesthetic-related death in dogs. J Am Vet Med Assoc. 2008;233(7):1096–104.
15. Brodbelt D, Pfeiffer D, Young L, Wood J. Risk factors for anaesthetic-related death in cats: results from the confidential enquiry into perioperative small animal fatalities (CEPSAF). Br J Anaesth. 2007;99(5):617–23.
16. Erkinaro T, Mäkikallio K, Acharya G, Päkkilä M, Kavasmaa T, Huhta JC, et al. Divergent effects of ephedrine and phenylephrine on cardiovascular hemodynamics of near-term fetal sheep exposed to hypoxemia and maternal hypotension. Acta Anaesthesiol Scand. 2007;51(7): 922–8.

Chapter 5

Chapter 6

Anesthetic complications

Even in patients deemed healthy, anesthesia is not always uneventful. In fact, when broken down by the American Society of Anesthesiologists (ASA) status (see Chapter 1), even patients considered ASA 1–2 have a risk of death of 0.05% (canine) to 0.11% (feline). This equates to roughly 1 in 2000 dogs and 1 in every 875 cats that are healthy enough to assign a low ASA score actually dying within 48 hours of anesthesia. When evaluating patients with higher risk (ASA 3–5), that number jumps significantly to between 1.33% (canine) and 1.4% (feline), or approximately 1 in every 75 dogs and cats that die within 48 hours of anesthesia (1). Given these odds, which are by far worse than human anesthetic risk, it stands to reason that even in the healthy patient, complications occur. This section describes complications encountered during anesthesia and recovery, their potential consequences, causes, and treatments. In the unhealthy patient, complications are expected. However, complications are mitigated when they are anticipated and appropriately addressed. To minimize adverse outcomes during anesthesia, it is recommended that a thorough preanesthetic workup is performed and a trained, experienced member of the veterinary team is dedicated to continuously monitoring anesthesia and recovery (see Chapter 1). It is important to have dedicated monitoring (even in the healthy patient) to help with early recognition of complications. The most common complications experienced during routine procedures include hypotension, hypoventilation, and hypothermia due to anesthesia's physiologically deregulating effects; it is imperative to monitor for these problems during any anesthetic event. Other aspects of the patient and the procedure will determine which complications the anesthetist prepares for.

I. Cardiovascular complications

Arrhythmias frequently present themselves in the anesthetized patient. Often, anesthetic and analgesic drugs, as well as preexisting cardiovascular disease, perpetuate arrhythmias. The use of an ECG to monitor the heart's electrical activity is important in identifying arrhythmias. A Doppler is a helpful tool as well. A systematic approach to ECG evaluation helps to determine which arrhythmia the anesthetist faces (see Table 6.1).

Small Animal Anesthesia Techniques, First Edition. Amanda M. Shelby and Carolyn M. McKune.
© 2014 John Wiley & Sons, Inc. Published 2014 by John Wiley & Sons, Inc.
Companion website: www.wiley.com/go/shelbyanesthesia

Table 6.1   Systematic evaluation of ECG.

Method:
1. What is the HR, and are the atria and ventricles beating at the same rate?
2. Are the atrial and ventricular rhythms regular?
3. What is the relation between the P wave (if present) and the QRS complex?
4. How are the P, QRS, and T waves configured?

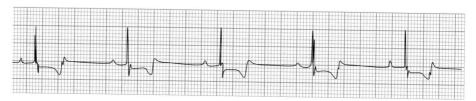

Figure 6.1   Sinus bradycardia in a dog, 25 mm/s, from an automated monitor.

A. Sinus bradycardia

Sinus bradycardia is one of the most common anesthetic complications experienced. This arrhythmia has a normal sinus rhythm (P wave for every QRS, QRS for every P), but the heart rate (HR) is slower than the patient's normal resting HR. Typically, in dogs, this is less than 60 beats per minute (bpm) and 100–120 bpm in cats; however, the patients' normal resting HR is considered when determining bradycardia.

1. Consequences

Sinus bradycardia is not always detrimental. However, bradycardia causes a reduction in cardiac output (CO), resulting in decreased blood pressure (BP) and organ perfusion. Additionally, if left untreated, it may develop into more adverse arrhythmias.

2. Causes

Sinus bradycardia is secondary to drugs used during anesthesia, including opioids, alpha$_2$ agonists, and beta blockers. Other causes include high vagal tone and hypothermia.

3. Treatment

Not all sinus bradycardias require treatment. The anesthetist determines if the bradycardia is affecting CO and perfusion. If CO and perfusion are compromised, immediate treatment is required. Anticholinergics (atropine or glycopyrrolate) are administered IV or IM depending on urgency (see Table 3.1). Atropine is faster acting but has a shorter duration than glycopyrrolate; however, glycopyrrolate produces less tachyarrhythmias. Anticholinergics are given preemptively for patients that are suspected to have high vagal tone (brachycephalic, gastrointestinal [GI] disease, etc.) and when sinus bradycardia is induced by opioids or beta blockers. Opioids are reversed if necessary. Caution is exercised in the administration of anticholinergics to treat sinus bradycardia caused by alpha$_2$ agonists. Reversal of the alpha$_2$ agonist is recommended to alleviate possible vasoconstriction (bearing in mind this will also reverse any analgesia and minimum alveolar concentration (MAC) sparing effects). If the HR does not increase following reversal, an anticholinergic is administered. Patients that are hypothermic (less than 92° F) are unlikely to respond to anticholinergics. Aggressive warming of the patient is warranted.

B. Atrioventricular (AV) block

AV block results from a delay or disruption in the conductance of depolarization between the sinus atrial (SA) node and the atrioventricular (AV) node. First degree AV block is characterized by a prolonged P-R interval; however, all atrial impulses are conducted to the ventricle. Second degree AV block is characterized by intermittent conduction from the SA node to the AV node, resulting in "dropped beats" or absent QRS complexes following P waves (see Figure 6.2). Second degree AV block is further classified into Mobitz Type I and Mobitz Type II based on assessment of the P-R interval. A progressively prolonged P-R interval is characteristic of Mobitz Type I, whereas an unchanged P-R interval but failure of normal conduction is characteristic of Mobitz Type II. Third degree AV block is a complete disassociation between the SA and AV node. The SA node has a consistent yet independent rate from the ventricle, which often conducts an escape rhythm (see Figure 6.2).

1. Consequences

Under anesthesia, any conduction disturbance results in a decrease in CO because the compensatory mechanisms present when a patient is conscious are diminished (if not

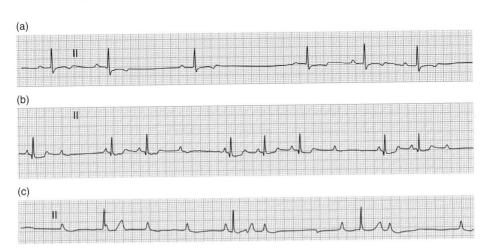

(a)

(b)

(c)

Figure 6.2 (a) First degree AV block, 50 mm/s, 10 mm/mV. (b) Second degree AV block, 50 mm/s, 10 mm/mV. (c) Third degree AV block 50 mm/s, 10 mm/mV in canine patient. Courtesy of Jorge L. Vila.

Chapter 6

then filtered by the AV node. Atrial flutter has a characteristic "saw tooth" baseline appearance of F waves. Atrial fibrillation has no distinguishable P waves, is irregularly irregular, and has a "wavy" baseline (see Figure 6.4b).

1. Consequences

Atrial flutter and fibrillation have some adverse outcomes, including decreased CO, stroke volume (SV), and perfusion, and sudden death (3).

2. Causes

The cause of atrial fibrillation and flutter in a patient may be unknown, but ruling out congestive heart failure (CHF), dilated cardiomyopathy (DCM), and digoxin toxicity is warranted with a thorough cardiac workup.

3. Treatment

If there is an underlying cause for the arrhythmia, it is prudent to address and resolve this prior to anesthesia. If the arrhythmia manifests itself under anesthesia, the HR and hemodynamic consequences will help to determine the need for intervention. If rate control is necessary, esmolol is a selective ultrashort acting beta$_1$ blocker metabolized by plasma esterases and thus has a short half-life. A bolus dose of 0.05–0.1 mg/kg is administered followed by a CRI of 6–24 mg/kg/h, if necessary. Cardio-conversion using a defibrillator is useful when atrial fibrillation is unresponsive to pharmacologic intervention.

E. Ventricular arrhythmias

The ventricles are capable of generating impulses to pace the heart, although this rate is much slower (40–60 bpm) than the rhythm generated by the SA node, as it does not use the normal conduction pathway but rather conducts from cell to cell. Simple ventricular premature complexes (VPCs) result in a wide, bizarre appearance to the QRS, with no P waves (see Figure 6.5b). VPCs are classified as uniform (similar in appearance) or multiform (varying in appearance). A ventricular rhythm with a rate above 150–180 bpm in dogs or 220 bpm in cats is classified as ventricular tachycardia (VT, see Figure 6.5a). Accelerated idioventricular rhythm (AIVR) is a ventricular rhythm with a rate between a normal sinus rate and VT (usually 100–140 bpm). Distinguishing between the two is important because VT may respond to lidocaine, whereas AIVR will not. Sustained VT lasts longer than 30 seconds, whereas nonsustained VT is less than 30 seconds, and thus may not require treatment.

1. Consequences

Runs of VPCs and sustainable VT result in a decrease in ventricular filling time, leading to a decrease in SV and CO. This compromises perfusion, leading to tissue hypoxia,

Chapter 6

(a)

(b)

(c)

(d)

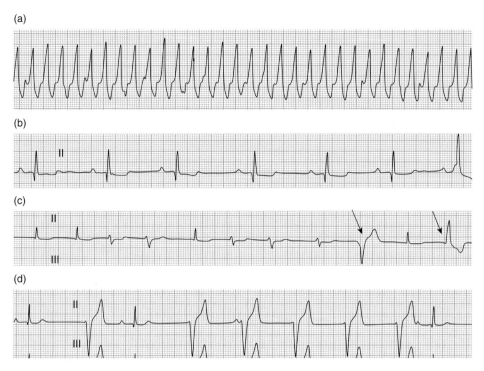

Figure 6.5 (a) VT 50 mm/s, 10 mm/mV. (b) Uniform VPCs 50 mm/s, 10 mm/mV. (c) Multiform VPCs (large arrow) 50 mm/s, 5 mm/mV. (d) AIVR 50 mm/s, 5 mm/mV. Courtesy of Jorge L. Vila.

Chapter 6

lactic acidosis, myocardial hypoxia, and additional cardiac arrhythmias. Sudden death may also result from sustained VT. Multiform VPCs and fast sustainable VT may deteriorate into ventricular fibrillation (VF), a life-threatening emergency.

2. Causes

Hypoxemia, electrolyte abnormalities (hypokalemia, hypomagnesemia, hypocalcemia), acid–base imbalances, pain, and sympathetic stimulation are leading causes of VPCs and VT under anesthesia. Primary cardiac disease, such as myocarditis, endocarditis, and cardiomyopathy may result in ventricular arrhythmias. Ventricular arrhythmias might also occur in patients with certain systemic diseases, such as splenic masses or GDV.

3. Treatment

The first step for most complications is to identify and correct any contributing cause. For example, VT or runs of VPCs from hypoxemia usually resolve if the patient receives supplemental oxygenation. AIVR or the occasional uniform VPC rarely requires treatment. VPCs only require treatment if they meet the certain criteria (see Table 6.2).

Table 6.2   Criteria for determining treatment of VPCs.

- Multiform in appearance
- HR is greater than 160 bpm
- Runs of VPCs occur (more than 30 in an hour)
- There is compromise to the rest of the hemodynamic system (such as low BP when VPCs occur)
- R on T phenomenon occurs.

Table 6.3   Treatment of ventricular rhythms.

| AIVR | VT, multiform or runs of VPCs | | VF or unresponsive/ sustained VT |
	Dogs	**Cats(6)**	
No treatment may be necessary	Lidocaine 1–2 mg/ kg IV followed by 3–6 mg/kg/h CRI or Procainamide 5–10 mg/kg IV followed by CRI 1.5–3 mg/kg/h CRI	Lidocaine 0.25– 0.5 mg/kg IV slowly; repeat up to twice more as needed or Esmolol 0.2–0.5 mg/ kg IV, CRI 1.5–12 mg/kg/h or Propranolol 0.02 mg/ kg slow IV; dose is repeated up to four times	Defibrillation: External 2–4 J/kg Internal 0.2–0.4 J/kg

Indeed, treatment of VPCs without the above criteria is often unsuccessful, because lidocaine (our first line of treatment for ventricular tachyarrhythmias other than ventricular flutter or fibrillation) relies on the presence of abnormal Na^+ channels to work effectively. Recommended treatments of ventricular rhythms are listed in Table 6.3.

F. Cardiac arrest rhythms: Asystole, pulseless electrical activity (PEA), and ventricular fibrillation (VF)

Cardiac arrest rhythms are terminal arrhythmias. Asystole, classically known as a "flat line," indicates there is no electrical activity occurring in the heart. PEA occurs when an ECG tracing is present—and may even look somewhat normal—but on palpation, there is no pulse present. In VF, there is no electrical organization to the heart creating a chaotic ECG (see Figure 6.6). Coarse VF will deteriorate into fine VF; however, coarse fibrillation responds better to electrical defibrillation. Therefore, rapid recognition and treatment is crucial to a successful intervention.

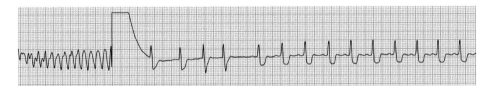

Figure 6.6 VF converted to ventricular rhythm following external defibrillation 25 mm/s. Courtesy of Jorge L. Vila.

1. Consequences

There is no mechanical function of the heart, and thus no circulation or perfusion to any organ, with all three rhythms.

2. Causes

Asystole and PEA have numerous causes, and occur without warning even in healthy patients under anesthesia. Heart disease (such as DCM), acid–base and electrolyte abnormalities, and sepsis are leading causes of VF.

3. Treatment

When perfusion to the body ceases, the brain no longer receives oxygen. Thus, immediate recognition and treatment (i.e., CPR) are critical components not only for a successful return to spontaneous circulation, but to discharging the patient. If asystole or PEA occurs, immediately palpate for a pulse at the site of a large artery (e.g., femoral artery). If no pulse is present, high quality CPR is implemented immediately (see Appendix C). Additionally, life-saving treatment for VF is electrical defibrillation (4). However, few veterinarians leave a defibrillator readily available and charged. Therefore, it is most practical if CPR is initiated immediately with high quality cardiac compressions, while the defibrillator is positioned and charged. It is important to understand that the action of the defibrillator is to stop electrical fibrillation of the heart so hopefully normal electrical conduction returns. It is the current recommendation in humans receiving defibrillation to deliver one large shock rather than incrementally increasing the dose delivered; this is because it is important to minimize the time between interruptions of chest compressions (5). Dose for external defibrillation is 2–4 J/kg or 0.2–0.4 J/kg internally. An immediate return to chest compressions is imperative to oxygenate the myocardium and increase success of resuscitation.

G. Isorhythmic dissociation

This conduction disturbance in the cat is often observed under anesthesia (6). Fortunately, it is rarely associated with any disease. The arrhythmia is characterized by a P and QRS which are unassociated, so one will observe the P wave "wandering" back and forth through the preceding or following QRS. The rate of the atria and ventricle are the same.

Chapter 6

1. Consequences

There are no pathologic consequences of this arrhythmia.

2. Causes

While this arrhythmia commonly manifests under anesthesia, it occurs in the awake feline as well. A definitive cause is unknown.

3. Treatment

This arrhythmia is benign and requires no treatment. There is some suggestion that increasing sinus rate by the use of anticholinergic may correct this.

II. Blood pressure

A. Hypertension

Hypertension is defined as a mean arterial pressure (MAP) over 100 mmHg, or in cases where a MAP is not obtained (i.e., when using only a Doppler and sphygmomanometer), a systolic arterial pressure (SAP) over 160 mmHg. Hypertension is rarely seen under anesthesia due the vasodilatory effect of most inhalant anesthetics. It is important to identify if the patient has preexisting hypertension, in order to work up the underlying cause.

1. Consequences

Prolonged hypertension damages many vital organs, such as the kidney and brain. High BP does not necessarily ensure improved perfusion. Hypertension as a result of increased SVR may cause states of decreased perfusion and tissue hypoxia.

2. Causes

Systemic diseases including renal disease, diabetes mellitus, intracranial diseases with a Cushing's reflex (see Chapter 5, "Neurological Disorders: Intracranial Disease" section), hyperthyroidism, hyperadrenocorticism (Cushing's disease), and pheochromocytomas, all result in hypertension. Hypertension occurring under anesthesia in a previously normotensive patient requires two primary rule outs: a light plane of anesthesia or response to noxious stimuli.

3. Treatment

IBP monitoring is recommended (see Chapter 2) to ensure accuracy of therapeutic interventions. Management of, or at the very least awareness of, diseases known to increase BP in a patient prior to anesthesia is crucial to understanding the management of hyper-

Table 6.4   Treatment options for hypertension.

1. Increase gas inhalant
2. Administer low dose of vasodilator such as 0.005–0.01 mg/kg acepromazine IV
3. Nitroprusside CRI 0.006–0.3 mg/kg/h

Note: One should use nitroprusside with extreme caution and only if necessary. See Chapter 3, "Nitroprusside" section.

tension during anesthesia. If hypertension persists from an underlying disease, and becomes severe, treatment may be necessary (see Table 6.4). If one is unsure whether a preexisting condition exists, it is helpful to watch for trends in BP. Patients that are hypertensive from a preexisting disease are usually consistently hypertensive. Using good technique to assess anesthetic depth (see Chapter 1) will allow the anesthetist to adjust the anesthetic plane accordingly. If the anesthetic depth is adequate, no preexisting disease exists, and the BP is still increased, noxious stimuli are addressed. Analgesia in the dog is provided with the use of either a bolus or CRI of opioids, local anesthetics, or an *N*-methyl-D-aspartate (NMDA) antagonist; or, if the patient is already receiving a CRI, the dosage is increased or something more potent is added. See "Noxious Stimuli" for information on the cat. Chapter 8 details regional analgesic techniques that are also beneficial for prevention of nociception.

B. Hypotension

Hypotension is one of the three most common complications experienced during anesthesia (with the others being hypoventilation and hypothermia) (7). It is defined as a MAP less than 60 mmHg; in cases were MAP is not evaluated (i.e., when using only a Doppler and sphygmomanometer), a SAP less than 90 mmHg. Perfusion to the body is dependent on oxygen content of the blood (see "Hypoxemia") and CO. CO is seldom measured in routine anesthesia cases; gold standards for CO measurement (i.e., dilutional techniques) require invasive equipment (i.e., pulmonary arterial catheter). Instead, knowing that CO is defined by HR, contractility, preload, and afterload, veterinarians often choose to measure a more readily available means of hemodynamic evaluation: BP, which gives information about afterload. It is important, however, that the anesthetist keep the "big picture" in mind—that during anesthesia we are ultimately striving for perfusion of organs, and BP evaluation is only one (albeit very important) part of the puzzle (see Figure 6.7).

1. Consequences

Hypotension results in decreased perfusion to vital organs (heart, brain, kidneys, skeletal muscle, etc.). This may lead to tissue hypoxemia, anaerobic metabolism, lactic acidosis, and organ damage. The kidneys are highly susceptible to this kind of damage, especially given the confounding nature of additional drugs administered around the perioperative period for patient comfort (e.g., NSAIDs).

Chapter 6

Table 6.6 Maximum blood loss estimations.

2 × 2 sponge/gauze	5 mL
4 × 4 sponge/gauze	10 mL
Laparotomy sponge	100 mL
Suction jar	See Equation 6.1

Note: These are estimations with sponges completely soaked. Weighing soiled sponges and subtracting weight of unsoiled is more accurate at estimating blood loss.

a normovolemic patient for a dog is 80–90 mL/kg or 8% of total body weight and 50–60 mL/kg or 6% of total body weight in the cat. The PCV of the patient may not reflect the total blood loss the patient has experienced. As well, a decrease in total proteins may result from dilution secondary to fluid therapy. Blood loss estimation is accomplished by evaluation of soaked gauze squares, lap sponges, and suction collection jars. Estimations are made by adding the number of soaked sponges following assumptions in Table 6.6 or more accurately by weighing the sponges and subtracting the weight of unsoiled sponges (1 g = 1 mL of blood).

$$\frac{\text{PCV of Suction Jar}}{\text{Pre-op PCV of Patient}} \times \text{Volume of Suction Jar} = \text{estimated mL of blood in suction jar}$$

(6.1)

1. Consequences

Intraoperative blood loss leads to reduced preload, decreased CO, decreased perfusion, and hypotension. Excessive blood loss may result in lactic acidosis and cardiovascular collapse.

2. Causes

Intraoperative hemorrhage results from unidentified source of bleeding, iatrogenic causes of hemorrhage, low platelet counts, coagulopathies, or toxicities affecting coagulation.

3. Treatment

If blood loss exceeds 20% of total blood volume or PCV falls below 20%, a transfusion is indicated. Whole blood (WB) is ideal; however, packed red blood cells (pRBCs) with fresh frozen plasma (FFP) are alternatives. The goal is to maintain adequate blood volume to provide adequate oxygen delivery to tissues. WB replaces deficit at a volume of 1 : 1. When delivering blood products in a nonemergent situation, start with a slow rate of 1–3 mL/kg/h for the first 15 minutes and evaluate patient for a transfusion reaction. Signs of an immediate transfusion reaction include hypotension, tachycardia, hives, and increased temperature. It is important to note these signs may be masked in the anesthetized patient. If no reaction is appreciated, the transfusion rate is adjusted to the patient's need. If a transfusion reaction is evident, discontinue the transfusion, and give diphenhydramine at 1 mg/kg IV. Blood products containing citrate as an anticoagulant are not administered with fluids that contain calcium (such as lactated Ringer's solution [LRS]), sodium bicarbonate, or positive inotropes.

III. Respiratory complications

A. Hyperventilation (hypocapnia)

Hyperventilation, or hypocapnia, is defined by $EtCO_2$ or $PaCO_2$ levels below normal range (less than 35 mmHg). If the anesthetist believes the patient is truly hypocapnic, an arterial blood gas sample is collected to evaluate $PaCO_2$.

1. Consequences

Brief episodes of hyperventilation or periods of low CO_2 are not detrimental. Prolonged hypocapnia results in respiratory alkalosis and decreased cerebral perfusion; this results in localized ischemic damage to areas of the brain. The brain will also begin to reset its own baseline CO_2 level when exposed to prolonged periods of hypoventilation (11).

2. Causes

The most common cause of hyperventilation is aggressive MV. Other causes include neurological disease, trauma, pain, noxious stimuli, or compensatory respiratory alkalosis. Hypoxemic patients may compensate by increasing respiratory rate (RR), thus sacrificing CO_2 to improve oxygenation.

3. Treatment

Treatment is focused on the underlying cause for hyperventilation; collection of an arterial blood gas guides therapy and helps with assessment of treatment. Adjustment of ventilation is required if hyperventilation is iatrogenic. If the patient is hyperventilating due to noxious stimuli during a surgical procedure, drugs to provide analgesia are indicated. When hyperventilation is secondary to a metabolic acidosis, the primary acid–base abnormality is corrected. Treatment for the hypoxemic patient is based on the cause of hypoxemia (see "Hypoxemia"). If the primary cause is not determined and treated, the patient can relapse or decompensate in recovery.

B. Hypoventilation (hypercapnia)

Hypoventilation is one of the three most common complications experienced during anesthesia (with the others being hypotension and hypothermia). Hypoventilation (hypercapnia) is present when the $PaCO_2$ is greater than 45 mmHg. Alveolar ventilation is defined in Equation 6.2.

$$V_A = (V_t - V_d) \times f \qquad (6.2)$$

Equation 6.2 Alveolar ventilation equation. V_A is alveolar ventilation, V_t is tidal volume, V_d is dead space, and f is frequency (RR).

Under general anesthesia, when the patient is intubated, V_d is fixed. Therefore, V_A is dependent on V_T and RR. In cases of hypoventilation, adjustments are made to V_T and RR.

1. Consequences

Mild increases in CO_2 levels are of little consequence in the healthy patient. As CO_2 increases, respiratory acidosis becomes evident, although the long-term impact of this is likely of little consequence, when the recovered patient resumes normal ventilation. As CO_2 levels exceed 95 mmHg, CO_2 may induce anesthesia, suggesting this level of CO_2 is certainly unacceptable. In patients with neurologic disease, hypoventilation results in increased intracranial pressure (ICP); if there is space occupying disease (e.g., a brain tumor) or intracranial hemorrhage, a brain herniation may result. CO_2 is carefully controlled in these patients. For patients with potential for a sudden increase in ICP, hyperventilation to maintain $PaCO_2$ levels near 32–35 mmHg may be beneficial until the ICP issue is directly treated (see Chapter 5, "Neurological Disorders: Intracranial Disease" section).

2. Causes

Typically, hypoventilation results from dose-dependent respiratory depressants (inhalant anesthetics) and worsens with a deep plane of anesthesia. Although rare, malignant hyperthermia (MH) will present itself as an increasing temperature and $EtCO_2$, and is a life-threatening condition. Neurological disease may affect the chemoreceptor's sensitivity to CO_2 and the respiratory muscle's mechanical function causing hypercapnia. Tight bandages restricting inspiratory efforts may also cause increase in CO_2. A rise in CO_2 is evident in cases of pneumothorax (with a concurrent decline in oxygenation). A rise in $PaCO_2$ without a rise in $EtCO_2$ suggests CO_2 is unable to diffuse out of blood efficiently; pulmonary thromboembolism (PTE) will lead to such a discrepancy (see "Pulmonary Thromboembolism").

3. Treatment

Identification of the cause of hypoventilation is key for treatment. RR, capnography, minute volume, and V_T are parameters used to monitor ventilation. Reducing excessive dead space (small or no "Y" piece for small patients) is helpful in minimizing hypoventilation. Check the patient's anesthetic plane and decrease the depth of anesthesia if possible. Supporting ventilation in the anesthetized patient is initiated by manual or MV (see Chapter 2). Reverse drugs that may cause respiratory depression (e.g., opioids), if hypoventilation is severe, especially during the recovery period. If there is a restrictive bandage, remove it until the patient is recovered and it can be loosely reapplied. If MH is the cause, treatment with dantrolene is indicated. Cases of PTE require extensive interventions (see "Pulmonary Thromboembolism").

C. Hypoxemia/inappropriate P:F ratio

Hypoxemia is defined as a PaO_2 less than 60 mmHg. PaO_2 is evaluated from an arterial blood sample, analyzed with blood gas analysis. If lung function is normal, PaO_2 is approximately four to five times the fraction of inspired oxygen (FiO_2). For example, in a patient breathing room air ($FiO_2 = 21\%$ O_2), PaO_2 should equal approximately 100 mmHg. If a patient is anesthetized and breathing 100% oxygen, PaO_2 equals approximately 500 mmHg. The ratio of PaO_2 to FiO_2 is referred to as the P:F ratio; as previously stated, normal P:F ratio is 5:1. A change in this ratio to less than 5:1 is important because of its impacts in recovery, when the patient returns to room air (21% O_2). For example, if a patient has severely compromised lung function with a PaO_2 of 100 mmHg when breathing 100% oxygen, that patient's P:F ratio is 1:1. This patient, while not currently hypoxemic (because the PaO_2 is not less than 60 mmHg), has a severely inappropriate P:F ratio. When that patient moves into recovery, 100% oxygen is discontinued, and 21% room air is breathed while the P:F ratio is unchanged; PaO_2 will fall to 21 mmHg—a severe and life-threatening hypoxemia. If blood gas analysis is unavailable, a pulse oximeter provides valuable information on oxygenation for patients' breathing room air.

As one can see from Figure 6.8, a pulse oximeter is of limited use in patients with normal lung function on 100% oxygen (i.e., under anesthesia); a patient must have

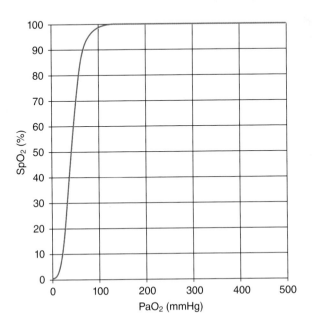

Figure 6.8   Oxygen hemoglobin desaturation curve.

severely compromised lung function before the pulse oximeter will read less than 98–100%. Even the previous example will have a PaO_2 of 100 mmHg and, thus, a pulse oximeter reading of 98–100% while on 100% oxygen.

1. Consequences

Inadequate oxygenation leads to tissue hypoxemia, lactic acidosis, and ultimately organ failure. Arrhythmias such as VPCs and VT followed by VF become evident if perfusion to the heart is compromised; organs like the brain and kidney are sensitive to reduced perfusion, and often this compromise is not detected until the postoperative period.

2. Causes

The causes of hypoxemia fall into one of five categories:

(a) Decreased FiO_2 (unlikely in anesthetized patients breathing an FiO_2 of 100%)
(b) Diffusion impairment (such as chronic fibrosis of the lungs or severe pulmonary edema)
(c) Right to left shunt (such as a reverse PDA)
(d) Hypoventilation (a common cause in patients breathing room air, but uncommon cause for hypoxemia in anesthetized patients with an FiO_2 of 100%)
(e) V/Q mismatch (the most common cause of hypoxemia under anesthesia)

Patients with diaphragmatic hernias, pneumothorax, foreign body (FB) airway obstructions, asthma, pneumonia, pleural effusion, large abdominal masses, ascites, or free fluid in the abdomen are at a high risk for hypoxemia.

3. Treatment

If the patient is hypoxemic or has increased respiratory effort prior to induction, preoxygenation will prolong the time before a patient desaturates (12). In the anesthetized patient, if the PaO_2 is less than expected (even if above 60 mmHg), the abnormality resulting in the low PaO_2 is addressed. For example, in cases of low FiO_2 (e.g., a patient receiving nitrous oxide), FiO_2 is increased. If the patient is recovering from anesthesia, supplemental oxygen options include placement in an oxygen cage or nasal oxygen cannulas for increased FiO_2. If diffusion impairment occurs because of a treatable cause, treatment is instituted; for example, evidence of pulmonary edema warrants the use of furosemide. While the primary indication for MV is hypoventilation, there are several maneuvers with MV that will improve oxygenation. First of all, it is imperative that the patient receives an adequate V_T for each breath. Increasing the I:E ratio allows a long duration of inspiration for oxygen exchange to occur; however, I:E ratio should not exceed 1:2, as that will not allow enough time for expiration to efficiently occur. A "sigh" breath is a recruitment maneuver intended to prevent collapse of marginally inflated alveoli. To deliver a sigh breath, one breath of every four to five breaths is delivered at a high peak inspiratory pressure (PIP) (25–$30 cmH_2O$). The use of peak end-expiratory

Table 6.7 Treatment of hypoxemia.

1. **Preoxygenate** with 100% oxygen for a minimum of 5 min up to point of intubation.
2. Initiate assisted ventilation[a] immediately.
3. Ensure adequate tidal volume (increase I:E ratio) and respiratory rate.
4. Administer sigh breath (PIP 25–30 cmH$_2$O) every 4–5 breaths.
5. Add PEEP valve.
6. Administer albuterol.
7. When the above fail: Maximize perfusion (positive inotrope for CO, appropriate fluid, or blood product therapy).

[a]See Chapter 2 for how to set up and ventilate using a mechanical ventilator.

Table 6.8 Supplemental oxygen methods.

Method of O$_2$ supplementation	O$_2$ Flow rate	Maximum FiO$_2$ (%)
Flow-by	2–3 L/min	20–40%
Oxygen mask	2–5 L/min	40%
Oxygen cage	Varies by cage size	40–60%
Nasal cannula	50–150 mL/kg/min	30–70%
Endotracheal intubation	200–300 mL/kg/min on NRB system, 20–30 mL/kg/min RB system	100%

Chapter 6

pressure (PEEP) will not improve oxygen content, but it may prevent worsening P:F ratios by preventing marginal alveoli from collapsing. PEEP valves come in different sizes, typically 5, 7.5, and 10 cmH$_2$O. Large PIP and PEEP valves will decrease CO by decreasing preload secondary to increased and sustained positive pressure in the chest. Benefits are compared to risks when deciding to use these tactics to reduce the V/Q mismatch. The use of an inhaled bronchodilator (i.e., albuterol) may also improve oxygen exchange in the lungs; contraindications include the presence of tachycardia, which may worsen secondary to the use of a bronchodilator. In cases where in spite of all attempts to improve oxygenation there is no improvement in PaO$_2$, the anesthetist's efforts move to improving perfusion by focusing on CO and maintaining normal hemodynamics while the procedure is rapidly concluded.

D. Pulmonary thromboembolism (PTE)

A PTE is an obstruction in the lung's vasculature, thus severely reducing or eliminating perfusion to the section of lung tissue that would normally be perfused. This is the most severe form of V/Q mismatch in that there is little to no perfusion to an area of ventilation. This is identified under anesthesia by a sudden and drastic drop in EtCO$_2$, and possible desaturation of the patient (drop in SpO$_2$). Blood gas analysis demonstrates a large gradient between $PaCO_2$ and $EtCO_2$. A decrease in PaO_2 will also be present if compared with a pre-thromboembolism.

1. Consequences

The anesthetist will struggle with hypoxemia and possibly bradycardia (if emboli lodge in the coronary vasculature). Respiratory arrest is a possible consequence of a PTE. A thrombotic patient likely has more systemic problems than the anesthetist may appreciate, in that it is unlikely the lung is the only organ affected. For example, if a thrombus reached the brain, neurologic signs may not be evident until recovery. Ultimately, recovery is complicated as the patient may require MV for support while the thromboembolic disease is addressed.

2. Causes

Patients that are hypercoagulable, such as those with Cushing's disease, septicemia, or heartworm disease, are predisposed. There is some evidence that laparoscopic procedures may result in air emboli to the lungs (13).

3. Treatment

Unfortunately, treatment is limited. Supportive ventilation and diligent monitoring of blood gases are instituted. Treatment of side effects is warranted. Anticholinergics cause bronchodilation (14) as well as increase HR if patient becomes bradycardic. Very few therapies, however, will eliminate an embolism once it is formed and thus, recovery maneuvers are supportive rather than curative.

E. Pneumothorax

A pneumothorax occurs when air enters the pleural space and reduces lung volume due to a loss of negative pressure. In the dog, there is no functional communication between sides of the thorax via the mediastinum, meaning pneumothorax on one side does not appear to affect the other (15); it appears this is true for the cat as well. Under anesthesia, a spontaneous pneumothorax presents itself as increased resistance during inspiration, decrease in the SpO_2, increase in RR, and initial decrease in $EtCO_2$. If the patient is on a ventilator, the V_T will decrease significantly while the PIP will drastically increase. A blood gas analysis will demonstrate an inappropriate P:F ratio (see Chapter 6, "Hypoxemia" section) or hypoxic PaO_2, a V/Q mismatch, and an increase in $EtCO_2$.

1. Consequences

A pneumothorax results in hypoxemia and hypoventilation by limiting lung expansion, reducing compliance, and increasing resistance to ventilation. A severe pneumothorax may result in respiratory distress or arrest.

Chapter 6

2. Causes

Iatrogenic causes of pneumothorax include any thoracoscopic or thoracotomy procedures; these intentional pneumothoraxes must be managed the same way postoperatively as a spontaneous pneumothorax. Trauma and ruptured bullae are leading causes of spontaneous pneumothorax. Additionally, pneumothorax is caused by extreme overinflation of the lung such that occurs when the pop-off valve is left closed or overly aggressive ventilation is used. The anesthetist must exercise caution when ventilating a patient with potential trauma to the thoracic cavity, such as a patient hit by car, as damaged lung tissue is fragile and susceptible to rupture.

3. Treatment

If a pneumothorax is present prior to surgery, the chest is tapped, and/or a chest tube is placed to allow for continuous drainage of air from the chest prior to induction of anesthesia (see Table 6.9). If a pneumothorax is intentionally created (i.e., during a thoracoscopy), use of a PEEP valve (which maintains a constant end expiratory pressure in the lungs) during the procedure will prevent the lung from collapsing down to residual volume (RV) and thus reduce the risk of trauma for reopening completely collapsed

Table 6.9   Traditional placement of chest tube.

Materials: Chest tube, clippers, aseptic preparation, sterile gloves, suture (Nylon), hemostats, Christmas tree adaptor, orthopedic wire, three-way stopcock, scalpel blade, bull dog clamp, or "C" clamp

Technique:
1. Clip large area over chest with intercostal spaces 7–9 in center; aseptically prepare.
2. Wearing sterile gloves, palpate rib spaces 7–9; select one of these rib spaces.
3. Stretch skin cranially over the site; make stab incision with the scalpel blade through the skin at the intercostal space selected on the cranial aspect of the rib.
4. Using hemostats, dissect down to the pleural lining.
5. Hold the chest tube perpendicular to the chest wall. Hold chest tube with one hand at the selected intercostal space; with other hand, pop end of chest tube to deploy into the pleural space.
6. Rest chest tube parallel with the chest and advance into thoracic cavity.
7. Aspirate to ensure chest tube is in thoracic cavity. Remove any air or fluid from chest (quantify amounts) until negative pressure is achieved.
8. Relax skin to "normal" position over chest tube.
9. Secure in place with a mattress knot or Chinese finger trap. A bull dog or "C" clamp is placed on the tube to prevent air from entering the chest should the stopcock become dislodged.
10. A Christmas tree adaptor is commonly placed on the end of the chest tube with a three-way stopcock to maintain a seal. The stopcock and Christmas tree are soundly secured to the tube with orthopedic wire.

Note: Negative pressure is not always achieved. If the chest is "open" (meaning there is a wound leading from the outside into the chest), negative pressure is not achieved. These patients' surgical closures are placed on a vacuum system. Alternatively, commercial chest tube kits are available which simplify the process.

alveoli; the use of positive pressure may improve oxygenation intraoperatively as well (16). Treatment of a spontaneous pneumothorax involves immediate decompression of the air within the thorax. This is achieved by a chest tap or placement of a chest tube. Manual or MV with positive pressure is required to preserve adequate ventilation, as the animal will no longer have negative pressure to expand the lung, thus making its own attempts to breath inadequate. Goals of ventilation include maintaining CO_2 levels within normal (35–45 mmHg) and providing adequate oxygenation ($PaO_2 > 60$ mmHg). When ventilating these patients, use of longer inspiratory times and low PIP are helpful. Blood gas analysis is part of routine monitoring and patient assessment well into the recovery period.

F. Respiratory distress or arrest

Respiratory distress or arrest occurs for a variety of reasons but ultimately leads to cessation of breathing, either because the patient is unable to breath or incapable of taking adequate breaths. Under anesthesia, respiratory characteristics such as effort and rate are very important to monitor as well as SpO_2, PaO_2, and capnography. Because the patient is vigilantly monitored, it is unlikely this complication would occur during anesthesia; the anesthetist usually notes hypoventilation and either manually or mechanically assists the patient. However, respiratory arrest is one of the three major causes of postoperative morbidity and mortality (1), indicating the need for careful monitoring in the postoperative period.

1. Consequences

Respiratory distress or arrest may result in fatality of the animal.

2. Causes

Respiratory fatigue, pneumothorax, and increased intra-abdominal pressure from diseases such as a gastric dilation and volvulus (GDV), pregnancy, large mass or foreign body, and diaphragmatic hernia may all result in respiratory distress or arrest. Additionally, an animal that is inadequately recovered from anesthesia in the postoperative period and not appropriately monitored may have respiratory distress or arrest that is unnoticed.

3. Treatment

Recognizing the cause of respiratory distress or failure is important in treatment. MV is indicated in a patient that may have compromised respiratory effort under anesthesia or postoperatively. If a pneumothorax is suspected, tapping the chest is indicated (see Table 6.10). Continuous monitoring of the patient's respiratory effort, blood gas or SpO_2 is important throughout the recovery period. Supplemental oxygen may be necessary and the patient must be observed for at least 3 hours postoperatively (17).

Table 6.10 Chest tap.

Materials: Over-the-needle catheter (16–18 g) or butterfly catheter, three-way stopcock, large syringe, sterile gloves, clippers, aseptic prep
Technique: 1. Clip area over intercostal spaces 7–9 (toward the dorsum for air, more ventral for fluid). Aseptically prepare the site. 2. While wearing sterile gloves, insert the catheter between the intercostal spaces of choice, on the cranial aspect of the rib. A "pop" is felt when entering the pleural space. If using an over-the-needle catheter, advance catheter into chest and remove stylet. 3. Attach three-way stopcock to end of catheter. 4. Place syringe on end of stopcock. Turn stopcock off to room air, withdraw until negative pressure is obtained with syringe. It is important to not place extremely negative pressure on the syringe, or damage to the lung tissue could result. Once the syringe is full of air or fluid, turn the stopcock off to the patient and empty syringe. This process is repeated until negative pressure is obtained. Record total quantity of air removed. 5. When negative pressure is achieved, the stopcock is turned off to the patient.

Table 6.11 Simple acid–base disorders and compensatory mechanism.

Primary disorder	Change in pH	Primary cause	Compensatory mechanism
Respiratory acidosis	Decreased	Increased $PaCO_2$	Increased HCO_3
Respiratory alkalosis	Increased	Decreased $PaCO_2$	Decreased HCO_3
Metabolic acidosis	Decreased	Decreased HCO_3	Decreased $PaCO_2$
Metabolic alkalosis	Increased	Increased HCO_3	Increased $PaCO_2$

Chapter 6

IV. Acid–base disturbances

Acid–base disturbances are common complications under anesthesia, especially in the critical patient. Knowing the patient's clinical history allows the anesthetist to differentiate between a primary problem and compensation. The ability to measure blood pH is essential to detecting an acid–base disorder. This is done as part of a routine blood gas analysis obtained with point of care monitors or bench top lab equipment. There are two approaches to diagnosing an acid–base disturbance: a traditional approach based on the Henderson–Hasselbalch equation and the Stewart approach. The traditional approach is described. For those interested in the Stewart approach and other new models evaluating acid–base disturbance, additional resources are available (18).

To evaluate changes in pH, other components of a blood gas, including $PaCO_2$, bicarbonate (HCO_3), and base excess (BE), are necessary. The first step is to evaluate pH—is it normal (7.35–7.45), acidotic (less than 7.35), or basic (above 7.45)? $PaCO_2$ and HCO_3 changes will indicate whether pH changes are because of a respiratory or metabolic disorder. The primary disorder follows the change in pH (see Table 6.11). For example, in a patient with acidosis, $PaCO_2$ is elevated (respiratory acidosis), or HCO_3 is decreased

Table 6.12 Acid–base examples.

Acid–base disorder	pH	PaCO$_2$ (mmHg)	HCO$_3$ (mmol/L)	BE (mmol/L)
Metabolic acidosis	7.28	21.8	10.2	−17
Metabolic alkalosis	7.55	52.6	27.8	9
Respiratory acidosis	7.23	58.6	25.1	−5
Respiratory alkalosis	7.49	20.3	18.5	5
Mixed/complex	7.38	19.9	30.4	Highly variable

(metabolic acidosis). In a patient with alkalosis, PaCO$_2$ is decreased (respiratory alkalosis), or HCO$_3$ is increased (metabolic alkalosis). The compensatory mechanism attempts to "correct" this problem. In disturbances with mixed/multiple issues, the pH is often normal with values of PaCO$_2$ and HCO$_3$ in opposite directions. One "rule of thumb" is the body will never *over*correct. In other words, it is not possible to have a pH that is acidotic or alkaline because the body has overcompensated for a disease. Arterial whole blood or heparinized samples (depending on the analyzer) are used for accurate acid–base analysis. Air has its own level of PaCO$_2$ (that is, zero) and PaO$_2$, and therefore is removed from the syringe, and the sample analyzed immediately for accurate results. If an arterial sample is not collected, a blood sample from the tongue (considered a mixed arterial and venous sample) is the next most accurate sample for acid–base analysis.

A. Metabolic acidosis

Metabolic acidosis is characterized by a pH less than 7.35 with a low HCO$_3$, negative BE, and decreased PaCO$_2$ (see Table 6.12).

1. Consequences

Acidosis, regardless of origin, causes a decrease in myocardial contractility, a decrease in CO, and vasodilation. It also leads to arrhythmias, including VF. During anesthesia, acidosis makes the patient less responsive to catecholamines. The conscious patient with metabolic acidosis will hyperventilate, which leads to respiratory exhaustion requiring support. However, under anesthesia, this compensatory mechanism is diminished.

2. Causes

When using a traditional approach to blood gas analysis, anion gap is evaluated to determine, from a list of rule outs, the cause of metabolic acidosis. One particularly concerning rule out is lactic acidosis caused by hypoperfusion, resulting in cells undergoing anaerobic metabolism and producing lactate. Acquiring a lactate value helps to eliminate lactic acidosis as a cause. Other causes include liver or renal failure, diabetic ketoacidosis, GI losses of HCO$_3$, and a variety of toxicities.

(a) Calculation of anion gap: Anion gap is the difference between measured cations and measured anions; the size of this difference assists in determining the cause of metabolic acidosis. A normal anion gap is usually less than or equal to 10 mEq/L. A low anion gap is unlikely. A high anion gap results from increase in unmeasured anions, such as lactate or ketones.

$$\text{Anion gap (mEq/L)} = (Na^+ + K^+) - (Cl^- + HCO_3^-)$$

An alternative to anion gap is the use of Stewart's equation, a mathematically complex formula using serum biochemistry values; the reader is referred elsewhere for further information.

3. Treatment

Treatment depends on identifying the primary problem causing metabolic acidosis. However, under anesthesia, the anesthetist's goals include maximizing perfusion with fluids or blood products, cardiovascular support drugs such as positive inotropes to increase CO, and supporting the patient's ventilation (usually, hyperventilation). For most cases, hemodynamic and ventilation support prevents the metabolic acidosis from becoming extreme. For life-threatening cases of metabolic acidosis while under anesthesia (pH less than 7.1), supplementation of sodium bicarbonate is used to increase pH for temporary preservation of life, while continued efforts are made to identify and correct the primary cause of the acid–base abnormality (see Chapter 3, "Sodium Bicarbonate" section). If sodium bicarbonate is supplemented, additional CO_2 is produced; augmentation of ventilation to adjust for this is necessary.

B. Metabolic alkalosis

Metabolic alkalosis is characterized by an increase in HCO_3, positive BE, and compensating increased $PaCO_2$ (see Table 6.12).

1. Consequences

Alkalosis (whether metabolic or respiratory in origin) results in impaired cerebral and coronary blood flow that ultimately leads to seizures, obtundation, and/or death. Cardiovascular consequences include vasoconstriction and possible ventricular arrhythmias. Conscious patients compensate with hypoventilation (increase in $PaCO_2$). Severe metabolic alkalosis leads to calcium binding to albumin causing hypocalcemia precipitating muscle weakness and decreased contractility. Other common electrolyte abnormalities seen with alkalosis include hypochloremia and hypokalemia.

2. Causes

Leading causes of metabolic alkalosis include patients with significant renal insufficiencies that affect the reabsorption of bicarbonate, excessive vomiting causing a loss of hydrogen and chloride ions (as occurs with a proximal obstruction of the duodenum),

Chapter 6

and hypovolemia. Oversupplementation of sodium bicarbonate also leads to metabolic alkalosis.

3. Treatment

Adequate volume resuscitation with possible supplementation of chloride and potassium is most important when treating or stabilizing this patient.

C. Respiratory acidosis

Respiratory acidosis is characterized by a low pH with a high $PaCO_2$ (see Table 6.12).

1. Consequences

This is the most frequent cause of acidosis under anesthesia. It is usually of little long-term consequence; however, cardiac arrest and hypoxemia may result if it is severe and left untreated. Acidosis, regardless of origin, causes a decrease in myocardial contractility, a decrease in CO and hypotension, as well as possible arrhythmias, including VF. During anesthesia, acidosis causes decreased responsiveness to catecholamines.

2. Causes

The leading cause of respiratory acidosis under anesthesia is hypoventilation due to a deep anesthetic plane or drug overdose. Other causes include airway obstruction, pleural effusion, MH, and chest wall disruption.

3. Treatment

Respiratory acidosis is most commonly the result of hypoventilation from excessive anesthetic depth. Depth of anesthesia is adjusted initially. Assisted ventilation is started once the anesthetic plane is addressed effectively. Assisted ventilation is achieved either by manually supplementing breaths or placing the patient on a ventilator (see Chapter 2 for directions on ventilator setup). If the patient is currently on a ventilator, increasing the RR or V_T will usually decrease $PaCO_2$.

D. Respiratory alkalosis

Respiratory alkalosis is characterized by a low $PaCO_2$ and resulting increase in pH typically above 7.45 (see Table 6.12).

1. Consequences

Severe alkalosis (pH greater than 7.6) regardless of metabolic or respiratory origin results in similar consequences, including decreased cerebral blood flow, seizures, possible ventricular arrhythmias, compensatory hypoventilation, and thus, intentional hypercarbia. Electrolyte abnormalities may also include hypocalcemia and hypokalemia.

2. Causes

The most common cause of respiratory alkalosis is iatrogenic hyperventilation. Other causes may include central nervous system injuries, pregnancy, hyperthermia, and pain.

3. Treatment

Identifying the primary causes of respiratory alkalosis and treating the underlying cause is most effective. Under anesthesia, the most effective treatment involves controlling ventilation so $PaCO_2$ may increase, correcting pH. Typically, decreasing the V_T or RR will allow $PaCO_2$ to increase, correcting the acid–base abnormality. It is important to continue to try to identify and correct the underlying cause to avoid relapse at recovery.

IV. Electrolyte disturbances

Electrolyte disturbances have negative ramifications if left unmonitored or without treatment. As with all patient complications, correction of these imbalances occurs prior to anesthetizing the patient when possible. Some diseases, such as obstructed or ruptured bladder, are surgical emergencies, and correction of electrolyte abnormalities are attempted during anesthesia. Normal values are influenced by the electrolyte analyzer. The normal ranges listed are general guidelines to follow; however, the anesthetist must be familiar with the reference ranges specific to his or her own laboratory.

A. Calcium

Calcium plays an important role in muscle contraction, with the anesthetist's primary concern being myocardial contractility. Changes in albumin levels (which occurs with fluid therapy) do not impact ionized calcium, and therefore under anesthesia, ionized calcium levels are used for therapeutic decisions.

1. Hypercalcemia

Hypercalcemia is defined in dogs as an ionized calcium value greater than 6 mg/dL or 1.5 mmol/L in the dog and 5.7 mg/dL or 1.4 mmol/L in cats. Very young animals may have slightly lower calcium values, whereas immature animals (especially large breed dogs) may have higher calcium values. Hypercalcemia is often a marker for malignant diseases or toxins.

(a) Consequences: The acuteness of hypercalcemia will determine if a patient has any consequences from it. For example, a patient that gradually becomes hypercalcemic from

Table 6.14   Treatment of hyperkalemia.

1. For anesthetic maintenance or bolus, 0.9% NaCl is the crystalloid fluid of choice.
2. Administer regular insulin at 0.1–0.2 IU/kg with or without a CRI of 0.01 IU/kg/h IV. It is prudent to administer a 50% dextrose bolus at 0.5–1 g/kg slow over 3–5 min diluted at least 1 : 3 with 0.9% NaCl, followed by 2.5–5% dextrose added to 0.9% NaCl ran at anesthetic fluid maintenance rate.
3. Calcium gluconate 0.2–0.4 mg/kg IV over 5–10 min may be "cardio-protective."
4. Sodium bicarbonate at 0.5–1.0 mEq/kg IV over 15–30 min will force potassium intracellularly.
5. Beta agonist such as dopamine or dobutamine will decrease K+ via the ATPase pump.

Note: While treating hyper- or hypokalemia, continuously monitor the ECG and serum potassium levels. If administering insulin, dextrose, calcium supplements or sodium bicarbonate, blood gas, blood glucose, and electrolyte values must be monitored closely.

following thromboembolism potentially result in hyperkalemia. Iatrogenic causes may include administration of expired pRBCs or oversupplementation of potassium.

(c) Treatment: Cardiac bradyarrhythmias are life threatening and require immediate treatment. Table 6.14 outlines guidelines for treatment of hyperkalemia.

2. Hypokalemia

Hypokalemia is characterized by serum potassium levels less than 3.5 mEq/L.

(a) Consequences: Muscle weakness, respiratory depression, and cardiac arrest (19).

(b) Causes: A decrease in potassium intake, vomiting, diarrhea, certain drugs (such as administration of loop diuretics, beta agonists, or insulin overdose), chronic renal disease or postobstructive diuresis without appropriate fluid supplementation, and diabetic ketoacidosis all potentially result in hypokalemia.

(c) Treatment: Supplementation of potassium is necessary; however, one is very careful when supplementing potassium under anesthesia. As with all complications, it is best to correct any potassium deficits prior to anesthesia. The authors suggest supplementing potassium if serum potassium is below 2.5 mEq/L. A general rule for supplementation is no faster than 0.5 mEq/kg/h IV; often during anesthesia, potassium supplementation is much less. Adding supplemental potassium to a bag of fluids to bring the total potassium concentration of the fluids to 20–40 mEq/L and administering at the surgical fluid rate is a conservative means of preventing an iatrogenic hyperkalemia, as long as one is careful not to bolus these fluids (separate, potassium free fluids are available to bolus, if needed). ECG and electrolyte values are continuously monitored for signs of hyperkalemia.

C. *Sodium*

Sodium is an important electrolyte in maintaining plasma osmolality and cellular hydration. Free water moves to areas of higher sodium concentrations. As serum sodium levels increase, water leaves cells, and the cells risk becoming dehydrated. As serum sodium decreases below the concentration in cells, free water moves into these cells, resulting in cellular edema. The kidney very tightly regulates sodium concentrations, with little fluctuations throughout the day.

1. Hypernatremia

Sodium concentrations above 165 mEq/L indicate hypernatremia.

(a) Consequences: As with other electrolyte imbalances, how quickly a change in electrolyte status occurs influences the severity of consequences. Altered neurological function, muscle tremors, seizures, and death can result from hypernatremia.

(b) Causes: Hypernatremia occurs due to severe dehydration (possibly due to lack of available water or exposure to high temperatures), vomiting, diarrhea, and renal failure. Iatrogenic causes include administration of solutions containing sodium, such as hypertonic saline or sodium bicarbonate. Diseases such as diabetes insipidus and neurological alterations may also cause increases in serum sodium.

(c) Treatment: Treatment includes diagnosing the underlying cause of hypernatremia and evaluating the patient's hydration status. The brain compensates for hypernatremia by accumulating its own osmolites to prevent dehydration. Rapidly decreasing sodium concentration does not allow the brain enough time to compensate, which leads to neuronal swelling and rupture. Care is taken to decrease serum sodium levels only 0.5–1 mEq/kg/h to avoid cerebral edema. If anesthesia absolutely must occur prior to sodium regulation, the anesthetist should administer a fluid solution that is the same milliequivalent per liter concentration of sodium as the patient's own serum sodium. This is achieved by taking a solution such as 0.9% NaCl and adding hypertonic saline to that fluid to raise sodium concentration (see Appendix B). This fluid is then used as the patient's maintenance fluid, and correction of the sodium imbalance begins in the postoperative period. Serum sodium levels are diligently monitored throughout anesthesia.

2. Hyponatremia

Hyponatremia is defined as serum sodium level below 130 mEq/L and is considered severe below 120 mEq/L.

(a) Consequences: Hyponatremia causes changes in mentation status, seizures, coma, and possibly death due to cerebral edema and increasing ICP. Rapidly correcting hyponatremia results in myelinolysis, making it advisable to slowly correct this abnormality before anesthesia.

(b) Causes: Causes of hyponatremia include fluid retention secondary to disease states (such as CHF), ascites or other body cavity effusions (i.e., uroabdomen or chylothorax), loss of sodium through the GI system or renal system, psychogenic polydipsia and hypoadrenocorticism, as well as iatrogenic causes, including excessive use of diuretics or hypotonic fluid administration.

(c) Treatment: Treatment involves correction with sodium supplementation no faster than 0.5 mEq/kg/h. If the patient is concurrently hypovolemic, rehydration with fluid therapy is also necessary. If anesthesia must occur, hypotension is likely and requires treatment (see "Hypotension").

V. Glycemic control

Serum blood glucose (BG) is regulated by a variety of hormones, including insulin (which lowers BG) and glucagon, epinephrine, cortisol, and growth hormones (which increase BG). Measuring BG concentrations is easily done with small, portable point of care monitors; however, one limitation of such monitors is their inaccuracy at very high or very low glucose concentrations. Familiarity with the analyzers' guidelines regarding sampling provides more accurate assessment of results.

A. Hyperglycemia

Hyperglycemia is defined as serum glucose greater than 250 mg/dL.

1. Consequences

Given the choice between hyper- or hypoglycemia in a patient, the anesthetist would prefer hyperglycemia. However, there is continued controversy about glycemic control under anesthesia in humans, with some studies demonstrating an improvement in morbidity for critically ill patients whose serum glucose is tightly regulated. This has lead to evidence-based literature reviews, which concluded that a target range of BG between 150 and 180 mg/dL may improve outcome in perioperative patients (20). However, the same review cautions vigilance for hypoglycemia and having the means to correct it in the event of aggressive glucose management. Additionally, patients that have a history of hyperglycemia (diabetics) that have had restricted access to water may be dehydrated or hypovolemic, worsening hypotension. Extreme hyperglycemia (greater than 600 mg/ dL) may cause a prolonged recovery, seizures, or coma.

2. Causes

Some diseases may perpetuate hyperglycemia or extreme fluctuations in glucose. The classic veterinary disease resulting in hyperglycemia is diabetes mellitus. Pancreatitis or acromegaly (felines) concurrently with diabetes may make BG more difficult to manage.

Stress causes increases in glucose, especially in the feline. Hyperglycemia also occurs in patients with adrenal abnormalities, such as hyperadrenocorticism (Cushing's disease) or pheochromocytomas, or from adrenal changes secondary to supplementation with glucocorticoids. Hyperglycemia occurs in septic patients as well. Iatrogenic hyperglycemia results from oversupplementation with dextrose.

3. Treatment

Regular insulin is ideal during anesthesia and is dosed at 0.25–0.5 IU/kg IV or at a CRI of 0.05–0.1 IU/kg/h. Glucose is closely monitored every 15–30 minutes to prevent hypoglycemia. Because of frequent blood draws to assess glucose, a sampling line is typically placed in these patients.

B. Hypoglycemia

Hypoglycemia is qualified by serum glucose less than 40–60 mg/dL.

1. Consequences

Glucose is a necessary energy source for cellular reactions and is critically important in the brain. Seizures will occur in the conscious patient; however, the neurologic damage that occurs is often masked in the anesthetized animal, until recovery. Generalized weakness is evident during recovery. Hypoglycemia prolongs recovery, especially in small, exotic animals and young patients.

2. Causes

The most common cause of hypoglycemia in patients that are not obtunded is an insulinoma, as these patients have become "tolerant" of their hypoglycemia. Other causes of hypoglycemia include liver insufficiencies (secondary to PSS), hypoadrenocorticism (Addison's disease), and sepsis (which results in hyperglycemia as well). Iatrogenic causes include overdoses of insulin and extended fasting, especially in young animals.

3. Treatment

It is important to know if a patient has an insulinoma before it is treated for hypoglycemia. If an insulinoma is present, aggressively supplementing dextrose will cause the insulinoma to release more insulin and further worsen hypoglycemia. Therefore, in the insulinoma patient, dextrose supplementation is used only if the patient is severely hypoglycemic (less than 40–50 mg/dL) and then usually as a CRI of a 2.5–5% dextrose solution in the fluids, with target BG levels between 50–60 mgL/dL. In patients with other reasons for severe hypoglycemia, especially iatrogenic reasons, a bolus of dextrose at 0.5 g/kg diluted (due to the highly osmotic nature of dextrose) at least 1:3 with saline, and administered IV slowly over 5 minutes, is warranted. In cases of mild to moderate

Chapter 6

hypoglycemia, the anesthetic fluids are supplemented with 2.5–5% dextrose and given at desired anesthetic fluid rate (usually 5–10 mL/kg/h).

VI. Other complications

A. Anaphylaxis/ anaphylactoid reaction

Anaphylaxis is a Type I (acute reaction mediated by immunoglobin E [IgE] attaching to mast cells resulting in degranulation) hypersensitivity. An anaphylactoid reaction is a reaction that, although clinically similar, is not mediated by IgE. Most reactions under anesthesia are anaphylactoid caused by mast cells and basophils releasing histamine in response to drugs and chemicals. Both reactions are treated in the same way.

1. Consequences

The degranulation of mast cells results in serious, adverse events including urticaria (hives), bronchospasm (although most patients are already intubated and so this is only evident at recovery), laryngeal and/or pulmonary edema, vasodilation, and tachycardia.

2. Causes

Drugs that prompt reactions include opioids (i.e., morphine), contrast media, antibiotics, and neuromuscular blocking agents. Blood products also have the potential to cause a reaction especially when used in an un-typed and un-cross-matched patient.

3. Treatment

Discontinue any drug suspected to result in the reaction. If the response has not become severe, diphenhydramine (0.5–2.0 mg/kg IV) may reduce symptoms (although it does not prevent further degranulation, as its action is to blockade H_1 receptors). Epinephrine (0.01 mg/kg IV) is warranted if symptoms progress or are initially very pronounced. As the patient recovers, the addition of a H_2 blocker, such as famotidine (1.0 mg/kg IV), is warranted to prevent the GI side effects of mast cell release. Other supportive measures (fluid therapy, inotropes, furosemide, etc.) are administered as needed.

B. Hyperthermia

Hyperthermia is defined as a body temperature above 103–104 F in dogs and cats.

1. Consequences

Increased body temperature causes an increase in metabolic rate and oxygen consumption, which increases workload of important organs like the heart, skeletal muscles, and brain. Severe hyperthermia (temperatures >107° F) may damage organs, including the brain, resulting in obtundation and seizures, ventricular arrhythmias, organ failure, and possibly, death.

2. Causes

The most common cause of intraoperative hyperthermia in the healthy patient is iatrogenic oversupplementation of heat, usually through the use of circulating water blankets or forced air-warming units. Hypermetabolic patients may present with hyperthermia. MH is a rare condition in which a defective ryanodine receptor allows for uncontrolled skeletal muscle activity, resulting in high temperatures, high $EtCO_2$, increased HR, RR, and muscle tone. While primarily occurring in pigs, this disease has been reported in dogs (21) in response to anesthetic drugs. With the advent of drugs such as tramadol, it is also important to note that serotonin syndrome, a syndrome reported in humans secondary to the use of drugs preventing serotonin reuptake, also results in hyperthermia. This syndrome is not reported in animals but may become more prevalent, especially if multiple drugs that inhibit serotonin reuptake are combined.

Postoperative hyperthermia is a unique phenomena that occurs in the cat secondary to the combination of the use of opioids and intraoperative hypothermia (22). Some feline patients reached temperatures greater than $107°$ F postoperatively, a situation that warrants aggressive intervention. While opioids such as hydromorphone resulted in postoperative hyperthermia in up to 40% of the cases (23), all opioids have at least some documented incidence of postoperative hyperthermia (24). Work by Posner's group identified the relationship between the degree of intraoperative hypothermia and postoperative hyperthermia in cats receiving opioids (22). This highlights the importance of thermoregulation and monitoring in the feline.

Chapter 6

3. Treatment

If the healthy patient has become hyperthermic under anesthesia, the anesthetist removes the source of heat. If using a forced air-warming device, ambient air ($68°$ F) is circulated. For extremely high temperatures ($>107°$ F), more drastic measures are taken. Oxygen supplementation is important in the face of hyperthermia due to the increased oxygen consumption. High flows (>300 mL/kg/min) will help cool the patient. Acepromazine at 0.01–0.03 mg/kg IV will cause vasodilation that will also assist with cooling. Cool ice-packs, particularly around the head with the intent of keeping the brain cool, are applied. Alcohol is applied to the foot pads as well. If severe hyperthermia is experienced under anesthesia along with an increase in $EtCO_2$ or $PaCO_2$, the anesthetist must rule out MH. The patient is disconnected from the current breathing circuit and placed only on oxygen, via a Bain circuit if available (injectable agents are used to maintain anesthesia if a procedure cannot be discontinued), in addition to the previously mentioned maneuvers. Controlling any arrhythmias and possible hyperkalemia are necessary steps as well. Definitive treatment includes the use of dantrolene at 1–5 mg/kg IV slowly, although this is infrequently available at most veterinary clinics, due to cost and short shelf-life. If a patient is suspected to have MH, dantrolene is obtainable from most human hospitals in advance of the procedure.

C. Hypothermia

Hypothermia is one of the three most common complications of anesthesia (with the others being hypoventilation and hypotension). In dogs and cats, normothermia is 99.5°F and 102°F, respectively. In the conscious human, body temperature rarely fluctuates more than 0.4°F (25); however, general anesthesia induces swings of 4–7°F (26). Mild hypothermia is somewhat beneficial to anesthetized patients in that myocardial and cerebral metabolic oxygen consumption is decreased, and inhalant requirement is reduced by approximately 5% for each 1.8°F decline (27). Hypothermia is possibly "neuroprotective" by limiting brain damage following cardiac arrest. As temperatures drift below 95°F (35°C), hypothermia requires intervention, unless deliberate hypothermia is utilized for anesthesia.

1. Consequences

Consequences of hypothermia depend on the degree of body heat loss. Generally, hypothermia causes decreased metabolism of drugs, mild metabolic acidosis, delayed wound healing, increased susceptibility to infection, and coagulopathies. Mild to moderate hypothermia results in vasoconstriction and decreased tissue perfusion. As hypothermia progresses, patients become bradycardic and unresponsive to anticholinergics, causing a decrease in CO resulting in hypotension, further worsening tissue perfusion. Cardiac arrhythmias such as AV block, VPCs, and VF are evident as temperature drops further. Below 85°F, the anesthetist will commonly see these arrhythmias, which are often unresponsive to defibrillation, should cardiac arrest occur. Hypothermia results in prolonged anesthetic recoveries and shivering. Although shivering may seem insignificant, it increases a patient's metabolic rate and oxygen consumption by 200–600% (28); this cost is profound to a patient with organ compromise.

2. Causes

Hypothermia most commonly results from lack of prevention. Small patients, neonates, debilitated, or emaciated patients are predisposed to hypothermia. In cases of cardiopulmonary bypass, hypothermia is deliberately induced; this is a complex procedure and is only taken on by an experienced anesthesia team.

3. Treatment

Treatment is aimed at prevention. If sedating the patient prior to induction, the patient is kept warm to avoid unnecessary losses in body temperature. Common equipment used to maintain patients' body temperature include circulating water blankets, forced air-warming blankets, electric warming units, plastic surgical drapes, and warmed intravenous fluids. Additional methods of warming the patient during a surgical procedure include warm abdominal lavage, decreasing oxygen flow rates to minimum requirement (rebreathing system 20–30 mL/kg/min, non-rebreathing system 200 mL/kg/min), preparation of surgical site with warm saline and chlorahexidine scrub (no alcohol), and minimizing anesthesia time. Aggressive warming and prevention is necessary in patients predisposed to hypothermia.

C. Regurgitation

Regurgitation is the passive flow of stomach contents or gastric secretions into the esophagus. Regurgitation is recognized by yellowish or brown fluid in the mouth or nares of the patient. Unfortunately, some dogs will silently regurgitate, meaning the anesthetist may not be aware of the regurgitation until the dog returns to the hospital at a future date with an esophageal stricture (29). Patients that have a history of vomiting, regurgitation, gastric obstruction such as a foreign body, or increased intra-abdominal pressure due to a mass or GDV are monitored closely for regurgitation; a "test suction" is done in patients were silent regurgitation is suspected. When positioning a patient for a procedure, care is taken to avoid positioning the head below the stomach if possible, especially in patients known to have regurgitated during previous anesthetic procedures.

1. Consequences

The pH of the stomach is extremely acidic. Over time, gastric contents in contact with the esophagus's lining result in endothelial damage and possibly lead to strictures. Aspiration pneumonia of gastric contents greatly increases morbidity and mortality.

2. Causes

Some predisposing factors include increased intra-abdominal pressure, gastric obstruction, positioning of patient, and light planes of anesthesia. In fact, many incidences of gastroesophageal reflux occurred immediately after anesthesia induction (30). There is some debate over the effect of preoperative fasting and the incidence of esophageal reflux, with some authors suggesting prolonged fasting may worsen the incidence of reflux (30).

3. Treatment

The esophagus is immediately suctioned and lavaged with normal saline if regurgitation is noticed. If normal saline is not available, tap water is used. Lavage of the esophagus is continued until the fluid removed is clear. It is important to always properly inflate the cuff of the endotracheal (ET) tube immediately following induction of anesthesia, as this decreases the chance of aspiration. Prior to extubation, the patient must be able to lift its head and swallow; the cuff is left inflated for removal of the tube. Instillation of sodium bicarbonate increases the esophageal pH (31), which may reduce the incidence of esophageal stricture.

D. Noxious stimuli

True pain is a conscious perception, and is defined as "an unpleasant sensory and emotional experience associated with actual or potential tissue damage, or described in terms

Chapter 6

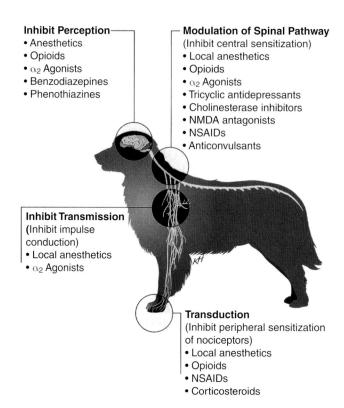

Inhibit Perception
• Anesthetics
• Opioids
• α_2 Agonists
• Benzodiazepines
• Phenothiazines

Modulation of Spinal Pathway
(Inhibit central sensitization)
• Local anesthetics
• Opioids
• α_2 Agonists
• Tricyclic antidepressants
• Cholinesterase inhibitors
• NMDA antagonists
• NSAIDs
• Anticonvulsants

Inhibit Transmission
(Inhibit impulse conduction)
• Local anesthetics
• α_2 Agonists

Transduction
(Inhibit peripheral sensitization of nociceptors)
• Local anesthetics
• Opioids
• NSAIDs
• Corticosteroids

Figure 6.10   Nociception pain pathways with analgesic drugs that target specific areas of pathway. Courtesy of Teton New Media.

of such damage" (32). Therefore, under anesthesia, upregulation of pain pathways is termed "noxious stimuli," to differentiate it from the cognizant perception that is pain. Nociception is the body's physiological response to pain.

1. Consequences

Upregulation of noxious pathways—even under anesthesia—result in modulation of the pain processing centers, which sets the stage for chronic pain, should treatment remain inadequate. Long-term consequences of mismanaged pain (i.e., postoperatively) are the subject of much debate, but ultimately, the presence of pain undeniably reduces quality of life.

2. Causes

Primary causes of pain under anesthesia are a result of inadequate analgesia during a surgical procedure; that is, it is not enough to simply turn up the vaporizer.

3. Treatment

The target for treatment of pain is a preemptive and multimodal approach in the anesthetic plan. A multimodal approach is one that combines a variety of analgesic drugs which target different receptors—for example, an opioid targeting opioid receptors, ketamine for NMDA antagonism, and lidocaine to target abnormal sodium channels. Premedication typically involves including an analgesic and sedative (see Table 1.5). Ideally, if the patient has an anticipated surgery scheduled, such as an orthopedic correction or fracture repair, appropriate analgesia is instituted prior to the preanesthetic phase. In this day and age, it is highly inappropriate for a patient to "earn" its analgesia; it is up to the anesthetist to anticipate pain and preemptively attempt to address it.

It is difficult under anesthesia to differentiate noxious stimulation from a patient that is inadequately anesthetized. End-tidal agent analysis assists with this; if the end-tidal agent values are at or above surgical MAC for the agent and patient, and the patient has hypertension, increased HR, or RR, noxious stimuli is suspected, and responsiveness to analgesic drug administration (opioids, ketamine, etc.) is assessed. In the absence of an end-tidal agent analysis, the determination is much more speculative; however, responsiveness to analgesic drug administration (which, in dogs, will often reduce the need for inhalant) is also used. If the animal is responsive to a bolus of the agent, a CRI is begun to deliver a background of analgesic drug. Noxious stimuli are much more difficult to address in a cat under anesthesia. Very few drugs reduce their inhalant requirements. Indeed, administration of some opioids may actually *increase* their MAC values. Yet, when these same cats are assessed conscious, the opioids administered clearly reduce the amount of pain experienced (33). Therefore, it is advisable in the cat to assume an invasive procedure will be painful and to preemptively provide analgesia for such a procedure. See Appendix D for calculations and suggestions for CRI drug combinations. It is important to address pain following the procedure in the anesthetic recovery phase. Conscious pain is evaluated with the assistance of pain scoring techniques (see Appendix A).

Chapter 6

References

1. Brodbelt D, Blissitt K, Hammond R, Neath P, Young L, Pfeiffer D, et al. The risk of death: the confidential enquiry into perioperative small animal fatalities. Vet Anaesth Analg. 2008;35(5):365–73.
2. Sartor DM. Sympathoinhibitory signals from the gut and obesity-related hypertension. Clin Auton Res. 2013;23(1):33–9.
3. Chen L, Sotoodehnia N, Bůžková P, Lopez FL, Yee LM, Heckbert SR, et al. Atrial Fibrillation and the risk of sudden cardiac death. JAMA Intern Med. 2013;173(1):29–35.
4. Scapigliati A, Ristagno G, Cavaliere F. The best timing for defibrillation in shockable cardiac arrest. Minerva Anestesiol. 2013;79(1):92–101.
5. Xanthos T, Karatzas T, Stroumpoulis K, Lelovas P, Simitsis P, Vlachos I, et al. Continuous chest compressions improve survival and neurologic outcome in a swine model of prolonged ventricular fibrillation. Am J Emerg Med. 2012;30(8):1389–94.
6. Little SE. The Cat: Clinical Medicine and Management. First ed. St. Louis, MO: Elsevier Saunders; 2012.

7. Gordon AM, Wagner AE. Anesthesia-related hypotension in a small-animal practice. Veterinary Medicine. 2006:22–6.

8. Paige CF, Abbott JA, Elvinger F, Pyle RL. Prevalence of cardiomyopathy in apparently healthy cats. J Am Vet Med Assoc. 2009;234(11):1398–403.

9. Ilkiw JE, Pascoe PJ, Haskins SC, Patz JD, Jaffe R. The cardiovascular sparing effect of fentanyl and atropine, administered to enflurane anesthetized dogs. Can J Vet Res. 1994;58(4):248–53.

10. Pascoe PJ, Ilkiw JE, Pypendop BH. Effects of increasing infusion rates of dopamine, dobutamine, epinephrine, and phenylephrine in healthy anesthetized cats. Am J Vet Res. 2006;67(9):1491–9.

11. Curley G, Kavanagh BP, Laffey JG. Hypocapnia and the injured brain: more harm than benefit. Crit Care Med. 2010;38(5):1348–59.

12. McNally E, Robertson S, Pablo L. Comparison of time to desaturation between preoxygenated and nonpreoxygenated dogs following sedation with acepromazine maleate and morphine and induction of anesthesia with propofol. Am J Vet Res. 2009;70(11):1333–8.

13. Richter S, Matthes C, Ploenes T, Aksakal D, Wowra T, Hückstädt T, et al. Air in the insufflation tube may cause fatal embolizations in laparoscopic surgery: an animal study. Surg Endosc. 2013;27(5):1791–7.

14. Gal TJ, Suratt PM. Atropine and glycopyrrolate effects on lung mechanics in normal man. Anesth Analg. 1981;60(2):85–90.

15. von Recum AF. The mediastinum and hemothorax, pyothorax, and pneumothorax in the dog. J Am Vet Med Assoc. 1977;171(6):531–3.

16. Rubio J, Rodríguez A, Varela A, López L, Freixinet J, García C, et al. [Evaluation of 2 techniques for ventilation support during single-lung ventilation]. Rev Esp Anestesiol Reanim. 1992;39(1):14–8.

17. Brodbelt D. Perioperative mortality in small animal anaesthesia. Vet J. 2009;182(2):152–61.

18. Corey HE. Stewart and beyond: new models of acid-base balance. Kidney Int. 2003;64(3):777–87.

19. Kjeldsen K. Hypokalemia and sudden cardiac death. Exp Clin Cardiol. 2010;15(4):e96–9.

20. Jacobi J, Bircher N, Krinsley J, Agus M, Braithwaite SS, Deutschman C, et al. Guidelines for the use of an insulin infusion for the management of hyperglycemia in critically ill patients. Crit Care Med. 2012;40(12):3251–76.

21. Adami C, Axiak S, Raith K, Spadavecchia C. Unusual perianesthetic malignant hyperthermia in a dog. J Am Vet Med Assoc. 2012;240(4):450–3.

22. Posner LP, Pavuk AA, Rokshar JL, Carter JE, Levine JF. Effects of opioids and anesthetic drugs on body temperature in cats. Vet Anaesth Analg. 2010;37(1):35–43.

23. Niedfeldt R, Robertson S. Postanesthetic hyperthermia in cats: a retrospective comparison between hydromorphone and buprenorphine. Vet Anaesth Analg. 2006;33(6):381–9.

24. Posner LP, Gleed RD, Erb HN, Ludders JW. Post-anesthetic hyperthermia in cats. Vet Anaesth Analg. 2007;34(1):40–7.

25. Lopez M, Sessler DI, Walter K, Emerick T, Ozaki M. Rate and gender dependence of the sweating, vasoconstriction, and shivering thresholds in humans. Anesthesiology. 1994;80(4):780–8.

26. Støen R, Sessler DI. The thermoregulatory threshold is inversely proportional to isoflurane concentration. Anesthesiology. 1990;72(5):822–7.

27. Vitez TS, White PF, Eger EI. Effects of hypothermia on halothane MAC and isoflurane MAC in the rat. Anesthesiology. 1974;41(1):80–1.

28. Horvath SM, Spurr GB, Hutt BK, Hamilton LH. Metabolic cost of shivering. J Appl Physiol. 1956;8(6):595–602.

Chapter 6

29. Wilson DV, Walshaw R. Postanesthetic esophageal dysfunction in 13 dogs. J Am Anim Hosp Assoc. 2004;40(6):455–60.

30. Galatos AD, Raptopoulos D. Gastro-oesophageal reflux during anaesthesia in the dog: the effect of preoperative fasting and premedication. Vet Rec. 1995;137(19):479–83.

31. Wilson DV, Evans AT. The effect of topical treatment on esophageal pH during acid reflux in dogs. Vet Anaesth Analg. 2007;34(5):339–43.

32. IASP. Part III: Pain terms, a current list with definitions and notes on usage. Seattle: IASP Press; [cited 2009 12/11/2009]. Second edition:[Classification of chronic pain]. Available from: http://www.iasp-pain.org/AM/Template.cfm?Section=Pain_Definitions&Template=/CM/HTMLDisplay.cfm&ContentID=1728-Pain.

33. Brosnan RJ, Pypendop BH, Siao KT, Stanley SD. Effects of remifentanil on measures of anesthetic immobility and analgesia in cats. Am J Vet Res. 2009;70(9):1065–71.

Chapter 6

Chapter 7

Anesthesia and analgesia in the exotic patient

Exotic pet owners seek veterinary care when they observe an abnormal behavior in their pets. Often, these animals are not truly domesticated, which may take up to six generations. Therefore, handling for medical procedures often requires anesthesia. The infrequency and inexperience of the veterinary staff with exotic species may contribute to the increase in morbidity and mortality seen in these species (1). Previous chapters have outlined the preanesthetic recommendations that apply to all species in regard to anesthesia. This section is designed to give information regarding differences and suggestions for performing anesthesia and providing analgesia. The reader is referred to additional sources (see Appendix F) for a more extensive review on specific species.

I. Common exotic mammals

Metabolic rate scales allometrically by species; that is, the smaller the species, the greater its metabolic rate. This will influence drug metabolism. Other parameters influenced by a change in metabolic rate include body temperature and oxygen consumption.

A. Ferrets

1. Characteristics

(a) Ferrets are often treated like cats in regard to drug dosing and intubation.
(b) If not descented, ferrets may spray scent glands when stressed or threatened.
(c) Ferrets have thick skin, requiring confidence when administering an SC injection.
(d) Ferrets produce copious respiratory secretions, making inclusion of an anticholinergic a suitable choice for anesthesia when not contraindicated.

2. Anesthetic considerations

(a) Handling and restraint: Squeeze cages are helpful in restraining the unfriendly ferret. They have very sharp teeth and inflict severe bites. For the tame ferret, scruffing the nape of the neck and supporting the lower half of the body with the other hand works well for restraint (see Figure 7.1).

Small Animal Anesthesia Techniques, First Edition. Amanda M. Shelby and Carolyn M. McKune.
© 2014 John Wiley & Sons, Inc. Published 2014 by John Wiley & Sons, Inc.
Companion website: www.wiley.com/go/shelbyanesthesia

Chapter 7

Table 7.1 Exotic small mammal vital normals.

Species	Adult weights (kg)	HR[a] (bmp)	RR[a] (breaths/ min)	Temp (F)	Fasting recommendation
Ferret	0.7–3.0	200–275	30–35	100–104	6–8 h (unless the patient has a suspected insulinoma)
Hedgehog	0.3–1.2	200–280	25–50	95–99	Not recommended
Pot belly pig	40–90	70–120	25–35	101–104	12–24 h
Rabbits	1–6	130–325	30–60	99–103	2–4 h for food only
Rats	0.25–0.5	250–450	70–130	99–100	Not recommended
Mice	0.02–0.04	350–800	60–200	98–100.5	Not recommended
Hamster	0.085–0.15	250–500	40–140	101–103	Not recommended
Gerbil	0.05–0.10	250–500	90–150	99–102	Not recommended
Guinea pig	0.7–1.2	230–380	50–100	101–103	2–4 h
Chinchilla	0.4–0.6	200–350	45–80	102–103	Not recommended

Sources: See Appendix F.
[a]Respiratory rates and heart rates may be lower during anesthesia.
Bpm, beats per minute; RR, respiratory rate.

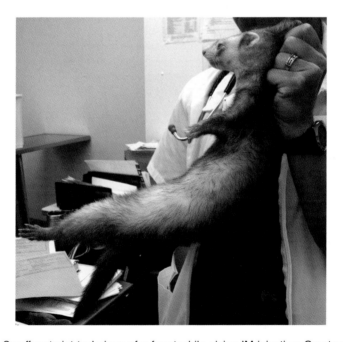

Figure 7.1 Scruff restraint technique of a ferret while giving IM injection. Courtesy of Meagan Putnam.

(b) Premedication: Agents that sedate and provide preemptive analgesia help facilitate catheter placement and reduce induction and maintenance drug requirements; a variety of agents are suitable in the healthy ferret (see Table 7.2). The hind limb muscles are common locations for IM injections; sadly, for these little creatures, the patient is often sore on the limb and may limp where the injection was given, especially if large volumes are given. IV access includes the cephalic, jugular, and saphenous veins. It is helpful to nick the skin prior to attempting catheterization.

(c) Induction: If IV access is not achieved under premedication, mask or box inductions with isoflurane or sevoflurane is the most common approach. If IV access is available, IV induction agents are administered (see Table 7.2).

(I) INTUBATION: Intubation is achieved with small endotracheal (ET) tubes similar to intubating a cat. The patient is placed in sternal recumbency with the head and neck hyperextended by an assistant. Some individuals suggest extending the head toward the person intubating while keeping the body straight. Lidocaine is used on the arytenoids to minimize laryngeal spasms. The tongue is pulled gently out of the mouth and a laryngeal scope is used for visualization. Small ET tubes ranging from 2.0 to 3.5 mm ID cuffed or noncuffed are commonly used. Placement of the ET tube is verified by auscultation of lungs bilaterally for respiratory noises on inspiration or with the use of a capnograph.

(d) Maintenance: All of the modern inhalants are commonly used. Total intravenous anesthesia (TIVA) is also used if IV access is available.

(e) Monitoring during anesthesia: An ECG and Doppler are recommended. BP is obtained with a cuff and sphygmomanometer. Pulse oximetry is obtained by placing a probe over a foot. Anesthetic depth is monitored similarly to the average small animal patient. Assessment of jaw tone, eye position, and palpebral reflex are indicators of depth. Additionally, changes in respiratory rate (RR) and blood pressure (BP) may also indicate anesthetic depth.

(f) Recovery: Keep the patient warm in recovery and continue to monitor vital signs. Because ferrets have such a variety of endocrinologic disease requiring anesthesia and surgery, tailor each recovery to the specific patient. Additional analgesia is administered as warranted.

Chapter 7

3. Common complications

(a) Intraoperative hypothermia, making forced air warming units, circulating hot water blankets, or companion animal warming units helpful to maintain body temperature.
(b) Hypoglycemia occurs due to high metabolic rates; 2.5% dextrose is added to the anesthetic maintenance fluids to correct this. The ferret with an insulinoma is a particular challenge in this regard, as it is a balance between providing enough dextrose without triggering release of an insulin surge.

Table 7.2 Anesthetic protocol for ferrets.

	ASA I or II	ASA III, IV, or V
Premedication	1. Opioid option: (a) Hydromorphone 0.1 mg/kg IM or SC or (b) Butorphanol 0.4 mg/kg IM or SC or (c) Buprenorphine 0.02 mg/kg IM or SC 2. +/− Glycopyrollate 0.01 mg/kg IM or SC 3. Sedative option: (a) Acepromazine 0.01–0.03 mg/kg IM or SC or (b) Dexmedetomidine 0.003–0.01 mg/kg IM or SC	1. Opioid option: (a) Hydromorphone 0.1 mg/kg or 2. Sedative option: (a) Midazolam 1 mg/kg SC or IM
Induction	(a) Mask/chamber with gas inhalant or (b) Propofol 4–6 mg/kg IV or (c) Ketamine 10 mg/kg + midazolam 1 mg/kg IM or IV or (d) Tiletamine-zolazepam 1.5–3 mg/kg IV	(a) Propofol 2–4 mg/kg + diazepam 1–2 mg/kg IV or (b) Ketamine 7.5 mg/kg + midazolam 1 mg/kg IM or IV or (c) Fentanyl 0.02 mg/kg + diazepam 1–2 mg/kg IV
Maintenance **Intraoperative analgesia**	Gas inhalant (a) Hydromorphone 0.1 mg/kg IM or (b) Buprenorphine 0.01–0.05 mg/kg IM, SC	Gas inhalant Fentanyl CRI 0.012–0.042 mg/kg/h
Post-op analgesic	(a) Carprofen 4 mg/kg SC SID and (b) Buprenorphine 0.02 mg/kg SC	(a) Buprenorphine 0.02 mg/kg SC

B. Hedgehogs

1. Characteristics

(a) Some species of hedgehog (European) hibernate when conditions are extreme (unlikely in the household pet).
(b) Nocturnal (i.e., normally inactive during the day and active in the evening).
(c) Spines cover the dorsal aspect of body.

2. Anesthetic considerations

(a) Handling and restraint: Handling and restraint is difficult, especially if the patient rolls into a ball. Some will unroll if rump spines are stroked. Leather gloves are recommended. While these animals rarely bite, they are reclusive by nature and often resent handling, regardless of the degree of socialization.

(b) Premedication: Often patients are masked or boxed down without the use of injectable premedications. However, SC injections are given with the assistance of forceps to grasp a fold of skin between the spines over the flank of the patient. IM injections are given in the thigh. Soreness results if large volumes are administered IM.

(i) IV ACCESS: Catheters are placed in the jugular or saphenous vein. Intraosseous (IO) catheters are placed in the proximal femur.

(c) Induction: Patients are typically too small to intubate. Attempts at intubation are made using 1–1.5 mm ID ET tube; however, care is taken to avoid trauma to the larynx which causes swelling, bleeding, and airway obstruction.

(d) Maintenance: Most drug doses come from rodent research. Mask induction and maintenance with an inhalant anesthetic is common clinical practice, although little research examines the benefits and risks of this method in the hedgehog.

(e) Monitoring: A Doppler is vital for monitoring the heart rate (HR) in these animals. Pulse oximetry is useful if the probe is placed on a foot in the unrolled hedgehog. ECG provides information on HR, but most monitors are only capable for displaying up to 250 bpm. RR is monitored by watching chest excursions.

(f) Recovery: Recover hedgehogs in a quiet, nonstimulating environment. Keep the patient warm in recovery and continue to monitor vital signs. Additional analgesia is administered as warranted.

Table 7.3 Anesthetic protocol for hedgehog.

	ASA I or II	**ASA III, IV, or V**

Premedication	1. Opioid option:
	  (a) Hydromorphone 0.1 mg/kg
	  or
	  (b) Butorphanol 0.4 mg/kg
	  or
	  (c) Buprenorphine 0.02 mg/kg)+
	2. Sedative option:
	  (a) Midazolam 1 mg/kg
	  and/or
	  (b) Ketamine 5–10 mg/kg SC or IM
		1. Opioid option:
		  (a) Hydromorphone 0.1 mg/kg
		2. Sedative option:
		  (a) Midazolam 1 mg/kg SC or IM

Induction	Mask/chamber with gas inhalant	Mask/chamber with gas inhalant
Maintenance	Gas inhalant	Gas inhalant
Intraoperative analgesia		(a) Fentanyl CRI 0.012–0.042 mg/kg/h if IV or IO access available
Post-op analgesic	(a) Meloxicam 0.2 mg/kg SC SID and/or (b) Buprenorphine 0.02 mg/kg SC	(a) Buprenorphine 0.03 mg/kg SC

3. Common complications

Complications are typically a result of the hedgehog's high metabolic rate and the anesthetist's underestimation of the patient's requirements.

(a) Hypoglycemia is possible; do not fast and administer 2.5% dextrose in fluids for extended procedures.
(b) Hypothermia due to small body size, use of non-rebreathing (NRB) circuits, and decreased metabolism is common. Use of esophageal temperature probes for continuous monitoring and forced air warming units are helpful.

C. Pot belly pigs (PBPs)

1. Characteristics

(a) PBPs have small tracheas compared to body weight; additionally, there is a sigmoid curvature to the airway and a ventral diverticulum anteroventral to the arytenoid fold preventing a straightforward intubation.
(b) PBPs have a high fat to muscle ratio (anatomically present as a thick layer of subcutaneous fat), making the effect of drug injections less predictable and intra-fat (rather than IM) injection more likely.
(c) Pigs are cannibalistic.
(d) Twelve- to twenty-four-hour fasting of adult pigs is recommended.
(e) Difficulty accessing veins means most anesthetic plans are developed with minimal biochemical and hematologic information.

2. Anesthesia considerations

(a) Handling and restraint: Pigs are difficult to restrain due to their shape and size. Often chemical restraint is used to avoid stress. Large pigs are controlled with a board or cage door front "squeezed" against a wall while an IM injection is given, or snared just behind the canine teeth. Small pigs are manually restrained (see Figure 7.2).

(b) Premedication: Behind the ear is the most common site for IM injections. In young PBP, there is less fat in this area so the effectiveness of the drugs is more predictable. The epaxial muscles are avoided because of the large layer of back fat and the tradition of avoiding this muscle group in pigs for market. Injection in the semimembrananosus and semitendinosus with a 3.5-inch stylet from a catheter is a possible alternative. Intranasal midazolam, 0.5 mg/kg, may quiet the pig to a degree and facilitate limited handling. In general, pigs are less susceptible to the sedative effects of opioids, phenothiazines, and alpha$_2$ agonists. Butyrophenones, such as azaperone (2.5 mg/kg IM), are often used for sedation in noncompanion pigs and are potentially useful in the PBP.

(I) IV ACCESS: Veins are difficult to access. Easiest vessels for catheterization include the medial and lateral auricular veins (see Figure 7.3) and lateral saphenous veins, which are

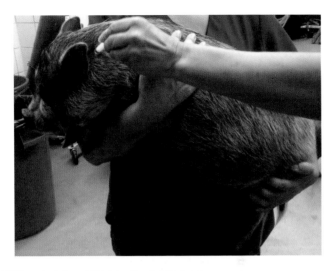

Figure 7.2 PBP restraint and IM injection behind ear.

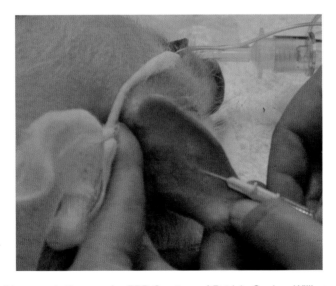

Figure 7.3 IV access in the ear of a PBP. Courtesy of Patricia Queiroz-Williams.

typically catheterized following induction. Cephalic veins are attempted, but venipuncture in this area is performed blindly, as these vessels are difficult to palpate and visualize.

(c) Induction: If IV access is obtainable following premedication, injectable agents are given to facilitate intubation. Otherwise, mask induction with isoflurane or sevoflurane is most common until the patient is intubated.

(i) INTUBATION: Intubation in pigs is a challenge for a number of reasons. The mouth does not open widely, and the larynx is at an angle to the trachea. Pigs have a pharyngeal diverticulum, as well as a tracheal bronchus; inaccurate placement of the tube in either of these areas results in trauma, swelling, or bleeding. Stylet or ET tube inadvertently placed in the tracheal bronchus cause pneumomediastinum and inadequate ventilation. Cuffed ET tubes of various sizes (smaller than for an equivalent sized canine patient) are used; for an average 60-kg PBP, an 8.0- to 9.0-mm ID ET tube is used. Place the patient in sternal recumbency. Gauze or dog leashes facilitate visualization, when placed behind the canine teeth and used to open the mouth. A long blade laryngoscope is helpful in visualizing the larynx by placing the blade at the base of the tongue and pressing down to displace the epiglottis. Lidocaine is placed on the arytenoids to minimize laryngeal spasms, which readily occurs. Introduce a long, thin stylet (crafted from small French urinary catheters connected together with tape or glue, approximately three times the length of the ET tube) into the trachea to assist intubation. If no resistance is encountered, an ET tube is passed over the stylet and gently rotated 180 degrees once it passes beyond the larynx. Laryngeal mask airways are used in pigs with success and may reduce the potential for airway trauma (2). Auscultation and capnography confirms appropriate placement. If resistance is encountered, rotating the stylet gently while advancing it forward may help; however, significant resistance warrants backing out of the trachea and trying again. Intubation attempts are minimized to prevent trauma.

(d) Maintenance: Inhalant anesthetics are most commonly used following intubation. IM injectable drugs, in combination with local blocks, facilitate adequate sedation and immobilization for minor procedures like castration, hoof trim, or tusk filing.

(e) Monitoring anesthetic depth: Palpebral reflex and jaw tone will give an indication of the depth of anesthesia. PBPs have small eyes, making ocular signs of anesthetic depth difficult to obtain. Vital parameters may also indicate changes in depth.

   An ECG and Doppler are recommended for monitoring the HR and rhythm. Pigs have little excess skin, so using sticky pads to monitor ECG is preferable to ECG clips. The Doppler crystal, BP cuff, and a sphygmomanometer give an indication of trends. The Doppler is often placed distal to the accessory claw, with the cuff below the carpus on the forelimb, or on the hind limb above the hock. Invasive blood pressure (IBP) is obtained from placing a catheter in the artery of the ear or dorsal pedal artery. It is also useful to monitor RR and EtCO$_2$. Pulse oximetry is obtained by placing a pulse oximeter probe on the tongue. Temperature is continuously monitored during anesthesia and into recovery.

(f) Recovery: Pigs are recovered without herd mates and only returned to the herd once completely recovered. Pigs are placed in sternal recumbency for recovery, if possible. Pigs may obstruct postextubation due to laryngeal swelling. It is important to ensure they are capable of swallowing and adequate independent ventilation is present prior to extubation. Nonsteroidal anti-inflammatory drugs (NSAIDs) are used, if not otherwise contraindicated, to minimize any airway swelling. Pigs experience postanesthetic sleep; although they appear conscious enough to extubate, once extubated, they sleep quite

Table 7.4 Anesthetic and analgesic drugs for PBP.

	ASA I or II	ASA III, IV, or V
Premedication	(a) Telazol 2–3 mg/kg IM or (b) Ketamine 7.5–10 mg/kg and dexmedetomidine 0.007 mg/kg IM	(a) Midazolam 0.2 mg/kg IM or (b) Midazolam 0.5 mg/kg intranasal
Induction	Mask until intubation	Mask until intubation
Maintenance	Gas inhalant	Gas inhalant
Intraoperative analgesia	Local blocks where possible	(a) Local blocks where possible
Post-op analgesia	(a) Flunixin 0.5–1.0 mg/kg SC or IV and (b) Buprenorphine 0.01–0.05 mg/kg IV or IM q 8 h or (c) Methadone 0.1–0.5 mg/kg IM q 4–6 h	(a) Fentanyl patch 50–100 mcg/h

heavily, which contributes to the possibility of postextubation obstruction. Temperature is monitored during and following recovery. Additional analgesic drugs are administered as warranted.

3. Common complications

(a) Airway obstruction at extubation is possible: The anesthetist is ready with additional induction agent (IV catheter remains in place until the patient is fully recovered) and a size smaller ET tube to intubate patient if an obstruction occurs.
(b) Hypoventilation, if not from excessive anesthetic depth, is often addressed with mechanical ventilation (MV).
(c) Hypothermia (especially in in small pigs) occurs intraoperatively and postoperatively. Use of circulating warm water blankets and forced air-warming units reduces the degree of hypothermia.

D. Rabbits

1. Characteristics

(a) Rabbits are obligate nasal breathers (require patency of the nares and nasopharnyx).
(b) It is common for rabbits to have inconspicuous respiratory infections; as a prey species, they are remarkably good at hiding signs of illness and pain.
(c) Rabbits do not regurgitate or vomit.

(d) Some rabbits have circulating levels of atropinesterase (3), which makes the use of atropine less effective. Glycopyrrolate is a suitable alternative.

(e) Rabbits have extremely powerful kick strength; their kick is strong enough to fracture their own spine if they are not properly restrained.

(f) Because rabbits are a prey species, they are remarkably efficient at hiding signs of pain and distress. Preemptive and appropriate postoperative analgesia is administered to these animals without expecting a behavioral qualification of pain.

2. Anesthesia considerations

(a) Handling and restraint: Rabbits are very easily stressed; it is wise to handle them in a quiet, dim environment to minimize stress until they are anesthetized. One method of restraint is to cradle the rabbit in one arm with the head tucked into the body of the handler. Alternatively, the handler grasps the patient by the scruff and supports the patient's hind end. Do not pick up by ears!

(b) Premedication: SC injections are an effective technique for premedication, and preferred, if possible, to IM injections. IM injections are administered in the muscular bodies on either side of the spine or hind limb. Squeeze boxes work nicely for IM injections in feral rabbits. Intranasal administration for soluble drugs, such as midazolam, is an alternative to a needle.

(c) Induction: Patients are often masked or boxed down. Because rabbits become stressed and excited, it is recommended that patients are sedated prior to boxing down with a gas anesthetic.

(I) INTUBATION: Intubation is a precarious maneuver in the rabbit (see Figure 7.4). For an average size rabbit, a 2.0- to 2.5-mm uncuffed ET tube or laryngeal mask airway (LMA) is used to secure an airway (4). Intubation is only attempted a maximum of two or three times. Traumatic or repetitive intubation attempts cause laryngeal swelling and airway obstruction after extubation. See Table 7.6 for intubation techniques.

(II) IV ACCESS: Catheterization is performed after induction in most cases. When clipping a site for catheterization, use gentle technique as the rabbit's thin skin is easily traumatized. The cephalic vein is suitable for venous access, and may reduce the possibility of damage to the ear. The lateral saphenous vein is accessible as well. In an emergency, the auricular artery is used to provide arterial access; however, this may result in sloughing of the ear due to reduced perfusion. Therefore, routine catheterization of the auricular artery is not advised. IO catheters are placed in the proximal femur, tibia, or humerus.

(d) Maintenance: The patient is typically maintained on gas inhalants, but a TIVA technique is possible if surgeon access to the airway is required and a catheter is in place.

(e) Monitoring: An ECG will display the patient's cardiac rhythm and HR; however, most monitors only read up to 250 bpm. A Doppler over the radial artery or directly over the

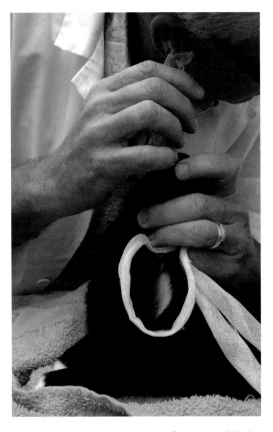

Figure 7.4   Blind technique for intubation in a rabbit. Courtesy of Anderson da Cuhna.

Chapter 7

heart works well to confirm mechanical (not just electrical) function of the heart. The forelimb is also a useful site for BP monitoring with a sphygmomanometer and Doppler crystal. Fluctuation in the volume of the Doppler may indicate changes in BP. Obtain RR by watching the chest rise and fall; if the patient is intubated, $ETCO_2$ confirms cardiac output and gives information about ventilation. Esophageal temperature probes are recommended for continuous monitoring of core body temperature.

(l) MONITORING ANESTHETIC DEPTH: Most reflexes are absent at a surgical plane of anesthesia; however, the palpebral reflex is maintained even at a deep anesthetic plane. A light plane of anesthesia is identified by response to a toe pinch, ear twitch, or response to surgical incision. A rabbit that is at a light plane of anesthesia may shake its head in response to painful stimuli. A deep plane of anesthesia is identified by fixed dilated pupils unresponsive to light with no corneal reflex, depressed ventilation, and minimal response to surgical stimulus.

(f) Recovery: Rabbits are recovered in a quiet, dim environment to prevent startling and kicking at arousal. Additional analgesia is administered as warranted.

Table 7.5 Anesthetic protocol for rabbits.

	ASA I or II	ASA III, IV, V

Premedication	1. Opioid options:
	  (a) Hydromorphone 0.2 mg/kg
	  or
	  (b) Butorphanol 0.4 mg/kg
	2. Sedative options:
	  (a) Midazolam 1 mg/kg IM, SC,
	    or intranasal
	  or
	  (b) Acepromazine 0.025–
	    0.05 mg/kg IM or SC
	  or
	  (c) Dexmedetomidine 0.003–
	    0.01 mg/kg IM or SC
		1. Opioid option:
		  (a) Hydromorphone 0.2 mg/
		    kg
		2. Sedative options:
		  (a) Midazolam 1 mg/kg IM or
		    SC or intranasal

Induction **Maintenance**	Mask/chamber with gas inhalant (a) Gas inhalant via mask or (b) Propofol 0.1–0.4 mg/kg/h	Mask/chamber with gas inhalant Gas inhalant

Intraoperative
analgesia
	(a) Local blocks where applicable	(a) Fentanyl CRI 0.010–
		    0.030 mg/kg/h
		(b) Local blocks where
		    applicable

Post-op
analgesia
	1. NSAID options:
	  (a) Flunixin 0.3–1.0 mg/kg SC or
	    IV SID
	  or
	  (b) Meloxicam 1.0 mg/kg PO SID
	and
	2. Opioid options:
	  (a) Buprenorphine 0.05–0.3 mg/
	    kg SC q 8h
	  or
	  (b) Hydromorphone 0.2 mg/kg
	    IM q 4h
		Opioid options:
		(a) Buprenorphine 0.05–0.3 mg/
		    kg SC q 8h
		or
		(b) Hydromorphone 0.2 mg/kg
		    IM q 4

3. Common complications

(a) Rabbits are very susceptible to corneal ulcers. The eyes cannot be lubricated enough; constant lubrication is recommended. Alternatively, some anesthetists tape the eyes shut.

(b) Fracture of the spine during improper restraint or boxing down occurs. Avoid boxing down the nonsedated rabbit.

(c) Hyperthermia is common during restraint and handling due to stress. Try to minimize stress during the preanesthetic and recovery phase.

(d) Hypothermia is common during anesthesia. The use of plastic surgical drapes, forced air-warming units, and circulating warm water blankets are helpful in maintaining body temperature.

Table 7.6 Blind intubation technique in rabbits.

Materials: Appropriate sized endotracheal tube (2–4 mm ID), laryngoscope with size 0–2 blade, umbilical tape or gauze to open mouth, a cotton tip applicator is helpful help extract tongue.

Blind Technique:
1. The patient is anesthetized adequately with a regular respiratory pattern.
2. Maintain the patient in sternal recumbency with the head and neck hyperextended. It is best if the patient is grasped from behind the head with the holder's thumb and forefinger by the ramus of the mandible. Nose is essentially directed toward the ceiling.
3. Place a lidocaine drop on the arytenoids to decrease spasms. However, some anesthetists find this diminishes the cough reflex, which is helpful in identifying location.
4. Advance the ET tube over the base of the tongue.
5. The anesthetist places his or her ear near the end of the ET tube and advances toward the larynx until respiratory noises are the loudest. Advance ET tube into trachea during the next breath; it is helpful to rotate the tube as you advance to pass between the arytenoids. Alternatively, the capnograph adaptor is placed on the end of the ET tube. When $EtCO_2$ is seen on the capnograph, advance the ET tube into the trachea during the next breath.
6. If no respiratory noise is ausculted with administration of a breath, the ET tube is likely in the esophagus and should be withdrawn.

(e) The thoracic cavity of the rabbit is quite small compared with the large abdominal cavity, thus worsening the chance of hypoventilation.

E. Rodents (chinchillas, gerbils, guinea pigs, hamsters, mice, rats)

1. Characteristics

(a) Many rodents are obligate nasal breathers.
(b) Undetected respiratory disease is common in rodents.
(c) Some species, such as hamsters, are nocturnal.
(d) Hamsters and guinea pigs have cheek pouches, for storage of food particles, which may result in aspiration pneumonia in the sedated or anesthetized animal.
(e) Rodents are prone to self-mutilation. Avoid giving IM injections especially with irritating solutions or in large volumes.
(f) Several species of rodent are capable of shedding their tails if picked up.
(g) Guinea pigs have a palatal ostium, which makes intubation of this species virtually impossible (5).
(h) Some species, such as the rat, mouse, and gerbil, do not vomit.

2. Anesthetic considerations

(a) Handling and restraint: Grasping the tail of rodents is avoided. If the rodent is tame, simply cupping it in the palm of a hand is ideal. Grasping the nape or scruff of the neck is the most acceptable means of restraint especially when giving injections.

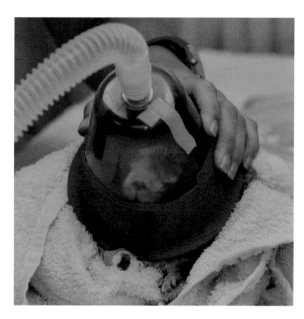

Figure 7.5   Masking rodent. Courtesy of Anderson da Cuhna.

(b) Premedication: A variety of premedications are suitable for rodents; in addition to the SC and IM routes, some medications are administered intraperitoneal (IP). Administration of drugs IP takes practice, so it is advisable for experienced personnel only to use this route (see Table 7.7). The muscle bodies for IM administration are small, and certain drugs may irritate tissues, so SC injection is often preferable. Generally speaking, the larger rodents (i.e., guinea pig) will require the lower dose range of agents listed in Table 7.8, while the small rodents (i.e., mouse) will require the higher end of the dosage range.

(c) Induction: Usually, rodents are masked or "boxed" down in a small enclosure with inhalants (see Figure 7.5). The patient is removed from the box when the "righting" reflex is absent and a face mask is placed until the patient is relaxed.

(i) INTUBATION: Larger rodents are intubated, but care is taken during the intubation process to avoid trauma, which may lead to swelling and subsequent airway obstruction. Minimal attempts are made especially in small rodents. Rats are intubated with the assistance of a modified #2 otoscope ear speculum to allow visualization of larynx. Lidocaine on the arytenoids will help minimize laryngeal spasms. Catheters (16–20 g) work well in place of ET tubes.

(ii) IV ACCESS: Catheterization in large rodents is accomplished in the cephalic or saphenous veins. IO catheters are commonly placed in the proximal femur, tibia, or humerus.

(d) Maintenance: Typically, gas inhalants are used to maintain anesthesia in nonlaboratory settings.

(e) Monitoring during anesthesia: HR is monitored with a Doppler over an artery or directly over the heart. ECG may be of limited use, as most monitors only read up to 250 bpm.

In small rodents, wire suture is placed in the skin of the animal to clip ECG leads to. Capnography is often inaccurate in small rodents but may assist with confirmation for placement of the ET tube. Instead, monitor chest wall excursions visually to obtain RR.

(I) ANESTHETIC DEPTH: Trends in HR and RR assist with assessment of depth of anesthesia. Responses to toe pinch, tail pinch, or skin incision all suggest too light a plane of anesthesia for surgery. A guinea pig may shake its head in response to surgical stimulus.

(f) Recovery: Continued thermal support is important in the recovery phase, as is oxygen supplementation and additional analgesic drugs as warranted.

Table 7.7   Intraperitoneal injection in rodents.

Materials: Second person to restrain, 25-g needle, drug for administration

Technique:
1. It is helpful for an additional team member to restrain the animal. This individual inverts the rodent with the head down, to displace abdominal viscera.
2. Enter the caudal quadrant of the abdomen at a 20-degree angle. The right caudal quadrant is used for most small rodents. The exception is the rat, where the left caudal quadrant is used.
3. Aspirate prior to drug administration.
4. Inject drug; maximum volume is 1–3 mL.

Table 7.8   Anesthetic protocols for rodents.

	ASA I or II	ASA III, IV, V
Premedication	1. Opioid options: 　(a) Buprenorphine 0.05–0.5 mg/kg SC 　or 　(b) Butorphanol 0.5–5 mg/kg SC 2. Sedative options: 　(a) Midazolam 0.5–2 mg/kg SC 　or 　(b) Acepromazine 0.5–5.0 mg/kg SC 　(c) Ketamine 5–10 mg/kg SC 3. Anticholinergic: 　(a) Atropine 0.05 mg/kg SC 　or 　(b) Glycopyrrolate 0.01–0.02 mg/kg SC	1. Opioid options: 　(a) Buprenorphine 0.05–0.5 mg/kg SC 　or 　(b) Morphine 2–5 mg/kg SC 　or 　(c) Oxymorphone 0.2–0.5 mg/kg SC 2. Sedative option: 　(a) Midazolam 0.5–1 mg/kg SC 3. Anticholinergic: 　(a) Atropine 0.05 mg/kg SC 　or 　(b) Glycopyrrolate 0.01–0.02 mg/kg SC
Induction	Mask/chamber with gas inhalants	Mask/chamber with gas inhalants
Maintenance	Gas inhalants	Gas inhalants
Post-op analgesia	(a) Carprofen 4–10 mg/kg SC SID and/or (b) Buprenorphine 0.05 mg/kg SC q6–8 h	1. Opioid options: 　(a) Buprenorphine 0.05 mg/kg SC q6–8 h 　or 　(b) Morphine 2–5 mg/kg SC q4 h

3. Common complications

(a) Hypoxemia may result because an airway is difficult to secure in several rodent species. Oxygenation by mask is a reasonable part of the plan.

(b) Hypoglycemia occurs in small rodent species that are used to free choice availability of food. Unfortunately, lack of venous access for administration of 2.5–5% dextrose complicates this. Therefore, preemptive steps, such as access to food prior to and immediately after anesthesia, are crucial to preventing hypoglycemia.

(c) Hypothermia occurs due to large surface area to body mass ratio, use of NRB circuits, and depressed metabolism. External heat support is necessary.

(d) Respiratory obstruction results from traumatic intubation; in some cases, it is preferable to use a mask as opposed to attempting intubation. Copious respiratory secretions may also obstruct the ET tube; look for increased respiratory effort, which may indicate the ET tube is obstructed.

II. Avians

A. Characteristics

1. Birds have a highly efficient respiratory system compared to mammals. Birds have higher V_T, lower RR, and larger minute ventilation. Inspiration and expiration are both active phases in the bird; that is, respiratory movements are accomplished by cervical, thoracic, and abdominal muscle contractions (there is no diaphragm to contribute to the active phase). Two complete respiratory cycles exchange inhaled gases via cross current gas exchange.

2. The trachea is longer and has an increased diameter when compared to mammals resulting in more dead space. Unlike mammals, the tracheal rings are complete. For this reason, the anesthetist utilizes uncuffed ET tubes. It is wise to review the specific species with regard to variations in respiratory anatomy—for example, some penguins have a double trachea and emus have a tracheal diverticulum.

3. The epiglottis is absent.

4. Birds have high metabolic rates which require higher substrate levels (blood glucose [BG] is greater than 200 mg/dL) and higher fluid rates (10–30 mL/kg/h).

5. Cardiovascular differences include larger stroke volume (SV), increased cardiac output (CO), and higher mean arterial pressure (MAP). HR varies considerably depending on the size of the patient.

6. Circulation influences the effect of various drugs. Birds possess a renal portal system. This network of vessels around the kidney, which selectively channels blood through or past it, results in a potential first pass effect of drugs administered in the caudal half of the body, altering the drugs intended effect. When a drug is given in the lower half of the body, it is metabolized by the renal portal system before reaching the central nervous system, the target site for effect.

7. Fasting is highly variable depending on the size of the bird; in general, fasting is usually less than 3 hours, but may not be performed at all for very small birds.

B. Anesthetic considerations

1. Handling and restraint

It is important to minimize stress while restraining birds. Ideally, a bird is allowed to acclimatize to the hospital environment before handling. In an emergency situation, acclimatization is not possible. Covering the eyes of the patient with a hood or towel helps to reduce stress. For smaller birds, utilize the hand technique: place the head gently between the thumb and forefinger with the body supported in the palm.

2. Preanesthetic assessment

The physical examination (PE) begins before the bird is removed from its housing. Visually assess RR and effort prior to handling. Look at the bird's posture and whether the feathers are "fluffed." When the bird is removed from its surroundings, a hands-on examination of the bird commences. This includes ausculting air sacs ventrally, lungs dorsally, and over the trachea for abnormal airway sounds. The heart is ausculted as well. Obtaining an accurate body weight is key to drug dosages and fluid rates; palpation of the keel gives an indication of body condition of the bird to know whether this weight is appropriate for the patient. Color of the urate is helpful in suggesting liver dysfunction when preoperative blood work (BW) is unavailable. Hydration status is assessed by moistness of the cloaca, ocular mucous membranes, and elasticity of skin. Sunken eyes and cold extremities suggest dehydration and/or shock.

3. Premedication

Anticholinergics are controversial for use in the bird; while an increase in HR is desirable, increased thickness of respiratory secretions increases the chance of ET tube occlusion. Additionally, some herbivorous birds may possess atropinesterases.

The pectoral muscles are utilized for IM injections, although consideration is given to a captive bird that may be released, as soreness may result and limit flight activity. However, when administered into the lower half of the body, the drugs pass through the portal venous system, which may result in altered drug metabolism.

4. Induction

Preoxygenate if possible. The most common means of induction is masking the patient down with an inhalant (see Figure 7.7). In the small avian, the mask is made with a syringe casing so the whole head of the patient fits in the "mask." An examination glove with a hole cut in the end is used as a diaphragm to create a sealed fit. The patient's HR and RR are monitored closely during induction because there is a tendency to achieve an excessive depth resulting in hypoventilation and bradycardia. Injectable agents are used if an IV catheter is available.

Chapter 7

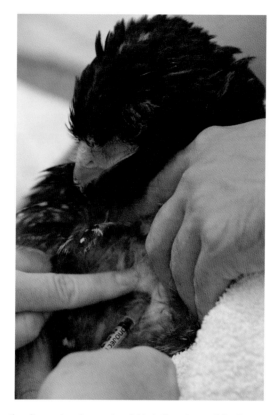

Figure 7.6 IM injection in pectoral muscle of bird. Courtesy of Anderson da Cuhna.

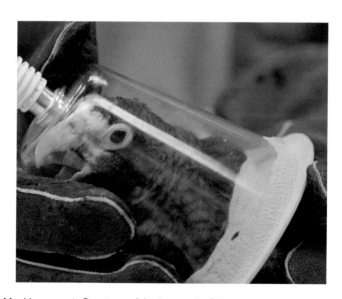

Figure 7.7 Masking parrot. Courtesy of Anderson da Cuhna.

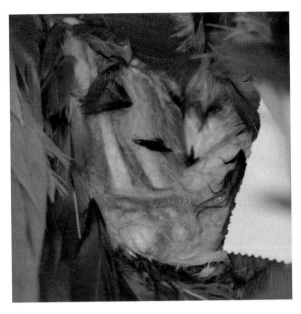

Figure 7.8 Brachial vein for IV catheterization in bird. Courtesy of Anderson da Cuhna.

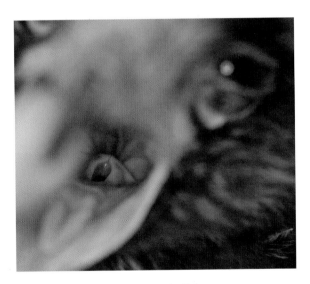

Figure 7.9 Avian larynx. Courtesy of Anderson da Cuhna.

(a) IV access: Vessels suitable for catheterization include the brachial vein, medial metatarsal, or jugular vein. Preference is given to upper half of body due to the circulatory pattern and its influence on drug metabolism. IO catheters are placed in the proximal ulna or cranial tibiotarsus; other bones are pneumatic (see Figure 7.8).

(b) Intubation: The glottis is readily visible for intubation (see Figure 7.9). Uncuffed ET tubes are used.

5. Maintenance

Inhalants in oxygen or TIVA are the most common techniques.

(a) Analgesia: Local techniques are used when possible. The toxic doses for lidocaine is about 2.5 mg/kg. Eutectic mixture of local anesthetic (EMLA) cream is used but is limited to small areas. In some species of birds, there is a prevalence of kappa receptors, making kappa agonists such as butorphanol or nalbuphine suitable analgesics in birds. However, new information suggests that pure mu agonists, such as hydromorphone or tramadol, may alter a bird's response to nociception (6, 7). Further clinical testing is necessary.

(b) Monitoring suggestions: A Doppler is considered essential monitoring for assessing HR; while an ECG is useful, many ECG units only count up to 250 bpm. Additionally, the thin skin of the bird makes ECG clips unsuitable for use, so small wire suture or a needle is placed in the skin as an alternative site for clips. An esophageal stethoscope is a suitable means of HR monitoring as well. Use of a Doppler and sphygmomanometer, with a BP cuff, allows the anesthetist to obtain BP trends. Additionally, in large birds, arterial access is possible. The brachial or carotid arteries are accessible; the use of EMLA cream may facilitate arterial line placement. Respiration is monitored. Ideally, there are minimal respiratory noises in the intubated patient, although the intubated bird, unlike mammals, has the ability to vocalize due the caudal location of the syrinx. Apnea for a period greater than 10–20 seconds warrants a manual breath; most birds benefit from MV under anesthesia. Capnography is helpful in assessing quality of ventilation and confirming that perfusion of the lungs is occurring; however, birds are one of the few animals where the $EtCO_2$ is possibly greater than $PaCO_2$. The benefits are considered in light of the possible increase in dead space or oversampling of a capnograph adapter. Pulse oximeters are not accurate in birds, due to the difference in avian hemoglobin. A cloacal or esophageal temperature is monitored to guide thermoregulatory management.

(I) MONITORING ANESTHETIC DEPTH: Reaction to toe pinch, cere pinch, cloacal pinch, or feather plucking, and increased jaw tone are all indications of a light plane of anesthesia. Muscle tone, such as neck or wing tone, may give an indication of depth as well. Slight palpebral and corneal reflexes are typical in the surgical plane of anesthesia. Decrease in HR, BP, RR, and apnea are indications of a deep plane of anesthesia.

6. Recovery

Indications of recovery include wing and leg movement. Jaw tone returns as anesthetic depth decreases and the patient is extubated when this occurs. Continued oxygen supplementation is administered after extubation. Additional analgesics are administered as warranted.

C. Common complications

1. Hypothermia occurs due to large surface area to body mass ratio, use of NRB circuits, and depressed metabolism. External heat support is provided.

Table 7.9 Common anesthetic and analgesic protocols in birds.

	ASA I or II	ASA III, IV, or V
Premedication	1. Butorphanol 1.0 mg/kg IM and 2. Midazolam 1–2 mg/kg IM and/or 3. Ketamine 10–20 mg/kg IM	1. Butorphanol 1.0 mg/kg IM and 2. Midazolam 1 mg/kg IM
Induction	Mask with gas inhalant	Mask with gas inhalant
Maintenance	Gas inhalant	Gas inhalant
Intraoperative analgesia	Local blocks where appropriate	Local blocks where appropriate
Post-op analgesia	1. Butorphanol 1.0 mg/kg IV or IM and 2. Carprofen 1 mg/kg IM SID or 3. Meloxicam 1.0 mg/kg PO SID	1. Butorphanol 1.0 mg/kg IV or IM

2. ET tube occlusions secondary to mucus plugs are extraordinarily common in birds; any resistance to administering a breath or difficulty ventilating a patient warrants an exchange of ET tube due to the possibility of occlusion.
3. Hypoventilation which is prevalent in this species often necessitates MV.

III. Reptiles

A. Characteristics

1. The heart has three chambers (two atria, one ventricle). This allows for mixing of oxygenated and deoxygenated blood with changes in vascular resistance under anesthesia. This "shunting" significantly worsens perfusion of vital tissues.
2. Reptiles are ectothermic; therefore, body temperature influences drug metabolism and clearance, as well as physiologic parameters.
3. Prior to anesthetizing a reptile, the reader is advised to review the individual species variations in regard to respiratory anatomy and physiology, as this is beyond the scope of this chapter. For example, many reptiles do not possess a diaphragm. Instead, abdominal, pectoral, and pelvic muscles control ventilation (like the bird, inspiration and expiration is active as well as passive). However, crocodilians have a nonmuscular tissue which functions as a rudimentary diaphragm. Most snakes possess a single elongated right lung, although boas possess the left lung lobe in addition to the right. Most reptiles have simplified sacs with folds allowing for respiratory gas exchange, but there is a whole spectrum of complexity. The trachea in a turtle is short and bifurcates early compared with most reptiles. Some reptiles, such as turtles, possess complete tracheal rings.
4. A renal portal system is present in reptiles as it is in birds. This network of vessels around the kidney, which selectively channels blood through or past it, results in a

potential first pass effect of drugs administered in the caudal half of the body, altering the drug's intended effects.

5. Although fasting is often not required, timing of last large meal (especially for snakes) is important to know. A recent large meal affects the patient's ability to adequately ventilate.

B. Anesthesia considerations

1. Restraint and handling

This varies greatly by species restrained. All reptiles are capable of biting; many have claws and tails that are used in defense. Leather gloves are useful in preventing trauma to the handler for large reptile species. Nonpoisonous snakes are grasped at the base of the head with one hand while the other hand supports the body. Lizards are similarly handled, although the body is often tucked under the arm of the handler to assist in restraint (see Figure 7.10). Turtles and tortoise are held at the shell; the length of the neck determines how far caudal on the plastron the animal is restrained. Some species of turtles have extremely long necks and deliver a powerful bite to an unsuspecting restrainer.

2. Preanesthetic assessment

In nonpoisonous and tame species, perform a PE prior to anesthesia to obtain a baseline HR, RR, body temperature, and accurate body weight. Physical parameters such as HR are greatly influenced by body temperature, environmental stress, and presence of noxious

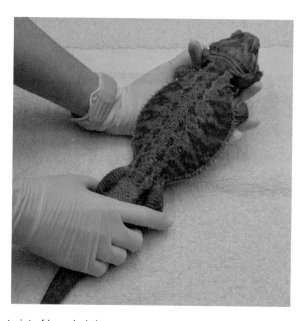

Figure 7.10   Restraint of bearded dragon.

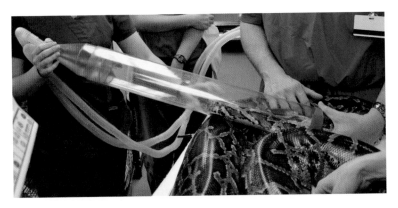

Figure 7.11   Masking a snake. Courtesy of Anderson da Cuhna.

stimuli. Due to the large variation in reptilian species, normal physical parameters are based on species-specific reference material and the patient's examination.

3. Premedication

Benefits of a premedication in animals include reduced dosages of induction drugs, analgesia, and sedation. However, clearance is prolonged in reptiles compared to mammals. Therefore, reversible drugs are chosen when possible. Some reptiles have mu opioid receptors, making morphine an effective analgesic option although significant respiratory depression may result (8). Any injectable premedication is administered in the cranial portion of the animal if possible; however, safety of the handler is prioritized over concern regarding the renal portal system.

4. Induction

Typically, reptiles are induced with inhalants via mask or chamber (see Figure 7.11). Inhalants are administered to the patient until it is relaxed and intubation is accomplished. Turtles and tortoises may be induced with IV induction agents by IV access or injection through the subcarapacial sinus under their shells (see Figure 7.12).

(a) Intubation of snakes and lizards: The position of the glottis is rostral, making intubation straightforward (see Figure 7.13). Noncuffed ET tubes, Cole tubes, or 16- to 19-g catheters for smaller reptiles are used. Typically, the best method of securing the ET tube is taping the tube to the patient's lower jaw.

In turtles (see Figure 7.14), the glottis is located at the base of the tongue. They have short tracheas so care is taken to ensure ET tubes are not advanced too far, causing an endobronchial intubation.

(b) IV access: In reptiles, IV access is infrequently achieved. In turtles and tortoises, catheterized vessels include the jugular or coccygeal veins; alternatively, IO catheters are commonly placed (see Figure 7.15).

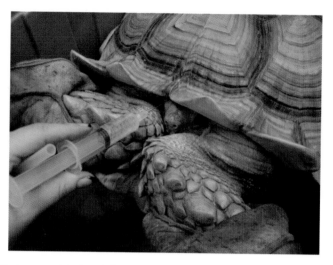

Figure 7.12 Subcarapacial sinus injection in a tortoises. Courtesy of Anderson da Cuhna.

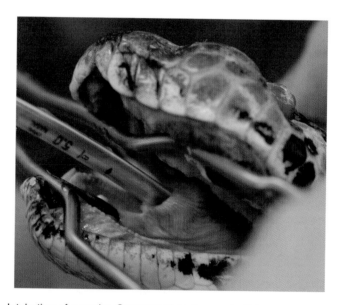

Figure 7.13 Intubation of a snake. Courtesy of Anderson da Cuhna.

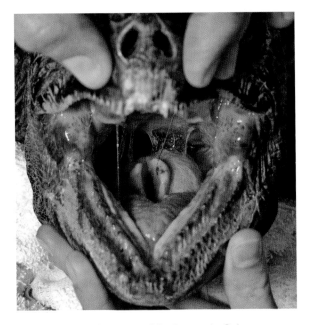

Figure 7.14 Larynx of a tortoise. Courtesy of Anderson da Cuhna.

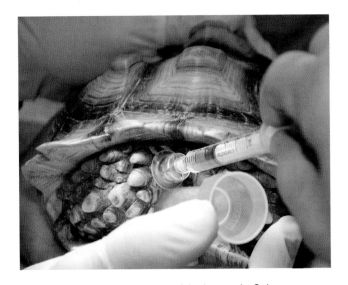

Figure 7.15 IO catheter in tortoise. Courtesy of Anderson da Cuhna.

5. Maintenance

General anesthesia is maintained primarily with inhalant anesthetics. Because these animals are ectothermic, external heat support is necessary throughout the anesthetic period to keep them in their optimal thermoregulatory range.

6. Monitoring under anesthesia

A Doppler is useful for monitoring HR; a pencil probe is ideal for the anesthetist to obtain HR via the ocular artery by placing this probe (well lubed) onto the eye. An esophageal stethoscope is also useful for obtaining HR. RR is visually observed. Assisted ventilation of one to four breaths per minute is recommended due to the long periods of apnea; MV is indicated for most reptiles. Capnography is not an adequate representation of ventilation due to intrapulmonary shunting (i.e., $EtCO_2$ is increased as compared to true $PaCO_2$), but does provide some evidence to the presence of CO. Pulse oximetry is not accurate in reptiles due to their alternative form of hemoglobin and difficulty placing the probe.

(a) Monitoring anesthetic depth: Muscle tone will decrease in the reptile as it becomes anesthetized. In the snake, relaxation occurs initially at the head, then through the torso, and proceeds caudally, lastly affecting the tail; recovery occurs in the opposite order. In snakes, the tongue retraction reflex will only subside in a deep plane of anesthesia. Palpebral reflexes may give an indication of anesthetic depth. Corneal reflexes are also lost in a deep plane. Toe or tail pinch is absent during the surgical plane of anesthesia. Jaw tone is also monitored in species where this is safe to assess.

(b) Recovery: Snakes typically take longer than lizards to recover; turtles, especially turtles that are capable of holding their breath, take an extraordinarily long time to recover. Maintaining optimal body temperature is critical to recovery. All reptiles are placed on room air to recover due to the downregulation of a reptile's respiratory system secondary to increased FiO_2. Continuing assisted ventilation is often necessary on room air. Extubation occurs once the patient is capable of spontaneous ventilation and pharyngeal reflexes have returned. Additional analgesia is administered as warranted.

C. Common complications

1. Hypothermia

Hypothermia is reduced by using circulating hot water blankets and forced air-warming units.

2. Hypoventilation

Hypoventilation secondary to apnea and respiratory depression is common in most reptiles, requiring assisted ventilation.

Table 7.10   Anesthetic protocol for reptiles.

	Snakes	Lizards	Turtle/Tortoise
Premedication (Note: No premedication in aggressive or poisonous species)	1. Butorphanol 20 mg/kg IM + and 2. Midazolam 1.0–2.0 mg/kg IM and/or 3. Ketamine 5–10 mg/kg IM	1. Morphine 0.4–1.5 mg/kg + and 2. Midazolam 1.0–2.0 mg/kg IM and/or 3. Ketamine 5–10 mg/kg IM	1. Opioid options: (a) Hydromorphone 0.5 mg/kg IM or (b) Morphine 0.4–1.5 mg/kg 2. Sedative option: (a) Midazolam 1.0–2.0 mg/kg IM and/or (b) Ketamine 5–10 mg/kg IM
Induction	Mask/chamber with gas inhalants	Mask/chamber with gas inhalants	1. Mask/chamber with gas inhalants or 2. Propofol via frontal sinus or IV 2–4 mg/kg to effect
Maintenance Intraoperative analgesia	Gas inhalants Local blocks where applicable	Gas inhalants Local blocks where applicable	Gas inhalants Local blocks where applicable
Post-op analgesia	1. Butorphanol 20 mg/kg IM and/or 2. Carprofen 1–4 mg/kg IM SID	1. Morphine 0.4–1.5 mg/kg IM and/or 2. NSAID options: (a) Carprofen 1–4 mg/kg IM SID or (b) Meloxicam 0.2 mg/kg PO or IV	1. Tramadol 5–10 mg/kg PO and/or 2. Carprofen 1–4 mg/kg IM SID

Chapter 7

References

1. Brodbelt D, Blissitt K, Hammond R, Neath P, Young L, Pfeiffer D, et al. The risk of death: the confidential enquiry into perioperative small animal fatalities. Vet Anaesth Analg. 2008;35(5):365–73.
2. Fulkerson P, Gustafson S. Use of laryngeal mask airway compared to endotracheal tube with positive-pressure ventilation in anesthetized swine. Vet Anaesth Analg. 2007;34(4): 284–8.
3. Tucker FS, Beattie RJ. Qualitative microtest for atropine esterase. Lab Anim Sci. 1983; 33(3):268–9.
4. Kazakos GM, Anagnostou T, Savvas I, Raptopoulos D, Psalla D, Kazakou IM. Use of the laryngeal mask airway in rabbits: placement and efficacy. Lab Anim (NY). 2007;36(4): 29–34.

5. Timm KI, Jahn SE, Sedgwick CJ. The palatal ostium of the guinea pig. Lab Anim Sci. 1987;37(6):801–2.
6. Geelen S, Sanchez-Migallon Guzman D, Souza MJ, Cox S, Keuler NS, Paul-Murphy JR. Antinociceptive effects of tramadol hydrochloride after intravenous administration to Hispaniolan Amazon parrots (Amazona ventralis). Am J Vet Res. 2013;74(2):201–6.
7. Guzman DS, Drazenovich TL, Olsen GH, Willits NH, Paul-Murphy JR. Evaluation of thermal antinociceptive effects after intramuscular administration of hydromorphone hydrochloride to American kestrels (Falco sparverius). Am J Vet Res. 2013;74(6):817–22.
8. Sladky KK, Miletic V, Paul-Murphy J, Kinney ME, Dallwig RK, Johnson SM. Analgesic efficacy and respiratory effects of butorphanol and morphine in turtles. J Am Vet Med Assoc. 2007;230(9):1356–62.

Chapter 8

Local analgesic techniques (regional blocks)

Local analgesic techniques are a beneficial adjunct to an anesthetic protocol. They reduce requirements of other anesthetics as well as provide analgesia. Although local anesthetics may have toxic effects at high doses, when used locally or in regional blocks, minimal systemic absorption takes place. Specific techniques are described in this section.

I. Bier block or intravenous block

A. Indications

Brief distal limb procedures.

B. Contraindications

Procedures exceeding 90 minutes.

C. Complications

1. Tourniquet pain.
2. Hypotension from rapid systemic absorption of large dose of local anesthetic.
3. Hypoperfusion of the limb distal to the tourniquet.

D. Practical points

1. Tourniquet is not used for longer than 90 minutes.
2. The tourniquet is released slowly, and the patient is monitored for hypotension and negative effects of rapid systemic absorption of lidocaine used in the block.

II. Brachial plexus block

A. Indication

Forelimb procedures below the elbow (e.g., radius or ulna fracture repair).

Small Animal Anesthesia Techniques, First Edition. Amanda M. Shelby and Carolyn M. McKune.
© 2014 John Wiley & Sons, Inc. Published 2014 by John Wiley & Sons, Inc.
Companion website: www.wiley.com/go/shelbyanesthesia

Chapter 8

Table 8.1 Bier block technique.

Materials: Intravenous (IV) catheter, lidocaine, tourniquet, Esmarch bandage, aseptic preparation

Drugs: Lidocaine 1–2 mg/kg. Bupivacaine is contraindicated (cardiovascular collapse may occur when tourniquet is released).

Technique:
1. Place IV catheter distal to proposed area for tourniquet, and then use an Esmarch bandage to desanguinate the limb, beginning at the distal aspect of the digit. Tighten the tourniquet on the proximal aspect of the limb, above the IV catheter following desanguination.
2. Administer 1–2 mg/kg lidocaine via the IV catheter. Do not release the tourniquet for at least 10–15 min.
3. Onset of analgesia is within 5–10 min.
4. Remove tourniquet within 90 min. Analgesia lasts for ~30 more minutes following the release of the tourniquet. If left in place longer than 2 h, muscle and nerve damage may result. There may be tourniquet-induced hypertension, secondary to tourniquet pain.

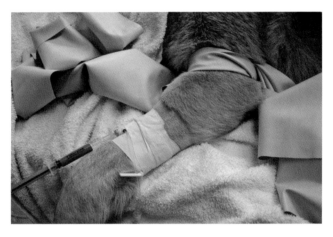

Figure 8.1　Bier block in the front limb of a canine patient. Courtesy of Patricia Queiroz-Williams.

B. Contraindications

1. Skin infection in area of injection.
2. Blocking of both front limbs (as patient may lose motor function and therefore ability to ambulate).

C. Complications

1. Accidental injection into the nerves or arteries: If there is resistance to injecting drugs, reposition needle, aspirate, and try injection again. If there is blood, reposition and reaspirate prior to injection.
2. Puncture of the thoracic cavity: Ensure negative pressure is present on aspiration prior to drug delivery.

Table 8.2 Brachial plexus block.

Materials: Spinal needle, local anesthetics, +/− nerve locator and appropriate insulated needle (may increase success of block), aseptic preparation
Drugs: Lidocaine 1 mg/kg + Bupivacaine 1 mg/kg or Bupivacaine 1–2 mg/kg alone
Technique: 1. Locate the point of the shoulder. 2. Clip a 5 cm × 5 cm area with the point of the shoulder in the center; prepare aseptically. 3. Insert the spinal needle at the point of the shoulder, through the skin. 4. The needle is placed lateral to the chest wall/medial to the scapula, and parallels the transverse processes of the cervical vertebrae, directed toward the scapula to avoid entering the thorax. The needle tip is slowly advanced caudal to the second rib. 5. With the blind technique, once the needle is inserted, attach the drug syringe, aspirate, and if no blood or air is present, approximately one-third of the drug volume is injected. The needle is withdrawn 1–2 cm, aspirate, and another third of the drug volume is administered. This continues until all drug is administered. 6. With the nerve finder and insulated locator needle technique, one lead is placed on the skin and the other on the needle. With the needle caudal to the second rib, the current begins relatively high (1.0–2.0 mA), and the needle is slowly advanced and retracted until a strong twitch is located. Reduce the current to the lowest possible setting with a detectable twitch (usually about 0.4 mA). 7. Connect syringe of drug to needle and aspirate. A small volume is injected; it is normal for twitching to disappear during injection. To ensure effectiveness, some anesthesiologists advocate depositing local anesthetic as the needle is slowly removed.

D. Practical points

1. The authors' preference is to combine lidocaine and bupivacaine, which may provide faster onset with longer duration of analgesia (empirical).
2. Stay below local anesthetic toxic dose range (see Table 3.7).

III. Digit block or ring block (radial, ulnar, and/or medial nerves)

A. Indication

Procedure requiring desensitization of distal branches of radial, ulnar, and medial nerve for areas distal to the carpus. Examples include declaws, digit amputations, orthopedic, or soft tissue surgeries.

B. Contraindication

Infection at the site of block.

C. Complications

Injection into a nerve, artery, or vein (always aspirate).

Chapter 8

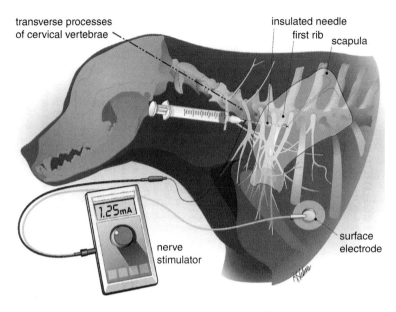

Figure 8.2 Diagram demonstrating brachial plexus block with a nerve locator and insulated needle. Courtesy of Teton New Media.

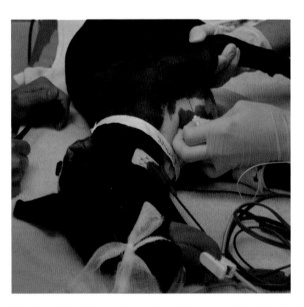

Figure 8.3 Brachial plexus block in canine patient. Courtesy of Patricia Queiroz-Williams.

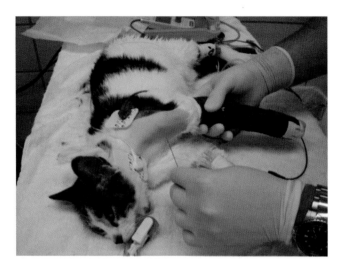

Figure 8.4   Brachial plexus block in feline patient.

Table 8.3   Radial/ulnar/medial nerve block.

Materials: 22- to 25-g needles, 3-mL syringe, examination gloves, aseptic preparation
Drugs: Bupivacaine 1.5 mg/kg and Lidocaine 2 mg/kg *per cat* (divide this between limbs if procedure involves multiple limbs)
Technique: 1. The forelimb is prepared for the procedure. (Remember to avoid alcohol for preparation if *laser* declaw method is used.) 2. The median nerve courses down the medial, palmar aspect of the paw. The palmar branch of the ulnar nerve runs alongside it. Insert a 25-g needle at the level of the first digit, below the carpal pad. 3. Aspirate, and if no blood is present, deposit a quarter of the volume of local anesthetic for *that* paw (volume is divided between limbs undergoing procedures). 4. The radial nerve is desensitized on the dorsal aspect of the paw, just above the first digit, on the medial side. 5. Aspirate, and if no blood is present, deposit a quarter of the volume of local anesthetic for *that* paw. 6. The dorsal branch of the ulnar nerve is desensitized on the palmar side of the paw, just dorsal to the carpal pad. 7. Aspirate, and if no blood is present, deposit a quarter of the volume of local anesthetic for *that* paw. Additionally, another quarter volume is placed as the radial nerve courses over the lateral, dorsal side of the paw at the level of the fifth digit. 8. Repeat this procedure on each limb undergoing surgery.

Chapter 8

D. Practical points

1. This block is also commonly completed as a ring block. Simply infuse local anesthetic around the distal aspect of the limb by connecting the "blebs" similar to the line block.
2. 0.9% NaCl is added to increase volume if needed.
3. Avoid diluting bupivacaine below 0.25% (2.5 mg/mL), as it may result in a poor block.
4. Stay below local anesthetic toxic dose range (see Table 3.7).

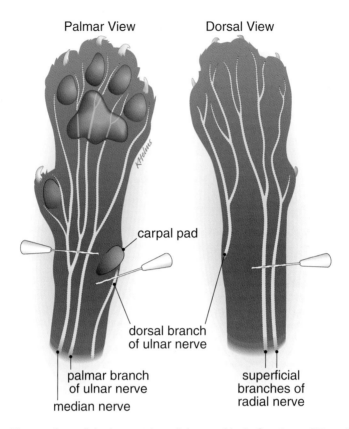

Palmar View   Dorsal View

carpal pad

dorsal branch
of ulnar nerve

palmar branch
of ulnar nerve
median nerve

superficial
branches of
radial nerve

Figure 8.5   Diagram for radial, ulnar, and medial nerve block. Courtesy of Teton New Media.

IV. Epidural

A. Indications

Performed in the anesthetized or heavily sedated patient undergoing noxious procedures of the caudal abdomen, hind limb, or thorax. Epidurals with morphine and a local anesthetic may provide long duration (12–24 hours) of analgesia. Epidurals are also used to reduce requirements of gas inhalants (1).

B. Contraindications

Skin infection, sepsis, hypovolemia/hypotension, urinary tract surgery (due to urine retention if morphine is included in the epidural), abnormal epidural space confirmation (e.g., pelvic fracture), coagulopathy.

C. Complications

Hypotension, hypoventilation, and apnea, cardiovascular collapse/reduction in sympathetic tone, infection/meningitis, urinary retention, delayed hair grown, pruritus (1).

D. Practical points

1. Express the bladder following the procedure.
2. Stay below local anesthetic toxic dose range.
3. For cranial abdominal or thoracic procedures use only morphine.
4. Preservative free (PF) drugs are recommended.
5. Opioids in the epidural space travel cranially affect ventilation during procedure and in recovery.

Table 8.4 Epidural placement with patient in lateral recumbency.

Materials: Aseptic preparation, sterile gloves, spinal needle of appropriate diameter and length, drugs, +/− glass syringe, +/− nerve stimulator and appropriate insulated needle

Drugs: Morphine PF 0.1 mg/kg +/− Bupivacaine PF 0.5–1.0 mg/kg or Lidocaine PF 0.5 mg/kg not to exceed calculated total volume[a]

Technique:
1. Once patient is sedated/anesthetized, place animal in lateral recumbency and pull hind limbs ventral (forward).
2. Clip a 10 × 10-cm square over the lumbosacral (LS) space; aseptically prepare site.
3. Open gloves and place necessary materials in a sterile manner on glove paper; glove carefully avoiding contaminating materials.
4. Palpate the iliac wings with thumb and middle finger. Use index finger to palpate the LS junction (usually just caudal to a line drawn between the two iliac wings).
5. In the canine, on midline, insert the needle perpendicular to the skin, approximately halfway between the spinous process of L7 and the sacrum. In the feline, the junction is slightly more caudal.
6. Feel for two "pops" (resistance which dissipates abruptly). The first minor pop is passage through muscle facia. The next, more prominent pop signifies passing through the ligamentum flavum. (If bone is encountered while advancing the needle, withdraw the needle to just below the surface of the skin, reassess location, and redirect the needle if no blood is present in the needle hub.)
7. Remove the stylet from hub and inspect for cerebral spinal fluid (CSF) or blood. If CSF is present, reduce the dose of drugs by 50%. If blood is present, remove needle and use an alternative analgesic technique. Obtaining CSF is more likely in cats because the spinal cord ends (L7) more caudally than in dogs.
8. Place 1–2 mL of air in a glass syringe (if a glass syringe is unavailable, a 3-mL regular syringe may work but will not be resistance-free like that of the glass syringe) and secure to spinal needle. Test for loss of resistance by injecting air to see if the plunger of the syringe advances smoothly. There is no resistance if in the epidural space. Remove glass syringe.
9. A 1-mL air bubble placed in the drug syringe helps to confirm that the needle remained in the epidural space (during injection of drugs, the air bubble will not collapse). Some anesthesiologists recommend aspirating prior to drug injection for blood or CSF. Inject drugs slowly over 60–90 seconds; injections should be smooth (no resistance).
10. At this point, some anesthesiologists advocate putting the affected limb down to encourage epidural spread to that region especially if local anesthetics were used.

[a]Total volume calculation options: (1) 1 mL/10 kg for perianal, 1 mL/7 kg for hind limb procedures, 1 mL/5 kg for thoracic/abdominal procedure. Avoid total volumes over 6–8 mL. Sterile 0.9% NaCl is used to add volume if desired. (2) 0.2 mL/kg (see example in Appendix G).

Chapter 8

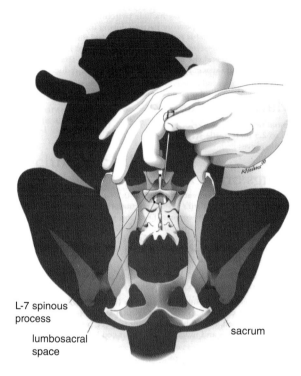

L-7 spinous
process

lumbosacral
space

sacrum

Figure 8.6 Diagram demonstrating landmarks for epidural placement. Courtesy of Teton New Media.

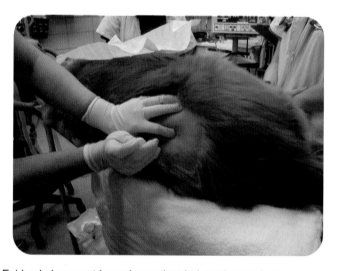

Figure 8.7 Epidural placement in canine patient in lateral recumbency.

Table 8.5 Sternal position epidural/hanging drop technique.

Materials: Aseptic preparation, sterile gloves, spinal needle of appropriate diameter and length, drugs, +/− glass syringe, +/− nerve stimulator and appropriate insulated needle

Drugs: Morphine PF 0.1 mg/kg +/− Bupivacaine PF 0.5–1.0 mg/kg or Lidocaine PF 0.5 mg/kg not to exceed calculated total volume[a]

Technique:

1. Once patient is sedated/anesthetized, place animal in sternal recumbency and pull hind limbs forward.
2. Clip a 10 × 10-cm square over the lumbosacral (LS) space; aseptically prepare site.
3. Open gloves and sterilely place necessary materials on glove paper; glove carefully, avoiding contaminating materials.
4. Palpate the iliac wings with thumb and middle finger. Use index finger to palpate the LS junction (usually just caudal to a line drawn mediolaterally between the two iliac wings).
5. In the canine, insert the needle perpendicular to the skin, approximately halfway between the spinous process of L7 and the sacrum, on midline. In the feline, the junction is slightly more caudally.
6. Remove stylet once through the skin and place sterile 0.9% NaCl in needle hub.
7. Feel for two "pops" (resistance which dissipates abruptly). The first minor pop is passage through muscle facia. The next, more prominent, pop signifies passing through the ligamentum flavum. At this point, the saline is pulled into the epidural space ("sucked") from the hub of the needle. (If bone is encountered while advancing the needle, withdraw the needle to just below the surface of the skin, reassess location, and redirect the needle if no blood is present in the needle hub.)
8. Inspect for CSF or blood. If CSF is present, reduce the dose of drugs by 50%. If blood is present, remove needle and use an alternative analgesic technique. Obtaining CSF is more common in cats due to location of where the spinal cord terminates (L7).
9. A 1-mL air bubble in the syringe of drugs may help to assess that the needle remains in the epidural space (during injection, the air bubble will not collapse if needle is correctly located). Some anesthesiologists recommend aspirating prior to drug injection for blood or CSF. Inject drugs slowly over 60–90 s; injections should be smooth (resistance free).
10. At this point, some anesthesiologists advocate putting the affected limb down to encourage epidural spread to that region especially when local anesthetics are used.

[a]Total volume calculation options: (1) 1 mL/10 kg for perianal, 1 mL/7 kg for hind limb procedures, 1 mL/5 kg for thoracic/abdominal procedure. Avoid total volumes over 6–8 mL. Sterile 0.9% NaCl is used to add volume if desired. (2) 0.2 mL/kg (see example in Appendix G).

Chapter 8

V. Femoral and sciatic nerve block

A. Indication

Hind limb procedures at the level of the stifle and below.

B. Contraindication

Skin infection in area of injection.

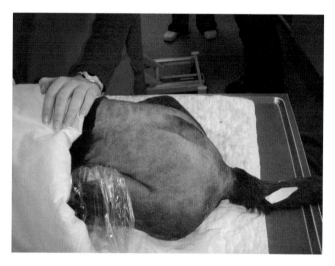

Figure 8.8   Canine patient in sternal positioning epidural technique.

C. Complications

1. Accidental injection into the nerves or arteries. If there is resistance to injecting drugs, reposition needle, aspirate, and try injection again. If there is blood, reposition and reaspirate prior to injection.
2. Hemorrhage if the femoral artery is punctured.

D. Practical points

1. The authors' preference is to combine lidocaine and bupivacaine to provide faster onset with longer duration of analgesia (empirical).
2. Stay below local anesthetic toxic dose range (see Table 3.7).
3. This block is best performed with a nerve stimulator.
4. There is a case report suggesting this is effective when combined with sedation as a way to avoid general anesthesia for hind limb procedures (2).

VI. Infiltrative or splash block

A. Indication

Infiltrative blocks are performed prior to incision to locally desensitize an area for minor surgical procedures. Splash blocks are performed prior to closure of an incisional site to provide local analgesia to the incised tissue.

B. Contraindications

1. Infection causes changes in the pH of the tissue, making local anesthetics less effective.

Table 8.6 Femoral and sciatic nerve block (2).

Materials: 20- to 22-g insulated needle (length depends on size of patient), nerve locator, syringe, local anesthetic, examination gloves

Drugs: Bupivacaine 1–1.5 mg/kg
Lidocaine 1–2 mg/kg

Technique:
1. Aseptically prepare the site once the patient is sedated or anesthetized.
2. Femoral nerve block: The patient is placed in lateral recumbency, with the limb for blockade up. The limb is extended slightly caudally with access to the medial side of the thigh. Palpate for the femoral artery in the femoral triangle. Cranial to the femoral artery, and caudal to the rectus femoris, lies the femoral nerve. An insulated needle is introduced through the quadriceps femoris targeting the location of the femoral nerve, and assessing for the twitch of the quadriceps muscle/extension of the stifle, which is achieved as low as 0.4 mA. Aspirate and then deposit local anesthetic.
3. Sciatic nerve block: After femoral nerve block, the leg is returned to its normal position. Identify by palpation the ischiatic tuberosity; insert the insulated needle just below the tuberosity, through the semimebranous and abductor muscles, medial to the biceps femoris. The nerve stimulator elicits either dorsiflexion or plantar foot extension at 0.4–1.0 mAs. Aspirate and then deposit local anesthetic.

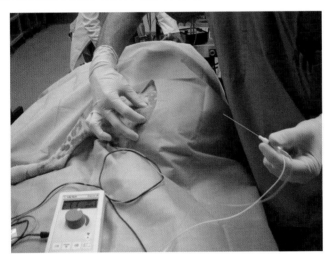

Figure 8.9 Palpation of landmarks for a femoral/sciatic nerve block with the assistance of a nerve locator and insulated needle.

Chapter 8

C. Complications

Accidental injection in an artery or vein; always aspirate prior to injection.

D. Practical points

1. Ensure infiltrative block will not affect tissue submission for histopathology.
2. Do not use infiltrative block for masses where malignant cells may be spread beyond margins by the needle used to administer the block.
3. Do not exceed the toxic doses for local anesthetics (see Table 3.7).

Table 8.7   Infiltrative or splash blocks.

Materials: 20- to 22-g needle, 3-mL syringe, local anesthetic, aseptic preparation, examination gloves
Drugs:[a]   Bupivacaine 1–2 mg/kg for dogs, 1 mg/kg for cats Lidocaine 2 mg/kg in dogs, 1 mg/kg in cats
Infiltrative technique: Area is clipped and aseptically prepped prior to block. An infiltrative block involves distribution of local anesthetic into tissue, usually subcutaneously, around a mass or area of incision.
Splash Technique: Splash block involves the "splashing" of local anesthetic over an incision after closure of the muscle layer, but prior to closure of the skin. The solution is given sterilely to the surgeon for administration or splashed sterilely into incision.

[a]The authors prefer a combination of bupivacaine (1 mg/kg) and lidocaine (1 mg/kg), for fast onset and longer duration (empirical).

VII. Intercostal block

A. Indication

For use in patients undergoing lateral thoracotomy, placement of chest tubes, or repair of thoracic trauma.

B. Contraindications

Avoid injecting directly into the nerve; instead, infiltrate around the nerve.

C. Complications

1. Accidental puncture of the thoracic cavity causing pneumothorax.
2. Accidental injection into nerve, artery, or vein. Always aspirate prior to injection. If blood is aspirated, redirect needle. If there is resistance upon injection, redirect needle.

D. Practical points

Two intercostal spaces cranial and caudal to the area affected are blocked for maximum effect.

VIII. Intrapleural block

A. Indication

Patients with intrapleural pain postoperatively, including pain secondary to the discomfort of a chest tube.

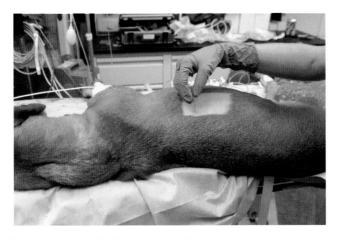

Figure 8.10   Intercostal nerve block in canine patient.

Table 8.8   Intercostal block.

Materials: 22- to 25-g needle, 3 mL syringe, examination gloves, aseptic preparation

Drugs:[a]   Bupivacaine 1 mg/kg
            Lidocaine 1 mg/kg

Technique:
1. Clip and aseptically prepare two cranial spaces, target space, and two caudal rib spaces for block.
2. Wearing examination gloves, palpate between the intervertebral foramen and the caudal border of each of the five rib spaces.
3. Place needle through the skin, just below the intervertebral foramen, caudal to rib. For appropriate depth, the needle must penetrate just below the intercostal muscles.
4. Aspirate and inject a portion of the volume in the intercostal space. Repeat at each space.

[a]The authors prefer the combination of bupivacaine (1 mg/kg) and lidocaine (1 mg/kg) for fast onset and longer duration (empirical).

B. Contraindications

Infection: There is also some controversy over the use of intrapleural infiltration in patients where pericardium has been removed.

C. Complications

Some animals may experience severe discomfort from the infiltration of local anesthetics, likely secondary to the drugs' low pH. Administer appropriate systemic analgesic drugs or heavily sedate the patient prior to administration of local anesthetics through a chest

Table 8.9 Intrapleural block (placement through a chest tube).

Materials: Local anesthetic, 60-mL syringe for aspiration of chest tube, 3- to 6-mL syringe of sterile saline, examination gloves

Drugs: Bupivacaine—initial dose in dogs not to exceed 2 mg/kg into chest; subsequent doses are 1 mg/kg repeated 4–6 h. This may be combined with sodium bicarbonate to reduce acidity (at a 1 : 2 dilution bupivacaine : sodium bicarbonate). It is common in cats to reduce the dose by half.

Technique:
1. Aspirate the chest tube prior to placement of drugs for air, fluid, or blood. Proceed once negative pressure is obtained (if possible).
2. Place dose of bupivacaine into chest tube followed by the smallest volume saline possible to flush drug through chest tube into chest.
3. The chest tube should not be aspirated for an hour to allow absorption of the drug.

---

tube; drug administration is also done very slowly in case of an adverse reaction. Respiratory distress may occur if too large a volume of drug is infused.

D. Practical points

1. If placing local anesthetic through the chest tube, aspirate chest tube to remove any exudate or air first. Ensure chest tube is sealed after drug administration to prevent pneumothorax.
2. Sterile technique is required if placing a drug through a chest tube.

IX. Intra-articular block (joint block)

A. Indications

Patient undergoing a procedure where the joint capsule is incised.

B. Contraindications

Infected joint or local infection involving the skin over site of injection.

C. Complications

Contamination of the joint if aseptic technique is not used. Additionally, local anesthetics may cause chondrocyte death.

D. Practical points

1. Typically, this block is done during surgery as the surgeon directly visualizes site for blockade.

Table 8.10 Intra-articular (joint) block of stifle.

Materials: 22- to 25-g needle, 1-mL syringe, morphine, aseptic preparation, sterile
gloves

Drugs: Morphine 0.1–0.3 mg/kg

Technique:
1. Clip and aseptically prepare the area over joint.
2. With the joint in flexion, palpate the lateral femoral condyle, tibial tuberosity, and
patella.
3. Insert needle from the lateral aspect between the femoral condyle and the lateral tibial
tuberosity, to the depth of the joint capsule (joint fluid is easily aspirated if placement
is correct).
4. Inject drug solution.

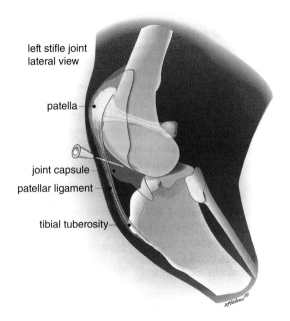

left stifle joint
lateral view

patella

joint capsule

patellar ligament

tibial tuberosity

Figure 8.11 Diagram showing intra-articular block in canine stifle. Courtesy of Teton New
Media.

Chapter 8

X. Oral nerve block

A. Indications

Regional blocks used for targeted areas of the maxilla and mandible, providing loss of
sensation to the teeth and lips. Area of desensitization depends on which block is used.

B. Contraindications

Infected gingiva and teeth.

C. Complications

Injection into nerve, artery, or vein (always aspirate).

D. Practical points

1. Stay below local anesthetics toxic dose range (see Table 3.7).
2. Required drug volumes are small (0.1–0.5 mL) due to size and location of foramen blocked.
3. In cats, some of these foramens (such as the infraorbital foramen) are very short; place the needle at the opening of the foramen rather than in the canal to avoid complications.

E. Materials

25-gauge needles, syringe, and examination gloves.

F. Drugs

1. Local anesthetics including lidocaine, mepivacaine, and bupivacaine are commonly used.
2. Drug dosages based on patient weight are usually unnecessary due to anatomical volume limitations; however, toxic doses based on weight are calculated and not exceeded.

G. Infraorbital nerve block

Indication: Procedures of the maxillary dental arcade.

Table 8.11 Infraorbital nerve block.

Materials: 1-mL syringe, local anesthetic, 25-g needle, examination gloves
Drugs: Lidocaine 1 mg/kg, Bupivacaine 1 mg/kg, or Mepivacaine 1 mg/kg
Technique: 1. Palpate the infraorbital foramen (on the buccal side of the maxilla, usually above the 2nd premolar). 2. Place the index finger over the foramen to guide needle, and insert a 25-g needle into the opening of the foramen. Inserting the needle deeper into foramen increases chance of injecting into the nerve. 3. Aspirate; if no blood is present, inject local anesthetic solution around opening of and slightly within the foramen. Little to no resistance to injection is felt when the needle is correctly placed.

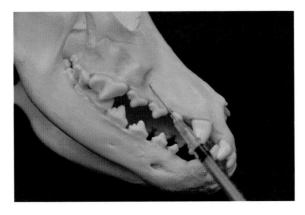

Figure 8.12 Infraorbital block in canine skeleton. Courtesy of Anderson da Cuhna.

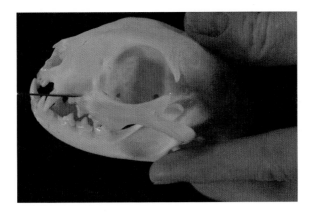

Figure 8.13 Infraorbital block in the feline skeleton. Courtesy of Anderson da Cuhna.

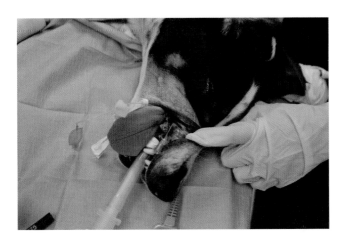

Figure 8.14 Infraorbital block in the canine patient. Courtesy of Anderson da Cuhna.

H. Maxillary nerve block

1. Indication: Procedures involving the maxilla, upper teeth, and lip
2. Complications: Apoptosis of eye if laceration of the maxillary artery.

I. Mandibular nerve block

Indication: Procedures involving the mandibular dental arcade.

Table 8.12   Maxillary nerve block.

Materials: 1-mL syringe, local anesthetic, 25-g needle, examination gloves

Drugs: Lidocaine 1 mg/kg, Bupivacaine 1 mg/kg, or Mepivacaine 1 mg/kg

Technique (inside mouth approach)
1. Palpate on midline (from rostrally to caudally along the hard palate) locating the caudal nasal spine of the palate. Laterally from the caudal nasal spine of the palate lies the pterygopalatine fossa and pterygoid process (the maxillary nerve passes through the pterygoid fossa); it is medial to the last molar if present.
2. Insert a 25-g needle into the area near the pterygoid fossa. See Figure 8.15 or Figure 8.16.
3. Aspirate; if no blood is present, inject 1–2 mL volume of local anesthetic.

Technique (from outside mouth):
1. A 25-g needle is inserted through the skin over the ventral border of the zygomatic process and 0.5 cm caudal to lateral canthus of eye. Direct the needle perpendicular to the arch.
2. Advance needle close to, but not in direct contact with, the pterygopalatine fossa.
3. Deposit 1–2 mL of 1% lidocaine (staying within the dosage limits for the patient).

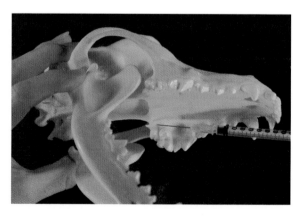

Figure 8.15   Maxillary block via internal approach in the skeleton of a dog. Courtesy of Anderson da Cuhna.

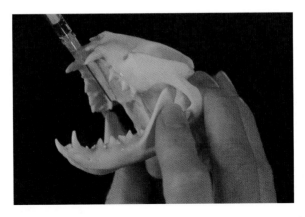

Figure 8.16 Maxillary block via internal approach in the skeleton of a cat. Courtesy of Anderson da Cuhna.

Table 8.13 Mandibular nerve block.

Materials: 1-mL syringe, 25-g needle, local anesthetic, examination gloves
Drugs: Lidocaine 1 mg/kg, Bupivacaine 1 mg/kg, or Mepivacaine 1 mg/kg
Technique:
1. Palpate the mandibular foramen on the caudal, medial (lingual) surface of the ramus (curve of the mandible) behind the last molar. The foramen is palpable both internally on the lingual side of the ramus, or externally (see Figure 8.17, Figure 8.18, or Figure 8.19).
2. Use index finger of the opposite hand to guide 25-g needle and a 1-mL syringe of local anesthetic near the foramen, between the mucosa and bone. If the approach is through the skin, the skin is first aseptically prepared.
3. Aspirate syringe. If no blood is present, inject local anesthetic around the mandibular foramen.

J. Mental nerve block

Indication: Procedures involving rostral lower lip of the mandible, mandibular canine and incisor teeth, and the mandibular symphysis.

XI. Paravertebral block

A. Indication

Forelimb procedures.

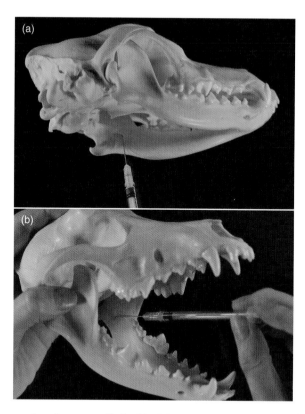

Figure 8.17 Approaches for a mandibular block in a canine skull. Courtesy of Anderson da Cuhna.

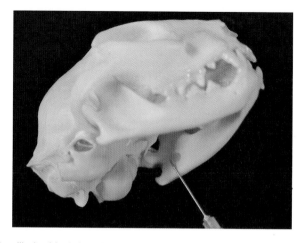

Figure 8.18 Mandibular block in a feline skull. Courtesy of Anderson da Cuhna.

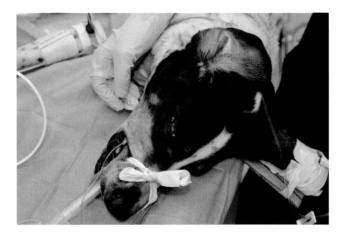

Figure 8.19 Mandibular block in canine patient. Courtesy of Anderson da Cuhna.

Table 8.14 Mental nerve block.

Materials: 1-mL syringe, 25-g needle, local anesthetics, examination gloves

Drugs: Lidocaine 1 mg/kg, Bupivacaine 1 mg/kg, or Mepivacaine 1 mg/kg

Technique:
1. Palpate the mental foramen on the buccal side of the mandible, just rostral the 2nd premolar tooth.
2. Insert 25-g needle in front of the mental foramen.
3. Aspirate syringe. If no blood is present, inject local anesthetic around the mental foramen.

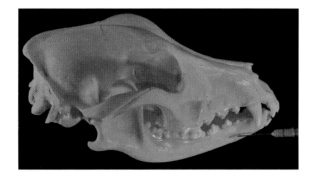

Figure 8.20 Mental block in canine skull. Courtesy of Anderson da Cuhna.

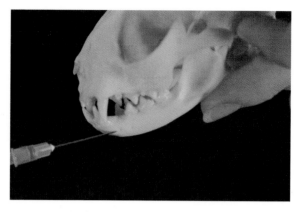

Figure 8.21   Mental block in a feline skull. Courtesy of Anderson da Cuhna.

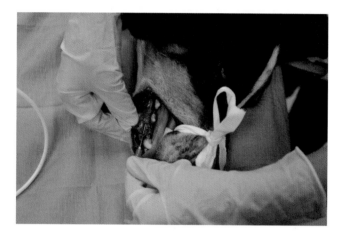

Figure 8.22   Mental block in a canine patient. Courtesy of Anderson da Cuhna.

B. Contraindications

1. Skin infection in area of injection.
2. Blocking of both front limbs (as patient may lose motor function and therefore ability to ambulate).

C. Complications

1. Accidental injection into the nerves or arteries. If there is resistance to injecting drugs, reposition needle, aspirate, and try injection again. If there is blood, reposition and reaspirate prior to injection.
2. Puncture of the thoracic cavity. Ensure you have negative pressure on aspiration prior to drug delivery.

Table 8.15 Paravertebral block (3).

Materials: 20- to 22-g spinal needles (length depends on size of patient), syringe, local anesthetic, examination gloves

Drugs: Bupivacaine 1–1.5 mg/kg
Lidocaine 1–2 mg/kg

Technique:
1. Aseptically prepare the site.
2. Blocking C6: By palpation, identify the transverse process of the sixth cervical vertebrae, and insert the needle just dorsal to this process. The needle is directed at sharp angle (30–45 degrees), in a dorsal ventral plane that parallels the transverse process.
   When contact is made with the transverse process, the needle is advanced cranially. Aspirate and deposit drug.
3. Blocking C7: After the blockade of C6, direct the needle caudally, aspirate, and deposit more drug.
4. Blocking C8: By palpation, identify the first rib, at a location dorsal to the spine of the scapula. Insert the needle parallel and cranial to the rib. Direct the need ventrally at a sharp angle (30 degrees). Deposit drug dorsal to the costochondral junction after aspiration.

D. Practical points

1. The authors' preference is to combine lidocaine and bupivacaine to provide faster onset with longer duration of analgesia (empirical).
2. Stay below local anesthetics toxic dose range (see Table 3.7).
3. In a study comparing three different techniques (blind, ultrasound guided, and nerve stimulator) for achieving blockade of the paravertebral brachial plexus, there was low success regardless of technique chosen. Therefore, the blind technique is described, as advanced techniques had no advantage.

XII. Retrobulbar blocks

A. Indication

Removal of the eye.

B. Contraindications

Infection of the tissue surrounding the globe.

C. Complications

Hemorrhage is possible resulting in proptosis of the eye. Subarachonoid injection or optic sheath injection will result in seizures and possibly death; if there is resistant to injection, *do not inject*. IV injection, if using bupivacaine, is life threatening. Always aspirate prior to injection.

Table 8.16   Retrobulbar block inferior temporal palpebral technique (4).

Materials: 22-g spinal needle (length is dependent on size of patient), 3-mL syringe, local anesthetic, aseptic preparation, sterile gloves

Drugs: Lidocaine 1 mg/kg or Bupivicaine 1 mg/kg

Technique:
1. Once animal is adequately anesthetized, aseptically prepare the injection site for the procedure.
2. Curve the needle to conform to the orbit.
3. Insert the needle at the 7 o'clock position, below the eyelid. When placing the needle, preferentially allow the needle to traverse along the bony orbit to avoid puncturing the globe and/or blood vessels.
4. The globe will rotate caudally until the conjunctival sac is breached, then the globe will rotate back to a standard position.
5. Advance the needle slightly further if there is no resistance. If any resistance is felt, immediately stop and withdraw the needle slightly.
6. Aspirate for blood, fluid, or resistance. If none is present, inject a test dosage (0.5 mL or less) of local anesthetic. If there is no resistance, and patient remains stable, continue with the rest of the injection.

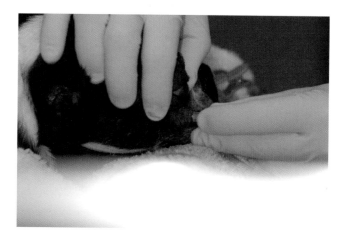

Figure 8.23   Retrobulbar block. Courtesy of Filipe Espinheira.

D. Practical points

There are several approaches with different complications depending on the experience of the individual performing the block.

References

1. Campoy L, Martin-Flores M, Ludders JW, Gleed RD. Procedural sedation combined with locoregional anesthesia for orthopedic surgery of the pelvic limb in 10 dogs: case series. Vet Anaesth Analg. 2012;39(4):436–40.

2. Campoy L, Bezuidenhout AJ, Gleed RD, Martin-Flores M, Raw RM, Santare CL, et al. Ultrasound-guided approach for axillary brachial plexus, femoral nerve, and sciatic nerve blocks in dogs. Vet Anaesth Analg. 2010;37(2):144–53.

3. Rioja E, Sinclair M, Chalmers H, Foster RA, Monteith G. Comparison of three techniques for paravertebral brachial plexus blockade in dogs. Vet Anaesth Analg. 2012;39(2):190–200.

4. Accola PJ, Bentley E, Smith LJ, Forrest LJ, Baumel CA, Murphy CJ. Development of a retrobulbar injection technique for ocular surgery and analgesia in dogs. J Am Vet Med Assoc. 2006;229(2):220–5.

Appendices

Appendix A: Instructions for using the CSU acute pain scale

The Colorado State University (CSU) Acute Pain Scale is intended primarily as a teaching tool and to guide observation of clinical patients. The scale has not been validated and should not be used as a definitive pain score. Use of the scale employs both an observational period and a hands-on evaluation of the patient. In general, the assessment begins with quiet observation of the patient in its cage at a relatively unobstructive distance. Afterward, the patient as a whole (wound as well as the entire body) is approached to assess reaction to gentle palpation, indicators of muscle tension and heat, response to interaction, and so on.

1. The scale utilizes a generic 0–4 scale with quartermarks as its base along with a color scale as a visual cue for progression along the five-point scale.
2. Realistic artist's renderings of animals at various levels of pain add further visual cues. Additional drawings provide space for recording pain, warmth, and muscle tension; this allows documentation of specific areas of concern in the medical record. A further advantage of these drawings is that the observer is encouraged to assess the overall pain of the patient in addition to focusing on the primary lesion.
3. The scale includes psychological and behavioral signs of pain as well as palpation responses. Further, the scale uses body tension as an evaluation tool, a parameter not addressed in other scales.
4. There is provision for nonassessment in the resting patient. To the author's knowledge, this is the only scale that emphasizes the importance of delaying assessment in a sleeping patient while prompting the observer to recognize patients that may be inappropriately obtunded by medication or a more serious health concern.
5. Advantages of this scale include ease of use with minimal interpretation required. Specific descriptors for individual behaviors are provided, which decreases interobserver variability. Additionally, a scale is provided for both the dog and cat.
6. A disadvantage of this scale is a lack of validation by clinical studies comparing it with other scales. Further, its use is largely limited to and is intended for use in acute pain (see Figure A.1 and Figure A.2).

Small Animal Anesthesia Techniques, First Edition. Amanda M. Shelby and Carolyn M. McKune.
© 2014 John Wiley & Sons, Inc. Published 2014 by John Wiley & Sons, Inc.
Companion website: www.wiley.com/go/shelbyanesthesia

Colorado State University
VETERINARY TEACHING HOSPITAL

Date _____

Time _____

Canine Acute Pain Scale

Rescore when awake	☐ Animal is sleeping, but can be aroused - Not evaluated for pain ☐ Animal can't be aroused, check vital signs, assess therapy

Pain Score	Example	Psychological & Behavioral	Response to Palpation	Body Tension
0	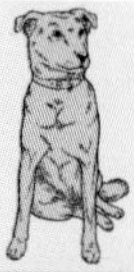	☐ **Comfortable** when resting ☐ **Happy, content** ☐ Not bothering wound or surgery site ☐ Interested in or curious about surroundings	☐ **Nontender** to palpation of wound or surgery site, or to palpation elsewhere	Minimal
1	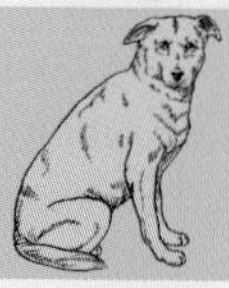	☐ **Content to slightly unsettled** or restless ☐ **Distracted easily** by surroundings	☐ **Reacts to palpation** of wound, surgery site, or other body part by **looking around, flinching, or whimpering**	Mild
2	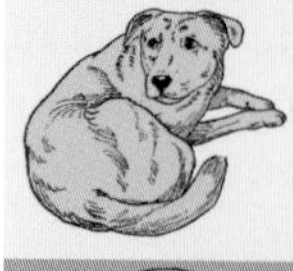	☐ Looks **uncomfortable** when resting ☐ May **whimper** or cry and may **lick or rub wound** or surgery site when unattended ☐ Droopy ears, **worried facial expression** (arched eye brows, darting eyes) ☐ **Reluctant to respond** when beckoned ☐ **Not eager to interact** with people or surroundings but will look around to see what is going on	☐ Flinches, whimpers cries, or guards/pulls away	Mild to Moderate **Reassess analgesic plan**
3	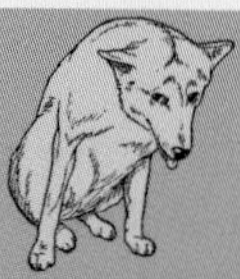	☐ **Unsettled, crying, groaning, biting or chewing** wound when unattended ☐ **Guards or protects** wound or surgery site by altering weight distribution (i.e., limping, shifting body position) ☐ **May be unwilling to move** all or part of body	☐ May be **subtle** (shifting eyes or increased respiratory rate) if dog is too painful to move or is stoic ☐ May be **dramatic**, such as a sharp cry, growl, bite or bite threat, and/or pulling away	Moderate **Reassess analgesic plan**
4	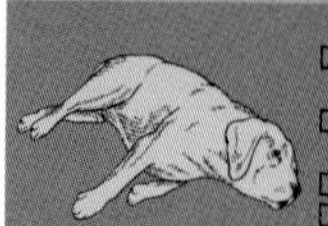	☐ **Constantly groaning or screaming** when unattended ☐ May bite or chew at wound, but unlikely to move ☐ **Potentially unresponsive** to surroundings ☐ **Difficult to distract** from pain	☐ **Cries at non-painful palpation** (may be experiencing allodynia, wind-up, or fearful that pain could be made worse) ☐ May react aggressively to palpation	Moderate to Severe **May be rigid to avoid painful movement** **Reassess analgesic plan**

RIGHT   LEFT

○ Tender to palpation
✕ Warm
■ Tense

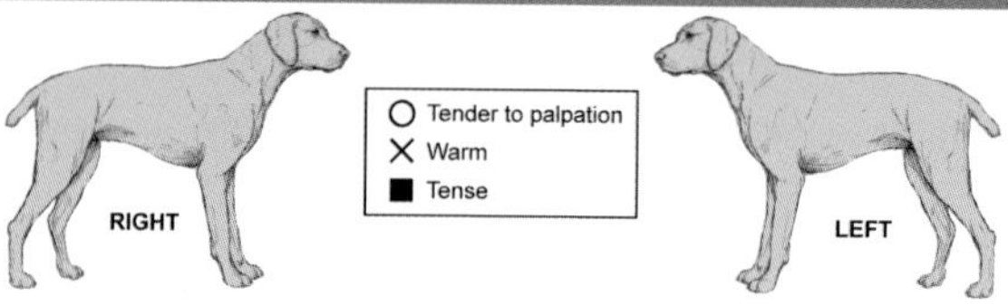

Comments _____

Figure A.1 Subjective and objective pain scoring sheet in dogs. Reprinted with permission from Dr. Robinson and Dr. Hellyer at Colorado State University.

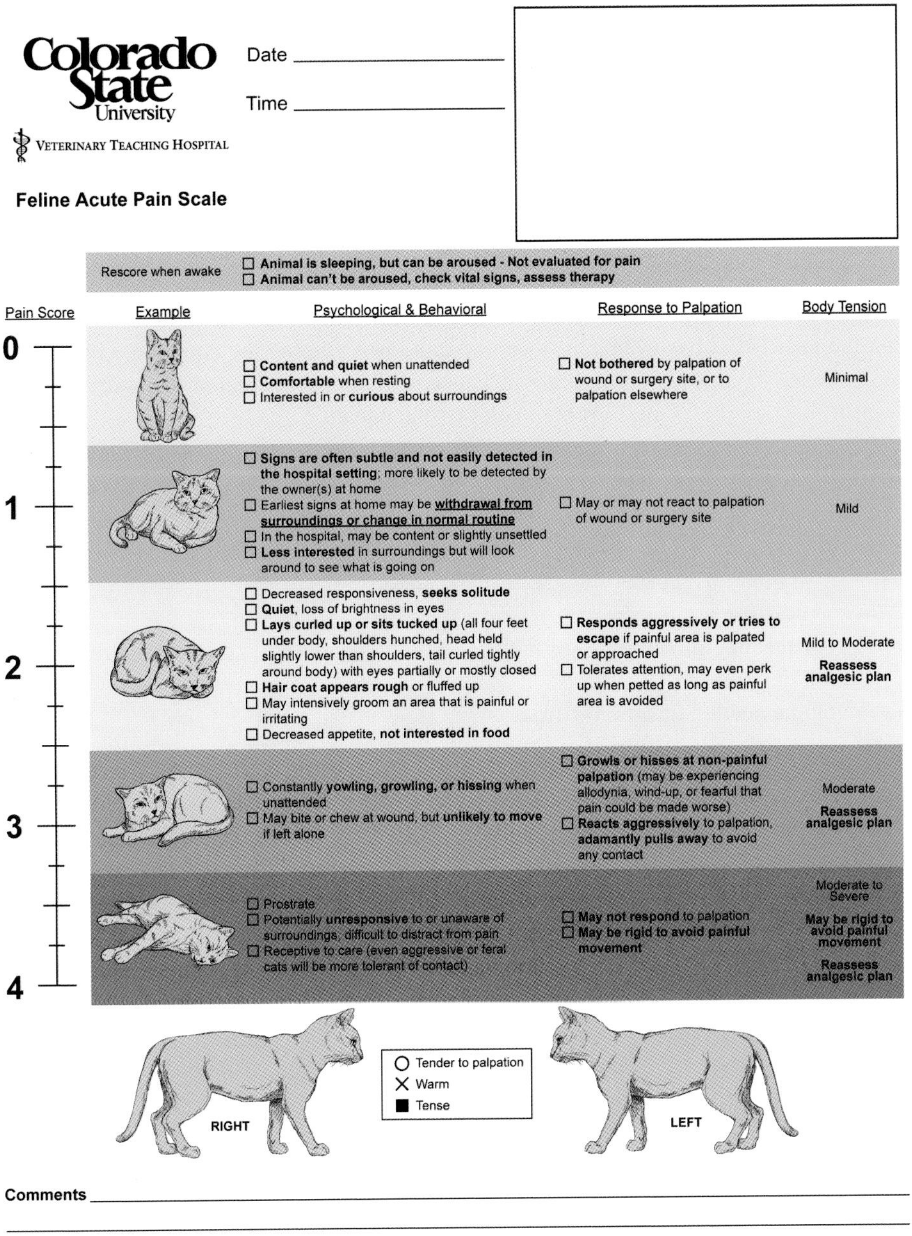

Colorado State University
VETERINARY TEACHING HOSPITAL

Feline Acute Pain Scale

Date _____

Time _____

	Animal is sleeping, but can be aroused - Not evaluated for pain
Rescore when awake	☐ Animal is sleeping, but can be aroused - Not evaluated for pain ☐ Animal can't be aroused, check vital signs, assess therapy

Pain Score	Example	Psychological & Behavioral	Response to Palpation	Body Tension
0		☐ **Content and quiet** when unattended ☐ **Comfortable** when resting ☐ Interested in or **curious** about surroundings	☐ **Not bothered** by palpation of wound or surgery site, or to palpation elsewhere	Minimal
1		☐ **Signs are often subtle and not easily detected in the hospital setting**; more likely to be detected by the owner(s) at home ☐ Earliest signs at home may be <u>withdrawal from surroundings or change in normal routine</u> ☐ In the hospital, may be content or slightly unsettled ☐ **Less interested** in surroundings but will look around to see what is going on	☐ **May or may not react** to palpation of wound or surgery site	Mild
2		☐ Decreased responsiveness, **seeks solitude** ☐ **Quiet**, loss of brightness in eyes ☐ **Lays curled up or sits tucked up** (all four feet under body, shoulders hunched, head held slightly lower than shoulders, tail curled tightly around body) with eyes partially or mostly closed ☐ **Hair coat appears rough** or fluffed up ☐ May intensively groom an area that is painful or irritating ☐ Decreased appetite, **not interested in food**	☐ **Responds aggressively or tries to escape** if painful area is palpated or approached ☐ Tolerates attention, may even perk up when petted as long as painful area is avoided	Mild to Moderate **Reassess analgesic plan**
3		☐ Constantly **yowling, growling, or hissing** when unattended ☐ May bite or chew at wound, but **unlikely to move** if left alone	☐ **Growls or hisses** at non-painful palpation (may be experiencing allodynia, wind-up, or fearful that pain could be made worse) ☐ **Reacts aggressively** to palpation, **adamantly pulls away** to avoid any contact	Moderate **Reassess analgesic plan**
4		☐ Prostrate ☐ Potentially **unresponsive** to or unaware of surroundings, difficult to distract from pain ☐ Receptive to care (even aggressive or feral cats will be more tolerant of contact)	☐ May not respond to palpation ☐ **May be rigid to avoid painful movement**	Moderate to Severe **May be rigid to avoid painful movement** **Reassess analgesic plan**

RIGHT

○	Tender to palpation
✕	Warm
■	Tense

LEFT

Comments _____

Figure A.2 Subjective and objective pain scoring sheet in cats. Reprinted with permission from Dr. Robinson and Dr. Hellyer at Colorado State University.

Appendix B: Creating dilutions and reconstituting solutions

$$C_1V_1 = C_2V_2 \tag{A.1}$$

A. Dilutions

Making dilutions is completed using a simple equation above. C_1 and C_2 are concentrations and V_1 and V_2 are volumes. C_1 represents what the anesthetist would like to obtain for the final concentration. V_1 is the volume available to work with. C_2 is the concentration the anesthetist has available. V_2 is the unknown volume the equation will solve to add to create the desired concentration. This equation is beneficial in that units are irrelevant if they are the "same" on both sides of the equation.

Example 1: Dextrose dilution

An anesthetist desires to make 5% dextrose in a 1000 mL bag of saline. Dextrose is available as a 50% solution.

$C_1 = 5\%$ dextrose
$V_1 = 1000$ mL bag of saline
$C_2 = 50\%$ dextrose
$V_2 =$ volume needed of 50% dextrose

$$(5\%)(1000 \text{ mL}) = (50\%)(V_2) \tag{A.2}$$

By solving the equation for V_2 (multiply 5% times 1000 mL then divide by 50%) the anesthetist determines that 100 mL of the 50% dextrose solution needs to be added to the 1000 mL bag of 0.9% saline. One should first remove 100 mL from saline bag then add the 100 mL of 50% dextrose thus creating 1000 mL of 5% dextrose in 0.9% saline.

Example 2: Diluting dopamine

Dopamine is available as a very concentrated solution (40 mg/mL) and is diluted prior to administration. The anesthetist would like 20 mL of 1 mg/mL dilution. See equation A.3 and solve for the unknown volume (V_2).

$$(1 \text{ mg/mL})(20 \text{ mL}) = (40 \text{ mg/mL})(V_2) \tag{A.3}$$

$C_1 = 1$ mg/mL
$V_1 = 20$ mL
$C_2 = 40$ mg/mL
$V_2 =$ Unknown volume of dopamine.

B. Reconstituting a solution

$$\text{Concentration of powder (mg)} \div \text{concentration of desired solution (mg/mL)} = \text{volume to add (mL)} \tag{A.4}$$

Some drugs (i.e., remifentanil) come as concentrated powders that reconstitute into a solution for administration. Equation A.4 is used to determine how much diluent is be added to create a desired concentration in solution. It is important to recognize that the "math" of any calculation is only correct when the units' cross-cancel and the answer are in the units desired (see Example 1).

Example 1: Reconstituting remifentanil

Remifentanil is available in 2 mg of powder per vial. Assume the desired concentration for administration is 50 mcg/mL. For this example, one needs to calculate how much diluent (V_1) to add to 2 mg powder (C_1) to get a concentration of 50 mcg/mL (C_2). It is important to convert units to equal powers (i.e., mg to mcg or mcg to mg). The desired concentration involves micrograms when the originating powder is in milligrams. First convert 2 mg into 2000 mcg (see Appendix I).

$$2000 \text{ mcg} \div 50 \text{ mcg/mL} = 40 \text{ mL} \tag{A.5}$$

Dissolving 2 mg powder into 40 mL creates the desired 50 mcg/mL solution.

Appendix C: CPR

A key goal in anesthesia is preventing the necessity of cardiopulmonary resuscitation (CPR), when possible. However, even in relatively healthy animals, cardiopulmonary arrest occurs (1). CPR is most successful when the team is prepared, the crisis is recognized early, and CPR is started immediately. Patients anesthetized that experience cardiac arrest have better survival rates because of early recognition, established patent airway, and IV catheter. It is important during a crisis to remain systematic in your approach to resuscitation (see Figure A.3).

1. Palpate for a pulse in a large accessible artery (i.e., femoral). If no pulse is present, go to Step 2.
2. Discontinue anesthesia (turn off vaporizer, CRIs, etc).
3. Begin basic life support with "CAB":
   (a) C = compressions. Compressions are started immediately, even before securing an airway in an unintubated patient, as the lack of forward blood flow makes ventilation a moot point. The patient is placed in lateral recumbency; compressions are targeted at 100–120 bpm. Compress 1/3 of the circumference of the patient. It is important to allow complete recoil of the chest before the next compression. Once begun, it is imperative to minimize interruption of chest compressions. The compressor is rotated every 2 minutes; the next compressor will place his or her hands over the current compressor's hands, and there is communication regarding the hand-off to new compressor, so transition is as seamless as possible. Use of appropriate compressor posture delivers effective compressions as well as reduces fatigue. Appropriate compressor posture includes elevation over the animal (using a stool if necessary), locking the elbows, interlocking the hands, and bending at the waist to utilize the entire upper body to deliver effective compressions.
   (b) A = airway. Compressions provide some ventilation. A second person obtains supplies to intubate the patient (ET tube, laryngoscope, oxygen and a securing tie). Again, interruption of compressions should be minimal. It is important for the most experienced and confident team member to quickly intubate the patient while compressions are occurring, if possible. If this is not possible, compressions are continued immediately once the ET tube is secured.
   (c) B = breathing. Once intubated, ventilate the patient at 10 breaths per minute with 100% oxygen. If a manometer is available, the PIP should be 20 cmH$_2$O per breath. Tidal volume is 10 mL/kg.
4. Monitoring during CPR:
   (a) Place monitoring equipment. A capnograph is now considered standard of care for use during CPR, with a target goal of 15 mmHg EtCO$_2$ or greater. Place ECG on patient; assessment of the rhythm is made during chest recoils, if possible, although a sudden rise in EtCO$_2$ may suggest a return of circulation and warrants an ECG assessment. Assess for pulse either by palpation of the femoral artery or by placing a gelled Doppler over the eye.
5. Drugs: Administer drugs via IV access closest to the heart (i.e., jugular catheter when available). Delivery of drugs is followed with a sufficient saline bolus, especially if a peripheral catheter is used.

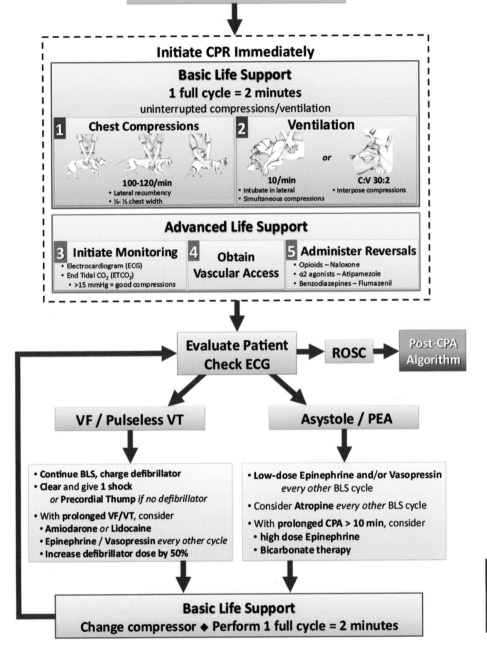

CPR Algorithm

Unresponsive, Apneic Patient

Initiate CPR Immediately

Basic Life Support
1 full cycle = 2 minutes
uninterrupted compressions/ventilation

1 Chest Compressions

100-120/min
• Lateral recumbency
• ⅓–½ chest width

2 Ventilation

or

10/min
• Intubate in lateral
• Simultaneous compressions

C:V 30:2
• Interpose compressions

Advanced Life Support

3 Initiate Monitoring
• Electrocardiogram (ECG)
• End Tidal CO₂ (ETCO₂)
• >15 mmHg = good compressions

4 Obtain Vascular Access

5 Administer Reversals
• Opioids – Naloxone
• α2 agonists – Atipamezole
• Benzodiazepines – Flumazenil

Evaluate Patient Check ECG → **ROSC** → **Post-CPA Algorithm**

VF / Pulseless VT

Asystole / PEA

• **Continue BLS, charge defibrillator**
• **Clear and give 1 shock**
   or **Precordial Thump** *if no defibrillator*
• With **prolonged VF/VT**, consider
  • **Amiodarone** *or* **Lidocaine**
  • **Epinephrine / Vasopressin** *every other cycle*
  • **Increase defibrillator dose by 50%**

• **Low-dose Epinephrine and/or Vasopressin**
  every other BLS cycle
• Consider **Atropine** *every other* BLS cycle
• With **prolonged CPA > 10 min**, consider
  • **high dose Epinephrine**
  • **Bicarbonate therapy**

Basic Life Support
Change compressor ◆ Perform 1 full cycle = 2 minutes

Figure A.3 CPR algorithm. CPR, cardiopulmonary resuscitation; PEA, pulseless electrical activity; VF, ventricular fibrillation; VT, ventricular tachycardia. Reprinted with permission from John Wiley and Sons, Daniel J. Fletcher, Manuel Boller, Benjamin M. Brainard, Steven C. Haskins, Kate Hopper, Maureen A. McMichael, Elizabeth A. Rozanski, John E. Rush, Sean D. Smarick, "RECOVER evidence and knowledge gap analysis on veterinary CPR. Part 7: Clinical guidelines," Journal of Veterinary Emergency and Critical Care, 2012 Jun; 22 Suppl 1:S102-31.

Appendices

(a) Epinephrine (0.01 mg/kg IV or 0.02–0.1 mg/kg diluted 1:1 with saline IT if no IV access is available) is administered for asystole or PEA; this is repeated every 4 minutes.
(b) Vasopressin (0.8 IU/kg IV/IO or 1.2 IU/kg IT) is an alternative for interchangeable use with the first dose of epinephrine.
(c) Atropine (0.04 mg/kg IV/IO or 0.08 mg/kg IT) is still recommended for use in the small animal, especially if high vagal tone is suspected, although it has lost favor for routine use in human CPR (2).
(d) Reverse any anesthetics or drugs administered for analgesia (reversal agents include naloxone, flumazenil, and atipamezole; see Table 3.13).
(e) Fluids during CPR: Use of IV fluids is reserved for patients considered hypovolemic prior to arrest.
(f) Sodium bicarbonate (1 mEq/kg, diluted 1:4, once) is considered for administration in cases of prolonged CPR.
6. Electrical defibrillation is delivered if it can be performed safely (i.e., without putting the CPR team members at risk) at 2–4 kJ/kg; chest compressions are begun immediately post defibrillation. In human CPR, there is a prevalence of ventricular fibrillation as the arrest rhythm and thus time to defibrillation is a major determinant of survival (3). In animals, it is still prudent to defibrillate early when possible.

If return of spontaneous return of circulation occurs, the veterinary team begins postresuscitative care. The reader is directed to a more thorough review of CPR and postresuscitative care in the companion animal, as this Appendix's target goal is that of an overview (2).

Table A.1 Emergency drugs.

Drug	IV (mg/kg)	IT
Epinephrine	0.01–0.02	0.1 (mg/kg)
Atropine	0.04	0.2 (mg/kg)
Vasopressin	0.4–0.8 (unit/kg)	1.2 (units/kg)

Appendix D: CRI calculations

CRIs are extremely beneficial for balancing the anesthetic technique. Often they are used to provide multimodal analgesia, minimum alveolar concentration (MAC) reduction, and supportive therapies (e.g., paralysis, inotropic support, electrolyte supplementation). The purpose of a CRI is to maintain a constant plasma level of the administered drug. A loading dose is used to fill the plasma compartment, followed by the start of the CRI to maintain this. Depending on the availability of equipment (e.g., syringe or fluid pumps), CRIs are routine practices in many clinics. Equation A.6 assists in calculating and administering CRIs from a bag of fluids. Steps in Table A.2 are followed when calculating CRIs:

$$\frac{\text{Dose (mg/kg/h)}}{\text{Rate (mL/kg/h)}} \times \text{Total Volume (mL)} = \text{mg of drug to add} \qquad (A.6)$$

As with any calculation, accuracy of the mathematics is assured when the units "cross-cancel" and the answer is delivered in the units desired.

Example 1: Hydromorphone, lidocaine and ketamine (HLK) CRI in a 20 kg dog undergoing a tibial plateau leveling osteotomy (TPLO)

This CRI is a combination of opioid, sodium channel blocker, and n-methyl-D-aspartate (NMDA) antagonist for painful procedures (e.g., orthopedic procedures, median sternotomy, total ear canal ablation and ventral bulla osteotomy [TECABO]). Hydromorphone is a common opioid administered but other opioids are also suitable.

Step 1. For this example, the patient will receive HLK during the procedure in the anesthetic maintenance fluids.
Total volume: 1000 mL LRS (1-L bag)

Step 2. Hydromorphone at 0.03 mg/kg/h, lidocaine at 3 mg/kg/h, and ketamine at 0.6 mg/kg/h intraoperatively will be used in fluids given at anesthetic maintenance of 5 mL/kg/h.

Step 3. Separate calculations are performed for each drug used. Calculations:

$$\text{Hydromorphone:} \frac{0.03 \text{ mg/kg/h}}{5 \text{ mL/kg/h}} \times 1000 \text{ mL} = 6 \text{ mg of drug to add}$$

$$\text{Lidocaine:} \frac{3 \text{ mg/kg/h}}{5 \text{ mL/kg/h}} \times 1000 \text{ mL} = 600 \text{ mg of drug to add} \qquad (A.7)$$

$$\text{Ketamine:} \frac{0.6 \text{ mg/kg/h}}{5 \text{ mL/kg/h}} \times 1000 \text{ mL} = 120 \text{ mg of drug to add}$$

Table A.2 Steps for calculating CRIs.

Step 1: Determine what total volume is desired (dependent on dose, duration, and size of patient).
Step 2: Select drug or drugs.
Step 3: Calculate (see Equation A.6).
Step 4: Create solution.

The answers to the calculations are in milligrams. The anesthetist divides by the concentration of the drugs used to determine the volume of each drug added to the bag of fluids.

$$\text{Hydromorphone: } 6 \text{ mg} \times \frac{\text{mL}}{2 \text{ mg}} = 3 \text{ mL}$$

$$\text{Lidocaine: } 600 \text{ mg} \times \frac{\text{mL}}{20 \text{ mg}} = 30 \text{ mL} \tag{A.8}$$

$$\text{Ketamine: } 120 \text{ mg} \times \frac{\text{mL}}{100 \text{ mg}} = 1.2 \text{ mL}$$

(d) Step 4. Creating: The total volume of drugs added is removed from the bag of LRS first. Then the drugs are added.

When this bag of LRS (now containing HLK) is administered to the 20 kg canine patient at the rate of 5 mL/kg/h, the patient receives 100 mL/h LRS with hydromorphone at 0.03 mg/kg/h, lidocaine at 3 mg/kg/h, and ketamine 1.2 mg/kg/h. Loading doses of these drugs are administered. A fluid pump is used to accurately deliver the 100 mL/h or additional fluid drip rate calculations are used to determine drop/sec for administion (see Appendix E).

Appendix E: Calculating fluid drip rates

$$\text{Body Weight (kg)} \times \text{Fluid Rate}\left(\frac{\text{mL}}{\text{kg/h}}\right) \times \text{conversion factor}\left(\frac{\text{h}}{3600 \text{ sec}}\right)$$
$$\times \text{Drip Set}\left(\frac{\text{drops}}{\text{mL}}\right) = \frac{\text{drops}}{\text{sec}} \qquad (\text{A.9})$$

1. Example 1. A 36 kg dog is undergoing anesthesia with a maintenance fluid rate of 5 mL/kg/h using a 10 drop/mL drip set. At how many drops/sec should the drip set be set?

$$36 \text{ kg} \times \frac{5 \text{ mL}}{\text{kg/h}} \times \frac{\text{h}}{3600 \text{ sec}} \times \frac{10 \text{ drops}}{\text{mL}} = \frac{0.5 \text{ drop}}{\text{sec}} \qquad (\text{A.10})$$

Appendix F: Supplemental texts for exotic animals

Carpenter J, Mashima T, Ruppier D. Exotic Animal Formulary. Second ed. Philadelphia: W.B. Saunders Company; 2001.

Hillyer E, Quesenberry K. Ferrets, Rabbits, and Rodents: Clinical Medicine and Surgery. Philadelphia: W.B. Saunders Company; 1997.

Johnson-Delaney C, Harrison L. Exotic Companion Medicine Handbook. Lake Worth, FL: Wingers Publishing, Inc.; 1996.

Appendix G: Epidural calculations

$$\text{Body weight (kg)} \times \frac{0.2\,\text{mL}}{\text{kg}} = \text{Total volume for epidural} \qquad (A.11)$$

First, calculate total volume desired for the epidural. A common total volume is 0.2 mL/kg. This will typically provide enough cranial migration of epidural solution to provide analgesia for hind limb, abdominal, or thoracic procedures. Lower volumes (0.1 mL/kg) may be used for exclusively hind limb procedures. Morphine is dosed at 0.1 mg/kg and bupivacaine at 0.5–1 mg/kg. Once these doses have been calculated and drawn, sterile saline is added to the drug solutions to equal the remaining volume from Equation A.12.

Appendix H: Abdominal tap

Table A.3   Abdominal tap.

Materials: Clippers, aseptic scrub, 16-g catheter, three-way stopcock, extension set, sterile gloves, 60 mL syringe, large container with volume markings, +/− **ultrasound**

Technique:
1. The patient is premedicated according to the anesthetic plan.
2. Maintain the patient in sternal recumbency or standing, if the patient tolerates it. Clip and prep the patient ventral medially on the right side of the abdomen (to avoid the spleen).
3. Open sterile gloves and, without contaminating the catheter, drop the catheter onto the gloves, along with one extension set.
4. In a sterile manner, carefully glove, taking care to not to contact the sterile catheter and extension set.
5. Palpate the fluid wave in the abdomen in the context of the clipped and prepped location. Grasp the catheter approximately 0.5–1.0 inch from the tip. Insert the catheter and stylet slowly through the skin and abdominal wall, watching for fluid flow from the catheter. The fluid should be of the expected composition (e.g., serosanguinous); if unexpected fluid is encountered (e.g., frank hemorrhage), pull out needle and apply direct pressure. Alternatively, an ultrasound probe is used to guide the needle into the fluid pocket.
6. When expected fluid flows back through the stylet, feed the catheter off the stylet. Minimal resistance is felt if the location is correct.
7. Attach the sterile extension tubing to the catheter hub; the other end is handed to an individual operating the syringe.
8. The individual operating the syringe attaches the three-way stopcock to the extension set and a 60-mL syringe to the three-way stopcock.
9. The stopcock is turned off to the environment, and the fluid is drained from the abdomen by pulling back on the syringe. When the syringe is full, the stopcock is turned off to the patient and emptied into the container.
10. Steps 8 and 9 are repeated until no more fluid is withdrawn; final volume is measured and recorded.

Appendix I: Conversions

Table A.4 Conversions.

1 kg = 2.2 lb
1 kg = 1000 g
1 g = 1000 mg
1 mg = 1000 mcg
1 L = 1000 mL
°C × 9/5 + 32 = °F
(°F − 32) × 5/9 = °C
1.36 cmH$_2$O = 1 mmHg
PSI × 0.3 = estimate of liters in oxygen tank
% = 1 g/100 mL

References

1. Brodbelt D, Blissitt K, Hammond R, Neath P, Young L, Pfeiffer D, et al. The risk of death: the confidential enquiry into perioperative small animal fatalities. Vet Anaesth Analg. 2008;35(5): 365–73.
2. Fletcher DJ, Boller M. Updates in small animal cardiopulmonary resuscitation. Vet Clin North Am Small Anim Pract. 2013;43(4):971–87.
3. Stokes NA, Scapigliati A, Trammell AR, Parish DC. The effect of the AED and AED programs on survival of individuals, groups and populations. Prehosp Disaster Med. 2012;27(5): 419–24.

Index

Note: Page numbers followed by "*f*" indicate figures; those followed by "*t*" indicate tables.

Index